Paediatrics
Lecture Notes

Simon J. Newell

MD FRCP FRCPCH
Consultant and Senior Clinical Lecturer in Paediatrics and Child Health
Leeds Teaching Hospitals NHS Trust and University of Leeds

Jonathan C. Darling

MD MRCP FRCPCH FHEA
Senior Lecturer and Honorary Consultant in Paediatrics and Child Health
University of Leeds and Leeds Teaching Hospitals NHS Trust

Ninth edition

WILEY Blackwell

Library of Congress Cataloging-in-Publication Data
Newell, Simon J., author.
  Lecture notes. Paediatrics/Simon J. Newell, Jonathan C. Darling. – Ninth edition.
    1 online resource.
  Paediatrics
  Includes bibliographical references and index.
  Description based on print version record and CIP data provided by publisher; resource not viewed.
  ISBN 978-1-118-81448-2 – ISBN 978-1-118-81449-9 (ePub) – ISBN 978-0-470-65707-2 (pbk.)
  I. Darling, Jonathan C., author.   II. Title.   III. Title: Paediatrics.
  [DNLM: 1. Pediatrics–methods.   2. Child Development–physiology. WS 100]
  RJ45
  618.9'2–dc23
                          2013030203
A catalogue record for this book is available from the British Library.

Cover image Sawayasu Tsuji / iStockphoto.com
Cover design by Grounded Design

Set in 8.5/11 pt Utopia Std by Aptara® Inc., New Delhi, India
Printed and bound in Malaysia by Vivar Printing Sdn Bhd

Paediatrics
Lecture Notes

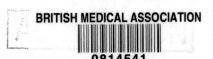

We dedicate this book to our students, past, present, and future.

Contents

OSCE stations

Preface

When *Lecture Notes: Paediatrics* began over 40 years ago, the notion of a weblink to watch a You-Tube video would have been science fiction. (Try **http://tinyurl.com/lnpcell** '*Inner life of the cell*' from Harvard and imagine trying to watch and believe this in 1973.) Looking back at the first edition, it tells of: high mortality from Rhesus disease; life-threatening infections, since abolished by immunization; lead poisoning; frequent admissions for accidental ingestion of drugs, before childproof containers and blister packs; and '*At present there is no cure for leukaemia…*'.

Paediatrics and child health have come a long way. Children are 20% of the population and are seen in 40% of general practice consultations. We have again set out to focus on the core of the paediatric curriculum that every medical student should learn. We hope our book will also be useful to other health professionals who care for children, especially our colleagues in advanced nursing roles.

In this new edition we have advanced the use of information boxes indicating *key points, practice points, treatment guides, learning logs,* and web-based support material. Each chapter begins with a chapter map and suggests practical ways of gaining experience in paediatrics in the learning log at the end. This edition offers many updated and new sections, as well as new chapters in adolescent health, genetics, safe prescribing and careers in paediatrics.

Students and teachers all want success in examinations. We have added more OSCE stations, along with OSCE tips at the end of each chapter, to be used alongside the section on *Preparing for Clinical Examinations in Paediatrics and Child Health* and the extended matching questions (EMQs). We hope you will find these useful.

We have amended the book to give it what we hope will be an easy-to-follow structure: Part 1 takes you through the essentials you need to know at the outset; Part 2 covers normal and abnormal from fetal life through to adolescence; then Part 3 moves to systems and specialties; and finally we explain in Part 4 what happens next – exams and (we hope) careers in paediatrics.

We both used *Lecture Notes* when we were medical students and it is a popular choice of text at home in the UK and abroad. We hope you will enjoy reading *Lecture Notes* during your paediatrics and that it will in some way contribute to still higher and better standards for children's health during your careers in the next 40 years.

Simon Newell
Jonathan Darling

Acknowledgements

This book was conceived by Professor Sir Roy Meadow and Professor Dick Smithells, whose teaching inspired many students in paediatrics.

We are grateful to the European Resuscitation Council for permission to use their illustrations, and algorithms in emergency paediatrics. We thank the focus groups of medical students, whose reflections on the previous edition were so helpful to us.

Further reading

Large comprehensive textbooks:

Kliegman RM, Stanton BMD, St Geme J, Schor NF (eds) (2011) *Nelson Textbook of Pediatrics.* 19th edition, Elsevier Saunders.

McIntosh N, Helms PJ, Smyth RL, Logan S (eds) (2008) *Forfar and Arneil's Textbook of Pediatrics*, 7th edition, Churchill Livingstone.

Rennie JM (ed.) (2012) *Rennie & Roberton's Textbook of Neonatology*, 5th edition, Churchill Livingstone.

We have included links to useful supplementary reading and resources throughout the text – look out for the **Resources boxes**.

How to use your textbook

Features contained within your textbook

Overview pages give a summary of the chapters in each part.

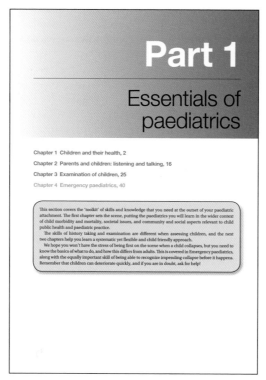

Every chapter begins with a **chapter map** showing the contents of the chapter and an **introduction** to the topic.

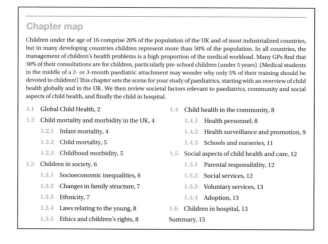

Treatment boxes give prescribing guidelines and advice.

 TREATMENT

Vitamin K is given to all newborns as an oral supplement or as a single IM injection. Oral vitamin K is repeated over the first month in breast-fed infants.

Key point boxes highlight important information about a topic.

 KEY POINTS

All children need:
- Self-esteem (we need to feel wanted)
- At least one good human relationship (we need to trust and feel trusted)
- Firm supervision and clear boundaries (we need rules).

A small change that helps to achieve one of these for a child may make a big difference.

OSCE tip boxes and **OSCE stations** help you prepare and revise for exams.

 OSCE TIP

In an exam, never do anything that is painful, likely to cause discomfort, or which is emabarassing. Some tasks are not practical in the OSCE settting. If you are going to omit part of the examination for these reasons, explain this to the examiner (e.g. in the cardiac examination, say that you would want to: plot growth centiles, measure BP with correct cuff, and examine femoral pulses).

Resource boxes point you to useful information in books and online.

 RESOURCE

- See the United Nations Development Programme website for the latest information on progress: **www.undp.org** and click 'Millenium Development Goals'.
- Health Metrics and Evaluation has a superb site to explore health and other data (**www .healthmetricsandevaluation.org**). Go to 'Tools' then 'Visualizations' and select 'GBD 2010' to review the global burden of different diseases by age and region.
- Visit **www.gapminder.org** for another great site to compare health and other data between countries and historically.

Practice point boxes give practical tips on how best to handle a specific scenario.

 PRACTICE POINT

- If a parent suspects a problem with their child, they are often right.
- Take the views and concerns of parents and other carers seriously.
- If in doubt, refer.
- Children at high risk of certain conditions may need additional screening tests.

Each chapter ends with a **Summary** and a section called **For your log** which suggests practical ways of gaining experience in paediatrics.

 # Summary

We have described how the paediatric history and consultation differs from adult medicine. There are different elements (such as birth, immunizations, development), but more importantly there is a different approach. This includes involving the child according to age, understanding the constraints of working through a third party (the parent), and being aware of the possibility of child abuse. There is no substitute for practice, and we hope you will enjoy taking and presenting many paediatric histories, and reviewing them with your teachers.

 OSCE TIP

- History of any common presenting symptom or problem.
- Counselling and explaining common and important paediatric problems, e.g. constipation, weaning, immunization, gastro-oesophageal reflux, asthma, febrile convulsions, epilepsy, enuresis.

 FOR YOUR LOG

Summarizing a history is key clinical skill. Write a brief (2–3 sentence) summary for every history you take. The process clarifies what is important in your mind, makes your verbal presentation clearer, and means you finish neatly. OSCE stations involving history taking or presentation will often ask for a summary.

The **Emergency** and **Paediatric symptom sorter quick reference guide** sections are clearly indicated for quick reference.

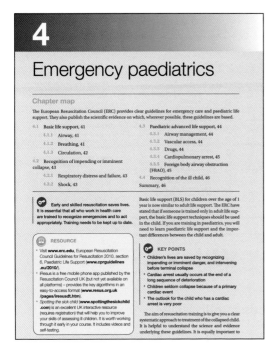

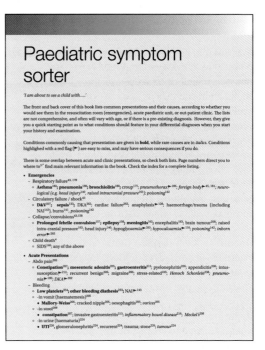

Don't forget to visit **www.lecturenoteseries.com/paediatrics** to download the **Symptom sorter** to your mobile device.

The anytime, anywhere textbook

Wiley E-Text

Your book is also available to purchase as a **Wiley E-Text: Powered by VitalSource** version – a digital, interactive version of this book which you own as soon as you download it.

Your **Wiley E-Text** allows you to:

Search: Save time by finding terms and topics instantly in your book, your notes, even your whole library (once you've downloaded more textbooks)

Note and Highlight: Colour code, highlight and make digital notes right in the text so you can find them quickly and easily

Organize: Keep books, notes and class materials organized in folders inside the application

Share: Exchange notes and highlights with friends, classmates and study groups

Upgrade: Your textbook can be transferred when you need to change or upgrade computers

The **Wiley E-Text** version will also allow you to copy and paste any photograph or illustration into assignments, presentations and your own notes.

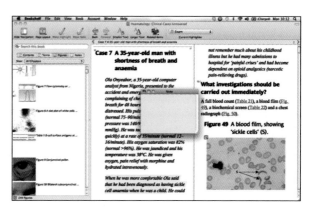

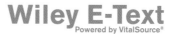

To access your Wiley E-Text:

- Visit **www.vitalsource.com/software/bookshelf/downloads** to download the Bookshelf application to your computer, laptop, tablet or mobile device.
- Open the Bookshelf application on your computer and register for an account.
- Follow the registration process.

The VitalSource Bookshelf can now be used to view your Wiley E-Text on iOS, Android and Kindle Fire!

- **For iOS:** Visit the app store to download the VitalSource Bookshelf: **http://bit.ly/17ib3XS**
- **For Android:** Visit the Google Play Market to download the VitalSource Bookshelf: **http://bit.ly/ZMEGvo**
- **For Kindle Fire, Kindle Fire 2 or Kindle Fire HD:** Simply install the VitalSource Bookshelf onto your Fire (see how at **http://bit.ly/11BVFn9**). You can now sign in with the email address and password you used when you created your VitalSource Bookshelf Account.

Full E-Text support for mobile devices is available at: **http://support.vitalsource.com**

CourseSmart

CourseSmart gives you instant access (via computer or mobile device) to this Wiley-Blackwell e-book and its extra electronic functionality, at 40% off the recommended retail print price. See all the benefits at: **www.coursesmart.com/students.**

Instructors…receive your own digital desk copies!

CourseSmart also offers instructors an immediate, efficient, and environmentally-friendly way to review this book for your course.

For more information visit **www.coursesmart.com /instructors**.

With CourseSmart, you can create lecture notes quickly with copy and paste, and share pages and notes with your students. Access your **CourseSmart** digital book from your computer or mobile device instantly for evaluation, class preparation, and as a teaching tool in the classroom.

Simply sign in at **http://instructors.coursesmart .com/bookshelf** to download your Bookshelf and get started. To request your desk copy, hit 'Request Online Copy' on your search results or book product page.

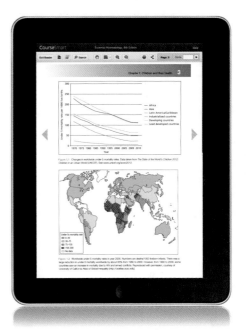

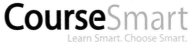

We hope you enjoy using your new book. Good luck with your studies!

About the companion website

Don't forget to visit the companion website:

 www.lecturenoteseries.com/paediatrics

The website contains a PDF of the **Paediatric symptom sorter** for you to download and view on your mobile device.

Part 1

Essentials of paediatrics

This section covers the 'toolkit' of skills and knowledge that you need at the outset of your paediatric attachment. The first chapter sets the scene, putting the paediatrics you will learn in the wider context of child morbidity and mortality, societal issues, and community and social aspects relevant to child public health and paediatric practice.

The skills of history taking and examination are different when assessing children, and the next two chapters help you learn a systematic yet flexible and child friendly approach.

We hope you won't have the stress of being first on the scene when a child collapses, but you need to know the basics of what to do, and how this differs from adults. This is covered in Emergency paediatrics, along with the equally important skill of being able to recognize impending collapse before it happens. Remember that children can deteriorate quickly, and if you are in doubt, ask for help!

1

Children and their health

Chapter map

Children under the age of 16 comprise 20% of the population of the UK and of most industrialized countries, but in many developing countries children represent more than 50% of the population. In all countries, the management of children's health problems is a high proportion of the medical workload. Many GPs find that 30% of their consultations are for children, particularly pre-school children (under 5 years). (Medical students in the middle of a 2- or 3-month paediatric attachment may wonder why only 5% of their training should be devoted to children!) This chapter sets the scene for your study of paediatrics, starting with an overview of child health globally and in the UK. We then review societal factors relevant to paediatrics, community and social aspects of child health, and finally the child in hospital.

1.1 Global child health

Children make up about 2 billion of the world's population. Health inequalities between nations are seen most starkly in childhood indicators, such as under-5 mortality rates (Figure 1.1). Most childhood deaths occur in sub-Saharan Africa and south Asia (Figure 1.2), and malnutrition causes or contributes to at least half of them, along with many other factors (Figure 1.3). There has been a sustained international effort in the last few decades to address inequalities, culminating in the Millenium Development Goals adopted in 2000 by all members of the United Nations. These set measurable targets to be achieved by 2015 in relation to poverty, maternal and child health and combating disease such as HIV and malaria. Progress has been made, but much remains to be done.

> **Under-5 mortality rate (rate/1000 live births)**
>
> The under-5 mortality rate is a useful measure of child health internationally. While similar to the infant mortality rate, it detects trends that the infant mortality rate might miss, because in some countries infants dying in the first few weeks are not recorded.

Paediatrics Lecture Notes, Ninth edition. Simon J. Newell and Jonathan C. Darling. © 2014 John Wiley & Sons, Ltd. Published 2014 by John Wiley & Sons, Ltd.

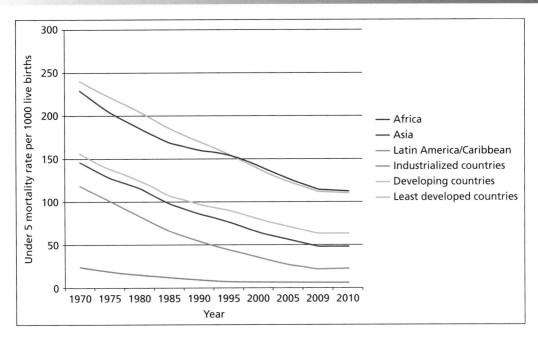

Figure 1.1 Changes in worldwide under-5 mortality rates. Data taken from *The State of the World's Children 2012: Children in an Urban World* (UNICEF). See www.unicef.org/sowc2012.

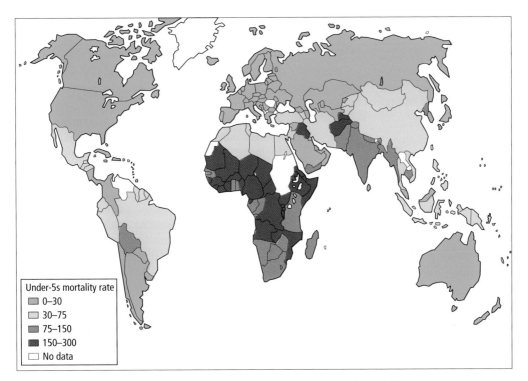

Figure 1.2 Worldwide under-5 mortality rates in year 2000. Numbers are deaths/1000 liveborn infants. There was a large reduction in under-5 mortality worldwide by about 65% from 1960 to 2000. However, from 1990 to 2000, some countries saw an increase in mortality due to HIV and armed conflicts. Reproduced with permission, courtesy of University of California Atlas of Global Inequality (http://ucatlas.ucsc.edu).

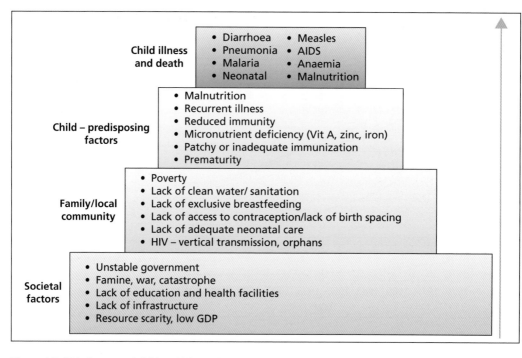

Figure 1.3 Global causes of child morbidity and mortality.

In developing countries:

20% lack food
20% lack safe drinking water
33% lack clothing, shelter, education and health services.

1.2   Child mortality and morbidity in the UK

The causes of death and the patterns of illness in children differ markedly from those in adults. They are influenced by a diversity of factors, which include sex, social class, place of birth and season of the year. The decline in child mortality in the past century has resulted more from preventative (public health) measures than from improved treatment. Today virtually the entire population of the UK has safe food and water, free immunization and easy access to local health care. This is not the case in non-industrialized countries.

In the UK, child mortality is concentrated in the perinatal period (Table 1.1). The only remaining scope for a major reduction in child deaths lies in better obstetric, neonatal and infant care.

1.2.1   Infant mortality

- UK infant mortality continues to fall (currently 4.3 per 1000 live births) (Figure 1.4).
  - But half the countries in the European Union have lower rates.

Table 1.1 UK mortality rates

Mortality indices	UK rate
Stillbirth rate (stillbirths per 1000 total births)	5
Early neonatal mortality rate (deaths in first 7 days per 1000 live births)	3
Perinatal mortality rate (stillbirths + first week deaths per 1000 total births)	8
Infant mortality rate (deaths in first year per 1000 live births)	6
Under-5 mortality rate (deaths in the first 5 years per 1000 live births)	7

Stillbirth: a child born dead after the 24th week of pregnancy
Abortion or miscarriage: a fetus born dead before 24 weeks of gestation
Live birth: Any newborn with signs of life (e.g. heart beat) at birth at any gestation.

- Several East European countries have infant mortality rates 2–3 times higher.
- Some non-industrialized countries have rates over 150.
- Improvement in UK infant mortality:
  - Mainly due to reduction in *neonatal* mortality
  - Less improvement in *post-neonatal* mortality (1 month to 1 year).
- Some deaths result from persistent, serious congenital abnormalities and perinatal problems, others due to accidents or diagnosable disorders, but many are infants who die at home, for whom no cause of death is found at postmortem (Section 15.3).

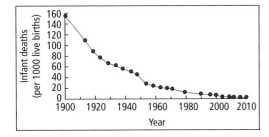

Figure 1.4 Infant mortality (0–1 years). By 2010, the infant mortality in England and Wales had fallen to a fraction of the level in 1900 (from 156 per 1000 live births to 4.3 per 1000). Even in the last 30 years it has fallen by over 60%.

1.2.2 Child mortality

- The major causes of childhood death are neoplasms and accidents.
- Deaths are concentrated in early life and are higher for boys at all ages, by a factor of 1.3 in the first month of life and by 1.6 for children of school age.
- For a schoolchild, death is more likely to be due to an accident, particularly a road accident with the child as pedestrian or cyclist, than to any disease (Figure 1.5).
- The decline in mortality from infectious diseases has made other serious disorders appear more common. Death from malignancy is now as common as from infection (Figures 1.5 and 1.6).

1.2.3 Childhood morbidity

- The pattern of morbidity in children is very different from that of adults (Figure 1.7):
  - Infections are common, especially of the respiratory, gastrointestinal and urinary tracts, as well as the acute exanthemata (e.g. chickenpox).
  - Degenerative disorders and cerebral vascular accidents are very rare.
- New forms of chronic disease are becoming relatively more important as formerly fatal childhood disorders become treatable (but not necessarily curable):
  - Children with complex congenital heart disease, malignant disease, cystic fibrosis and renal failure benefit from modern life-saving therapies but may not achieve a cure, and often have to live with the difficulties and side-effects of complicated treatment.

The hallmarks of childhood are growth and development, which influence both the kinds and the patterns of childhood illness. Congenital malformations, genetic disease and the consequences of problems in the perinatal period (e.g. cerebral palsy) are common. You do not need to spend much time looking after children to realize that disturbances of development and behaviour, and anxiety about normal variants, are both prevalent and important to parents.

It has been estimated that a British GP with an average practice would see a new case of pyloric stenosis every 4 years, childhood diabetes every 6 years, Down syndrome every 16 years, Turner syndrome every 60 years and haemophilia or Hirschsprung disease every 600 years! Hospitals may give a very false impression of the pattern of illness in the community at large.

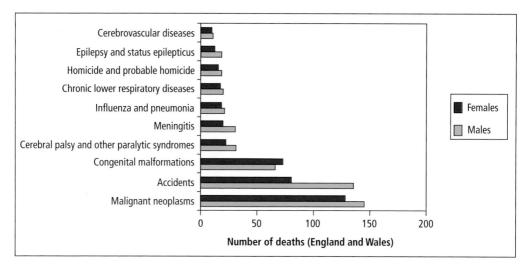

Figure 1.5 Causes of death in childhood. Mortality ages 1–14 in 2003.
Source: National Statistics Online at www.statistics.gov.uk.

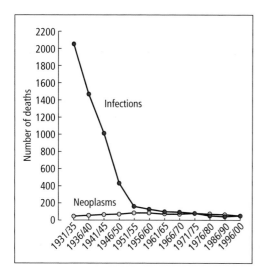

Figure 1.6 Child mortality from infections and neoplasms, per million children living (aged 1–4 years).

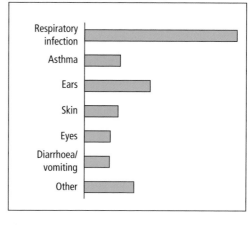

Figure 1.7 Most common reasons for a child to be seen by their GP.

1.3 Children in society

1.3.1 Socioeconomic inequalities

Socioeconomic status is a key determinant of child health. The health and educational progress of a child is directly related to the home and the environment. A child in social class V has a 50% greater chance of being born dead or with a serious physical handicap than one in social class I (see Table 1.2). The disadvantage is there at birth and continues throughout childhood. The social class IV or V child will have more accidents, more physical illnesses, will be smaller and will read less well than the child from social class I or II. At any age a child from social class V is twice as likely to die as one from social class I. In many developed countries, health inequalities have grown wider even as average health levels have improved.

The UK has one of the worst rates of child poverty in the industrialized world. The proportion of children living in poverty grew from 1 in 10 in 1979 to 1 in 3 in 1998. Today, 30% of children in Britain (nearly 4 million) are living in poverty. Since 1999, when the Government pledged to end child poverty, 550 000 children have been lifted out of poverty.

Table 1.2 Social class and childhood mortality: death rates per 100 000.

Age	Social class				
	I	II	III	IV	V
1–4	33	34	46	64	116
5–9	24	19	24	31	45
10–14	20	22	23	31	36

 RESOURCE

See **www.endchildpoverty.org.uk** for more information.

1.3.2 Changes in family structure

Family structure has become more fluid in the UK, reflecting changing societal attitudes to marriage, divorce and cohabitation. Children more often have to make transitions to new family structures. They are helped by: family stability; good relationships between partners; avoiding sustained exposure to conflict; and keeping children's needs paramount. Although marriage has declined and 40% of births are now outside marriage, 7 out of 10 families are headed by a married couple. Step-family combinations are increasing. With more single-parent families, and families where both parents work, grandparents play a significant role in childcare (at least weekly for 25% of families); 23% of dependent children live in single-parent families. Although UK teenage pregnancy rates have fallen recently, they are still among the highest across developed countries. Half of all teenage mothers live in the 20% most deprived areas.

Home factors that can adversely affect children's health and development include:

- Parental discord
  - Quarrelling
  - Separation and divorce
  - Domestic violence
- Parental illness
  - Death of a parent
  - Chronic disability
  - Physical illness
  - Mental illness
- Inability to cope with demands of parenting
- Abuse
- Financial hardship.

The complexity and multiplicity of the factors that cause a child to be disadvantaged sometimes makes us feel helpless. However, since adversities compound one another, much may be achieved by modifying even one adverse factor.

Extensive medical and social services exist, particularly for handicapped children, but all too often they are best used by well-informed, middle-class parents, while the parents of the disadvantaged child do not use them sometimes because they do not know about them. All medical and paramedical staff have a duty to recognize children in need or in distress, and to see that they benefit from the help that is available.

 KEY POINTS

All children need:
- Self-esteem (we need to feel wanted)
- At least one good human relationship (we need to trust and feel trusted)
- Firm supervision and clear boundaries (we need rules).

A small change that helps to achieve one of these for a child may make a big difference.

Twenty per cent of the world's population live in absolute poverty. Nearly half of them are children.

1.3.3 Ethnicity

Most countries have ethnic minority communities with particular needs. The UK continues to become more ethnically diverse. In the UK, 15% of the population (and one-third of newborns) are from ethnic minority groups. There is great regional variation. Consanguinity (marrying a blood relative) is more common in some cultures (e.g. some Muslim communities), increasing the risk of recessively inherited disease. Rickets is more common in some ethnic groups due to diet, pigmented skin and lack of exposure to sunlight. There remain significant health inequalities for many minority groups in Europe.

Find out about your own local situation and be aware of cultural and health differences. These range from what names to use, through to differences in patterns of disease, through travel (e.g. malaria), contact (e.g. tuberculosis) or racial susceptibility (e.g. sickle cell disease). Understanding the importance of racial background, family, cultural and religious beliefs improves paediatric care.

Ethnic composition – England and Wales (2011)	
White	86%
Asian/Asian British	7.5%
Black/Black British	3.3%
Mixed	2.2%
Other	1%

Situations where the withholding or withdrawal of life-prolonging treatment might be considered:

- Brain death: brain stem death despite life prolonging care
- Permanent vegetative state: reliant on others for all care and does not react or relate with the outside world
- 'No chance' situation: life-sustaining treatment simply delays death
- 'No purpose' situation: treatment may save life, but physical or mental impairment is too much to bear
- 'Unbearable' situation: further treatment is more than can be borne.

1.3.4 Laws relating to the young

For legal purposes, a child remains a 'child' up to the age of 18. However, many laws become operative at other ages. School education is compulsory for children aged 5 and over. Children may not leave education until they are 17.

Children may not be employed until they are 13. Then they may be employed only between the hours of 7 a.m. and 7 p.m., and for a maximum of 2 h on school days.

Children under 10 (under 8 in Scotland) are not considered 'criminally responsible' for their misdeeds, and may be dealt with by the juvenile courts. The court can make (1) a care order giving parental rights to the local authority; or (2) a supervision order which may be administered by the social services department or, if the child is over 14, by the probation department. At the age of 15 children can be sent to youth custody.

Adult courts deal with those over the age of 17. Although it is legally possible to be sent to prison for a first offence at the age of 17, in practice it is rare before the age of 20.

1.3.5 Ethics and children's rights

In 1989 the United Nations declared that children worldwide should have special rights due to their immaturity and vulnerability. This Convention on the Rights of the Child sets out what every child needs for 'a safe, happy and fulfilled childhood'. These include the right to health, family life, and to have his views taken seriously in matters affecting him. Consent and competence are covered later (Section 16.2). Once a child is deemed to be competent, then the doctor has the normal duty of confidentiality, including not disclosing information to a third party (including a parent). Sometimes this has to be overridden because of safeguarding concerns, but this should be explained to the child.

A challenging part of intensive care (whether paediatric or neonatal) is the decision to withdraw life-prolonging treatment. Decisions should be made by the treating team in partnership with the parents, taking time to ensure all relevant information is considered.

1.4 Child health in the community

1.4.1 Health personnel

1.4.1.1 Community paediatricians

Most paediatricians have a commitment to some services outside of the hospital. Community paediatricians specialize in working outside of the hospital. They work closely with health visitors and the staff of child health clinics, and also with GPs, social and educational services. The boundary between hospital general paediatrics and community paediatrics is increasingly blurred. Community paediatricians often specialize in one or more of the following:

- Child health surveillance
- Provision of children's services to a specific geographical sector
- Learning problems and disability
- Child protection (child abuse)
- Audiology
- Adoption and fostering
- School health.

1.4.1.2 Health visitors

These are registered nurses with additional training in health promotion and prevention of illness in all age groups. Many are attached to general practices and a few specialize (e.g. in diabetes) and have hospital attachments. They are responsible for family health, and particularly for mothers and pre-school children. Their job is to prevent illness and handicap by giving appropriate advice, by detecting problems early and by mobilizing services to deal with those problems. They have a key role in child health promotion.

1.4.1.3 School nurses

School nurses provide a variety of school-based services:

- Confidential health advice for children and young people
- Sex education
- Developmental screening
- Health interviews
- Immunization programmes
- Working with schools to create a health-promoting environment
- Enuresis management.

1.4.2 Health surveillance and promotion

1.4.2.1 Child health promotion

Child health promotion

- Primary and secondary prevention of problems.

Child health surveillance

- Part of child health promotion
- Secondary prevention through early detection of existing problems.

The core child health promotion programme in the UK includes (Table 1.3):

- Childhood surveillance
- Immunizations
- A systematic process to assess the individual child's and family's needs
- Early interventions to address those needs
- Health promotion.

The aim is a flexible, targeted approach in partnership with parents, to ensure that all children's health and developmental needs are addressed. The programme is a combined undertaking, starting at birth with the postnatal check by the paediatrician or midwife, and then involving the primary health care team: health visitor, GP and later school nurses.

PRACTICE POINT

- If a parent suspects a problem with their child, they are often right.
- Take the views and concerns of parents and other carers seriously.
- If in doubt, refer.
- Children at high risk of certain conditions may need additional screening tests.

1.4.2.2 Child health clinics

These clinics aim to be readily accessible to young families. They are often in GP surgeries, but may also be located in health centres, village halls or purpose-built accommodation. They are staffed by health visitors and GPs. About 90% of babies attend such a clinic during their first year, but thereafter attendance falls off.

Functions

- Child health surveillance
- Routine medical and developmental examinations for infants and pre-school children
- Immunization
- Health education
- Advice and support for those with special problems.

1.4.2.3 Parent-held child health record

Parents should be encouraged to take the 'red book' whenever the child attends clinic or hospital. It contains a permanent record of child health surveillance, the child's growth including a centile chart, hospital visits, health education and advice (Figure 1.8).

PRACTICE POINT

Whenever you see a young child, ask to see the red book. Thank the parent for bringing it.

1.4.2.4 Health education and preparation for parenthood

During the final years at school and in the antenatal period, there are numerous opportunities for health education and training in *parentcraft*. Effective and timely health promotion reduces fetal, infant and childhood morbidity and mortality.

Key messages for parents

- Regular antenatal care
- Avoid smoking and alcohol during pregnancy
- Breast feeding, and information on how to breast- or bottle-feed
- Reduce risk of SIDS (Chapter 15)
- Immunization
- The parent-held record (the red book)
- Good childhood nutrition
- Love, care, nurture and play
- Avoid parental smoking (respiratory disease in children)
- What action to take when your child is ill
- Reduce risks of accidents at home and on the road
- Good dental health.

Table 1.3 UK Child Health Promotion Programme

Age	Intervention (universal)	Intervention (progressive or targeted)

Antenatal	• Antenatal screening
	• Preliminary assessment of child and family needs
	• Preparation for parenthood
	• Advice on breast-feeding
	• Advice on general health and well-being
	  • Healthy eating and weight
	  • Smoking cessation
	• Plan transition from midwifery to health visiting service
		• Extra support and needs assessment for higher risk groups (at all stages below):
		  • Young first time mothers
		  • Learning difficulties
		  • Drug and alcohol abuse
		  • Domestic violence
		  • Serious mental illness

Birth to 1 week	• Infant feeding support
	• General physical examination
	  • Especially eyes, heart and hips
	• Vitamin K (im or drops)
	• Blood spot screening test (age 5–6 days) (Section 7.4.1).
	• Newborn hearing screen (within first month)
	• Assess child and family health needs
	• Give Personal Child Health Record
	• General information and support, e.g. SIDS advice (Section 15.3, p. 147), injury prevention
		• Immunization for at risk infants:
		  • BCG
		  • Hepatitis B
		• Advice on Healthy Start programme (including vitamin supplements) for low income groups
		• Extra support for infants with special problems (e.g. prematurity, low birth weight)

One to six weeks	• New baby review by 14 days (e.g. midwife, health visitor) and assess maternal mental health
	• Home safety advice
		• For children at risk of obesity
		  • Advice on exercise and nutrition for whole family
		• Extra support for:
		  • Maternal depression
		  • Difficult parental relationship
		  • Parental insensitivity to infant needs

Six weeks to six months	• General physical examination at 6–8 weeks
	  • Especially eyes, heart and hips (and testes for boys)
	  • Review growth
	• Immunizations at 2, 3 and 4 months (Table 14.1)
	• Review general progress
	• Deliver key messages about parenting and health promotion, e.g. promoting development, safety, SIDS
	• Weaning advice
		• Extra support for infants with special problems or parental issues as above
		• Smoking cessation interventions

Six months to one year	• Systematic assessment by health visiting team by one year:
	  • Child's physical, emotional and social development
	  • Family needs
	• Planning to address any needs and agree future contact with parents
	• Advice about dental health
		• As above

One to three years	• Immunizations at 12 and 13 months months (Table 14.1) • 2–2.5 yr review of health and development by health visiting team • Partnership with parents • Build on other contacts (e.g. immunization, visits to GP) • Dental health (avoid sugary food and drinks, teethbrushing)	• Health or developmental problems to be referred early to specialist team • For children at risk of obesity • Advice on healthy eating, portion size and mealtime routines • Smoking cessation support

Age	Intervention (universal)	Intervention (progressive or targeted)
3–5 years	<ul><li>Immunization age 3 yr months (Table 14.1)</li><li>Review general progress</li><li>Deliver key messages about parenting and health promotion</li></ul>Around time of school entry, check the following:<ul><li>Immunizations up-to-date</li><li>Access to primary and dental care</li><li>Appropriate interventions in place for physical, developmental or emotional problems</li><li>Child's height and weight</li><li>Hearing and vision test done</li></ul>	<ul><li>As above</li></ul>
Primary and secondary schools	<ul><li>Access to school nurse through drop-in sessions or clinics<ul><li>Self-referral</li><li>Parents</li><li>Teachers</li></ul></li><li>Referral to specialists for children causing concern</li><li>In-school nursing care for some medical needs/disabilities</li><li>Heaf test age 10 to 14 years +/- BCG</li><li>School-leaver immunization (Table 14.1)</li></ul>	

Further details of the UK health promotion programme can be found in the Department of Health publication *Healthy Child Programme – pregnancy and the first five years*. 2009. This can be accessed at www.dh.gov.uk (search there for the title).

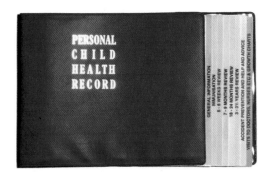

Figure 1.8 Parent-held record ('the red book'). It is useful to refer to the parent-held record during your history for further details about growth, development and immunizations

Government objective

To reduce rates of smoking throughout pregnancy to 11% or less (from 14%) by the end of 2015.

1.4.2.5 Immunization

Immunization is a key part of the programme (Chapter 14).

1.4.3 Schools and nurseries

1.4.3.1 Pre-school facilities

In the UK, all 3- and 4-year-olds are entitled to free part-time early education, which can be in school nurseries, day nurseries, playgroups or with approved childminders.

Nurseries or playgroups may be stand-alone or attached to primary schools. They aim to encourage a child's development and learning by play, stimulation and physical activity. Infants and younger children may attend day nurseries while their parents are at work, or parent–toddler groups with a parent. Pre-school facilities are particularly important for children from disadvantaged backgrounds. 'Surestart programmes' develop facilities for these children, and provide support for parents with young children.

> ### Incidence of some important problems
>
> **At 5 years:**
>
> - 7% have had at least one seizure
> - 5% have a squint
> - 5% have a behavioural problem
> - 5% have a speech or language problem
> - 2% have a substantial congenital defect.
>
> **At 7 years:**
>
> - 15% have eczema, asthma or hay fever
> - 13% require special education
> - 10% wet their beds
> - 2% have had a hernia repair
> - <1% have had an appendicectomy.

1.4.3.2 Healthy schools

Children spend a large amount of time in school, and the school environment affects their health. The 'Healthy Schools' initiative programme in the UK encourages schools to take positive steps towards promoting children's health.

> ### Promoting healthy schools
>
> - Healthy eating;
> - Physical activity;
> - Personal, social and health education (PSHE);
> - Emotional health and well-being.

Promotion of regular water-drinking and easy access to clean and well-maintained toilets reduces problems of constipation, urine infections and wetting.

1.5 Social aspects of child health and care

> ### Disability Living Allowance (DLA)
>
> - Care allowance from birth for levels of care in excess of those needed by healthy child
> - Mobility allowance is available from the age of 5 years.

1.5.1 Parental responsibility

Both parents have legal 'parental responsibility' if they are married at the time of the child's birth, or if both are registered on the birth certificate. Otherwise, the mother has parental responsibility, but there are legal mechanisms by which the father can acquire it.

1.5.2 Social services

The social services department of the local authority is responsible for the care and/or supervision of children up to 18 years if:

- Parents are unable to care for their children
  - e.g. illness, abuse
- No parent or carer for children
  - e.g. death of parent(s), child abandoned or lost.

In these situations, the local authority assumes parental rights in order to provide security and protection for the child.

Parental rights may be given to the local authority by the court (usually a family court or juvenile court), in which case a child is said to be the subject of a *care order*. The court must be satisfied that the child has suffered, or is likely to suffer, significant harm because of the standard of parental care or because of being beyond parental control. 'Harm' includes ill-treatment, sexual abuse, and the impairment of good physical and mental health and development.

The local authority tries to keep or place children with their own parents, relatives or friends. When this is not possible, the child is looked after by the local authority in:

- *Foster homes* (75%) in which a child is cared for in a family other than his own. There are an increasing number of schemes in which the foster parents are paid extra to look after children with physical and mental handicap or disturbed adolescents.
- *Residential placements:* Children's homes, residential schools and secure units (25%) aim to provide as normal an upbringing as possible, despite frequent changes of staff. They contain a higher proportion of difficult or handicapped children than foster homes. Of children in these homes, 95% still have a living parent, so that many are visited regularly or may be reunited with their parents for weekends or longer periods.

Children may be supervised in their own homes, either on a voluntary basis or as a result of a court *supervision order*. The social worker's prime aim is to prevent family break-up and to help with problems of care, both physical and emotional. He or she works as part of a team with others involved with the family, e.g. health visitors, doctors and teachers.

The social services department is responsible for supervising children placed privately with foster parents. People who look after other people's children, whether on a day (child day-care, childminder) or residential (foster) basis, must register with their local social services department, even if they are paid directly by the parent. Social services also provide advice about financial benefits available from the Department of Social Security.

> **Children Act 1989**
>
> The Act affects all aspects of the welfare and protection of children including day-care, fostering and adoption, child abuse and the consequences for children of marital breakdown. The spirit of the Act is reflected in the opening paragraphs:
>
> 'the child's welfare shall be the court's paramount consideration'
>
> 'any delay in determining the question (of the child's upbringing) is likely to prejudice the welfare of the child'
>
> 'a court shall have regard to … the ascertainable wishes and feelings of the child concerned'.

1.5.3 Voluntary services

The statutory services are supplemented by a large number of voluntary and charitable organizations, many of which were in existence before, and paved the way for, statutory provisions. Many of those offering services to children have a high level of professional expertise. The NSPCC (National Society for the Prevention of Cruelty to Children) and its Scottish counterpart continue their historic role of protecting children, and giving advice and support to families under stress. Barnardo's, the Children's Society and the National Children's Homes have adapted their activities to the changing pattern of child needs. The Save the Children Fund gives support to deprived inner cities in the UK as well as relief in developing countries. Many voluntary bodies receive some funding from central and/or local government.

1.5.3.1 Parent support groups

These exist for almost every chronic disorder of childhood (e.g. Cystic Fibrosis Trust). Their membership consists largely of parents of affected children who can offer advice to others from first-hand experience. They also raise money to support research, thereby augmenting the work of the major medical research charities.

1.5.3.2 The Family Fund

This gives financial help to less well-off families with very severely handicapped children. It is financed by the Department of Health, but administered by the Rowntree Trust in York. Charitable organizations can often minimize bureaucracy and cut administrative costs and delays.

1.5.4 Adoption

Couples wishing to adopt a child approach their local authority who will assess suitability. The process includes medical assessment of the child and parents. Once adopted, the child is a full member of the family; he or she takes their name and has all the rights of a natural child. It is best for parents to inform their child from the beginning that they are adopted.

1.6 Children in hospital

Health care for children has changed dramatically in the last 60 years. Children were separated from their parents for long periods with little appreciation of their particular needs. The birth and development of paediatrics as a medical specialty was largely attributable to the first children's hospitals. Now the special needs of children are recognized in the design and provision of services, e.g. unrestricted visiting, facilities for resident parents, play activities for younger children (Figure 1.9) and education for older children. Every effort is made to minimize a child's need to stay in hospital. Infants account for more than half of all paediatric admissions (Figure 1.10). The majority of admissions are due to respiratory conditions and infections (Figure 1.11).

Hospitals are not without risk to patients, especially child patients. The hazard of cross-infection is obvious: the hazard of mother–child separation is less obvious but can be more serious, especially among the 1–4-year-olds. At this age, children are old enough to grieve for a lost mother, but not old enough to understand the reason, or that the separation is temporary. 'Tomorrow' has no meaning for a toddler.

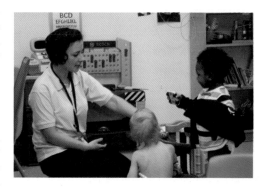

Figure 1.9 Children in hospital. The play specialist plays a vital role.

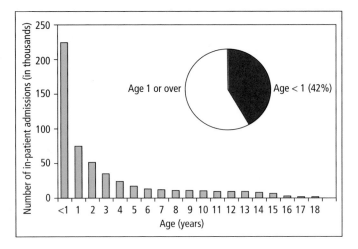

Figure 1.10 Number of paediatric in-patient admissions by age. Number of admissions per year in 1000s in the UK of children 0–18 years old. *Source:* Audit Commission 1993.

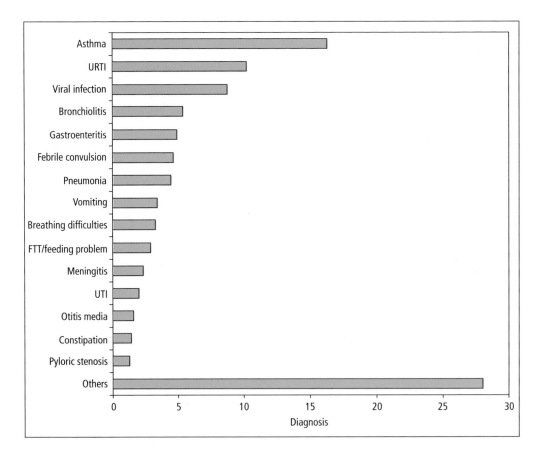

Figure 1.11 Causes of paediatric admissions. Based on a study of admissions to a District General Hospital. Respiratory problems (asthma, URTI, bronchiolitis, pneumonia and breathing difficulties) caused 57% of admissions, and infective illness 44%. FTT, failure to thrive; URTI, upper respiratory tract infection; UTI, urinary tract infection. *Source:* Y. Thakker, T.A. Sheldon, R. Long, R. MacFaul (1994). *Archives of Disease in Childhood* 70: 488–92.

Changes in hospital care

- The average stay in hospital is much shorter.
- There are similar numbers of medical and surgical admissions.
- More children are admitted – 1 in 4 by age 2 years, 1 in 3 by 4.5 years.
- Many medical and surgical procedures are done as day cases.
- Parents are actively involved in care.
- Outreach nursing teams and day assessment units reduce the need for admission.
- Neonatal care makes increasingly heavy demands on resources.

A young child separated from his mother may go through three stages:

Protest: he cries for her return.

Withdrawal: he curls up with a comfort blanket or toy and loses interest in food and play.

Denial: he appears happy, making indiscriminate friendships with everybody. This can be mistakenly interpreted as the child having 'settled', but the mother–child bond has been damaged and will have to be rebuilt. On returning home, he may exhibit tantrums, refuse food or wet his bed.

These problems can be avoided or minimized by:

- Avoiding hospital admission if possible
- Reducing the length of any admission to the minimum
- Performing operations (e.g. herniotomy, orchidopexy) and investigations (e.g. jejunal biopsy, colonoscopy) as day cases
- Encouraging parents to visit often and arranging for one to sleep alongside a young child.

Hospital organization can also help to reduce stress. Paediatric wards mean that children are looked after by staff specially trained and experienced in the care of children in a child-friendly environment. Teachers,

nursery nurses and play leaders organize education and play. The first impression of a children's ward should be of happy chaos, rather than of the highly technical medicine, which is in fact going on.

 # Summary

Although most of this book will focus on illness and disease in children, the issues we have covered in this chapter are vital to understanding child health, and need to underpin all your work with children and families. Most of the global burden of childhood disease is in developing countries, and the good news is that progress is being made to reduce this. Health inequalities are important to UK child health – if poverty could be eradicated, more than 1000 child deaths each year would be prevented. Health promotion is of great importance, as are the social aspects of child health. When you meet children and their families in hospital, a thoughtful, sensitive and child-friendly approach can transform a 'job to be done' into a positive and even therapeutic encounter.

 FOR YOUR LOG

- Find out about child health statistics for your local area – in the UK go to www.chimat.org.uk and explore the child health profiles and data atlas.
- Discuss local child health issues with paediatric (and if accessible) public health staff.
- Look up parent support group websites for some of the conditions you come across – *Contact a family* is a good place to start (www.cafamily .org.uk).
- Visit a pre-school or school catering for children with special health or learning needs if this can be organized within your course.
- Visit community health facilities and primary care – focusing on provision for children.

2

Parents and children: listening and talking

Chapter map

You will have already learnt the importance of good communication skills in adult medicine. In paediatrics, you need to extend and develop these skills, not only so that you can take an effective history, but so that you can conduct a whole consultation with children and parents together, reassure appropriately and break difficult news. This chapter will focus on history-taking, but will also cover some wider aspects of communication.

2.1 History-taking and diagnosis

> 🔑 Paediatric history-taking is vital because it usually holds the key to the diagnosis.

Diagnosis involves a recurring cycle where you formulate and test hypotheses. As you collect more information about the patient, you will reject some diagnoses, and come up with alternatives that were not on your original list (Figure 2.1). When you first begin paediatrics, it is useful to work through a list of standard questions. Once you are familiar with these, aim to move towards problem-orientated histories: generate mental lists of differentials for common presenting symptoms and then focus your history around these. This thoughtful, logical approach is much better than blindly asking a series of questions that you have learned by rote.

> **Differences from an adult history**
>
> **Triadic consultation: the child, their family and the doctor**
>
> **Indirect information from parents**
>
> **Child's contribution important but variable and unpredictable**
>
> **Different elements of history**
> * Perinatal and birth
> * Development
> * Immunization
> * Family and social history emphasis
>
> **Different illnesses and time courses**
>
> **Need to adapt to child's age and development**
>
> **Possibility of child abuse.**

Paediatrics Lecture Notes, Ninth edition. Simon J. Newell and Jonathan C. Darling. © 2014 John Wiley & Sons, Ltd. Published 2014 by John Wiley & Sons, Ltd.

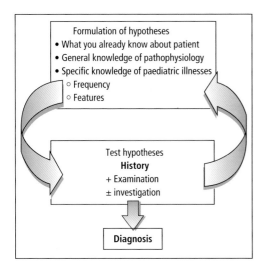

Figure 2.1 Reaching a diagnosis. It is important to start with a reasonable differential diagnosis (your hypotheses). The 'Paediatric symptom sorter' in this book can help. The history contributes much more than examination or investigations.

Table 2.1 **Fact and interpretation in history and examination.**

Fact	Interpretation
She cries and draws her legs up to her tummy	Our baby has colic
He has watery stools 6 times a day, whereas his normal stool is formed and once daily	He has bad diarrhoea
She gets wheezy when she runs	She has asthma
He falls asleep at school	He is lazy at school

2.1.1 Parents

Throughout most of childhood, parents act as the child's advocate and interpreter. Parents tell us about the child's symptoms – although the children contribute more and more as they grow older. Parents put into effect any treatments needed outside hospital.

Small children only survive because their parents are concerned about them. A few are less concerned than they should be, and their children suffer from neglect. Others are more than usually concerned. Do not regard overanxious parents as a nuisance. Instead, view their genuine concern for their child positively, and help them cope with their anxieties through patient reassurance. Parents' behaviour often reflects their own upbringing, as do excessive concerns with physiological functions, such as eating, sleeping and bowel habits.

Some parents seem easy to interview, and others difficult. If you are tempted to label someone a 'bad historian', remember that a historian is the person who collects and records the history!

Try to disentangle the facts from the parents' interpretation. Ask 'What exactly did you see that made you think that?' rather than accepting interpretations at face value (Table 2.1).

2.1.2 Involving the child

Children from about 2 years can hear, understand and say a lot. By 7 or 8 years, they are wise. Do not talk about them as if they had no understanding – and you may have to discourage parents from doing the same. Sometimes, if both are agreeable, it is useful to talk to the parent(s) and the child privately to allow them to express concerns, or to give particular advice. Older teenagers may prefer to be seen on their own first. Whatever the medical problem, the child is first a child. Not 'he is a diabetic' or 'she is an epileptic': he has diabetes, she has epilepsy.

2.1.3 History-taking

The child's history covers the same ground as that of an adult patient, with some important additions.

2.1.3.1 Approach

- Address the parents by name, not as 'mum' or 'dad'.
- Find out what the child is called at home and use that name.
- Begin your notes with the name, sex and the age in years and months – accurate age is essential and often defines the differential diagnosis.
- Note the name of the school, nursery, clinic or health centre she attends.
- Consider the child during the history:
  - A young child may be happiest on a parent's knee.
  - A more independent one may prefer playing with toys, which should be available.
  - An older child must be fully included in the discussion.
- Arrange the furniture to encourage a sense of partnership between parents and doctor and avoid confrontation over the top of a desk.

Standard paediatric history

(additions to adult history in italics)
Name/Age/Sex/Consultant/*Historian*
Presenting complaint
History of presenting complaint
Past medical history

- *Birth history*
- *Where*
- *Delivery*
- *Gestation*
- *Weight*
- *Ante/postnatal problems*
- *Neonatal problems (jaundice, SCBU, ventilation, antibiotics)*
- *Maternal health*
- *Illnesses, operations and accidents*
- *Feeding – neonatal, weaning, concerns about growth*
- *Immunizations*
- *Development*

Drugs
Allergies
Family and social history

- *Mother – name/age/occupation/health*
- *Father – name/age/occupation/health*
- *Siblings – name/age/health*
- *Inherited or genetic conditions*
- *Contact with common infections*
- *Nursery/school*
- *Pets*
- *Housing.*

PRACTICE POINT

If the parents do not speak English, insist on an interpreter. Do not try to use the child as an interpreter, except in emergencies.

2.1.3.2 History of the presenting condition

Begin with this because it is what they have come to tell you about. Let them tell it their own way first; then ask specific questions to fill in necessary details (Figure 2.2). Frequent interruptions or insistence on ordered chronology inhibit free speech.

Ask about patterns of eating, sleeping and activity. If these have not changed, serious illness is unlikely. A reduction in appetite or activity, or an increased need for sleep, are likely to be significant. Recorded weight loss is always important.

PRACTICE POINT

- Start with OPEN questions: How is she? Why are you worried?
- Add CLOSED questions: How often does he wheeze? Which inhaler do you use most?

PRACTICE POINT Always find out how the illness affects the child's life

- Normal activity, e.g. does acute asthma stop the child from running, walking and talking?
- School – for non-acute problems, how much school has been missed through illness?
- Social – is the child opting out of games or of leisure activities at home?

What are the parents' own ideas about what is the matter with the child? Sometimes this will alert you to an unnecessary anxiety; at other times it may lead to a correct diagnosis you had not considered. Mothers are more likely than anyone else to understand their babies' cries, and research shows that babies can 'talk'. They have different cries for hunger, pain, etc. The mother will usually know when the cry is abnormal and sometimes will be able to suggest a reason.

Listen to the mother – she will tell you the diagnosis.

It is often helpful, especially if psychological problems are suspected, to ask 'What kind of boy is he?' The answer may be 'a worrier', 'placid', 'never still', 'obsessional'. If you then ask 'Who does he take after?', it often provides useful insight for the parent. It is also helpful to know what the child does in his spare time and whether he is by nature gregarious or solitary.

PRACTICE POINT

Make a note of who gave you the history, who referred, and location.

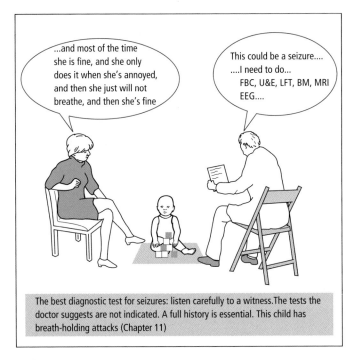

The best diagnostic test for seizures: listen carefully to a witness. The tests the doctor suggests are not indicated. A full history is essential. This child has breath-holding attacks (Chapter 11)

Figure 2.2 The best diagnostic test for seizures is a good history.

 OSCE TIP

Students often move on from the presenting complaint too quickly. Make sure you have understood precisely what is happening, impact on child and family, and details of any previous treatment (including name, dose, when given and by whom, and effect).

2.1.3.3 Previous medical history

- Illnesses, operations or hospital attendances.
- Allergies or drug sensitivities.
- Immunization history: it may help to exclude a suspected condition, and it identifies those families in need of advice about further immunization.
- Ask the parents for their child's parent-held health record (and thank them for having brought it) (see Figure 1.9). This includes details of previous weights, immunizations and other health events.

2.1.3.4 Family history

- The ages of the siblings and parents.
- Whether any other member of the family has had the same condition as the child, e.g.
  - A rash and fever (has the child caught the same infection?)
  - Six digits on each hand (an inherited condition).

- What illnesses the parents and close relatives have had, in order to identify familial and infective problems and allay needless worries. The parents may worry that their child's stomach ache is caused by stomach cancer, because a relative recently died with it.
- An enquiry regarding consanguinity, especially in Muslim families, because rare inherited conditions are more likely if the parents are related.

 PRACTICE POINT

Diagnostic signs on examination are rare; the child's diagnosis lies in the history.

2.1.3.5 Perinatal history

- Pregnancy
  - Gestation (normal is 40 weeks)
  - Illnesses
  - Medications
  - Smoking and alcohol
- Delivery
  - Place (hospital/home)
  - Presentation (head/breech)
  - Type (spontaneous, forceps, caesarean section)
- Birth weight

- Neonatal period
  - Abnormalities
  - Illnesses
  - Need for special/intensive care
  - Day of discharge home.

2.1.3.6 Developmental history

This is almost unique to paediatrics. It is important, particularly for young or disabled children. It includes details of the times at which skills such as walking and talking were acquired (Chapter 9).

2.1.3.7 Social history

After establishing rapport with the parents, talk with them about their life, their home, their work and their problems. Parental employment may give insight into particular pressures for the family, and level of understanding of health issues. Who looks after the child if both parents work? If the mother is now a housewife, what was her job before? If she was a nurse, she will have a different level of knowledge and a different need for information.

Explore the following areas, since they have a direct influence on the child:

- Family composition
  - Other children in the home?
  - Who are the main carers?
  - Do parents live together?
  - Other significant adults in the home or close to child (e.g. grandparents)?
- Family pressures
  - What do parents see as stressful for themselves or their children?
  - May include busy jobs, financial hardship, parental discord, neighbourhood harassment
- Housing
  - Stability – frequent moves can be unsettling and affect continuity of health care
  - Space – cramped or overcrowded accommodation is stressful for all and increases infection transmission
  - Specific needs – children with disability may need modifications to their home
  - Difficulties – some families struggle with housing problems which dominate family life.

 PRACTICE POINT

Preface these questions with an explanation that an understanding of the child's home and family can often help with diagnosis and management. Ask sensitively. Otherwise they can seem irrelevant or intrusive.

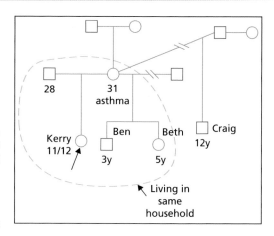

Figure 2.3 Family tree. The broken lines between parents indicate a separation. Ben and Beth live in the same household as Kerry (who is the presenting child, indicated with an arrow), but are her half-siblings, to mother's previous partner.

 PRACTICE POINT

Drawing out a family tree with the parents' help is a good way to understand complex family arrangements (Fig 2.3). This can be annotated with details of illnesses, names, dates (e.g. of bereavement/separation/divorce).

2.2 The consultation

Families are often anxious on arrival, waiting for the doctor's 'verdict'. Their fears are often worse than the reality.

 PRACTICE POINT

Each person who sees the family should introduce themselves, explain their role and what they are going to do.

As a student, you should check the parents are happy to speak to you, and clarify your task and the time available with the doctor supervising you. Once the history and examination have been completed, the remainder of the consultation often takes one of three directions:

- Explanation and reassurance
- Investigation and/or treatment but with a favourable outcome probable
- Bad news.

Students may be involved in discussing aspects of the first two under supervision, but should not attempt to break bad news. If a child or parent asks you questions when you do not know the answer, admit it. Offer to find someone who can help.

2.2.1 Reassurance

- Readily accepted by some parents who 'just wanted to make sure everything was all right'.
- Remember that the presenting condition may only be a pretext to visit, and that more serious concerns lie elsewhere.
- Some parents are very difficult to reassure.
  - Careful explanation is usually helpful – parents may stop worrying if they understand why the doctor is not worried.
  - A specific anxiety needs an equally specific reassurance, e.g. parents who fear their child's pallor is due to leukaemia may need to be told 'She has not got leukaemia', rather than just that the blood count is normal.

2.2.2 Investigations and treatments

- Explain honestly and in advance
  - Don't say it won't hurt if it will – but you can emphasize the things that will minimize anything unpleasant.
  - An MRI scan is noisy (or, for very young children, may require a general anaesthetic).
- Give results promptly with clear explanation and interpretation
  - Parents appreciate being told the results of tests, and their implications, promptly – a phone call often helps.
- Explain and give reasons for treatments
  - Some treatments are flexible and others not, and it helps if parents understand the rationale e.g. why four times a day?
  - Demonstrate techniques for use of inhalers for asthma, injections for diabetes or rectally administered anticonvulsants.

Parents are increasingly informed about health issues, through television, newspapers, magazines and the internet. Unfortunately the media tend to exaggerate or sensationalize, presenting an experimental new treatment as a 'breakthrough', or a particular clinic or hospital (often in another country) as 'the only one of its kind' and hence, by implication, the best. The accolade of TV hype is more impressive than holy writ, and it may be an uphill task to put things in perspective. We need special understanding for parents who have been offered hope when they had none before.

2.2.3 Bad news

This usually concerns:

- A birth defect in a newborn baby
- A serious handicap in a young child
- A serious, progressive or incurable disease.

The news that a baby is abnormal is a great shock to the parents. Even minor anomalies are seen as major tragedies. At the first interview, detailed explanations will not be grasped. Later, parents will need detailed explanation of the care needed and how to recognize any problems that are likely to arise.

 PRACTICE POINT

Parents want to know:
- Exactly what is the matter, in terms they can grasp
- What the doctors can do about it
- What the parents can do about it
- The outlook for this child
- The outlook for any other children that may follow
- Why it happened (did they cause it?).

2.2.3.1 Breaking bad news

- Both parents present if possible
- Unhurried (no mobiles or pagers)
- Ask what the parents understand
- Clear information
- Diagrams and/or printed materials for reference
- Regularly summarize and invite questions
- Make a clear plan.

Parents' self-help groups can provide information, leaflets and mutual support. Parents should be told about them.

 PRACTICE POINT

When transferring a baby to another hospital (e.g. for surgery, neonatal intensive care)
- Ensure mother sees her infant before transfer.
- Arrange frequent progress reports until mother is able to visit.

2.2.3.2   Genetic counselling

Parents of children with serious defects or handicaps need advice about the recurrence risks if they plan another child later on. For easily recognizable conditions in which a genetic (or non-genetic) basis is clearly established, the family doctor or paediatrician can provide this information. For more complex problems refer to a *genetic counselling* clinic.

Essentials of genetic counselling
- A firmly established diagnosis (often more difficult than it sounds)
- Knowledge of inheritance
- A full family history
- Ample time to elicit facts and anxieties, and to explain recurrence risks, prenatal tests and other relevant issues.

2.2.3.3   Parents' reactions to bad news (Figure 2.4)

- Recognizable pattern
- Time scale varies widely from one family to another
- Important for doctors to recognize this pattern
  - To help the family
  - To understand parents' negative reactions (e.g. anger towards the doctor).

The stages of adaptation to personal tragedy, which often overlap, are as follows:

1. Intellectual and emotional numbness
   - Information does not get in, emotions do not get out.
     - Health staff may be relieved that the parents have 'taken it so well'.
     - Don't be annoyed if parents later say 'nobody told us anything' when you spent hours telling them everything.

2. Denial
   - The message has got through but cannot yet be believed.
     - 'There must be some mistake' or 'But he will catch up, won't he?'
   - Resist the temptation to hedge or use woolly phrases (e.g. 'slow developer') – they may falsely encourage parents to believe that the problem is curable.

3. Guilt and anger
   - The truth has registered and blame must be apportioned.
     - Parents often blame themselves – for some act of commission or omission, real or imaginary.
     - Blame others – the feeling of guilt may be so intolerable that the parents blame someone else (the doctor) or something else (the tablets).

4. Grief
   - A natural and healing process.
   - Tears are healthy – the health professional who shares these moments should feel privileged, not embarrassed.

5. Reconstruction
   - The former pattern of family life has been demolished; the new must now be built.
   - Give parents a key, active role in any therapeutic programme.
   - Never say 'Nothing can be done' – it is not true.

2.3   Adolescence

Effective consultation with adolescents requires a different approach to that with younger children. See Chapter 16 for more details.

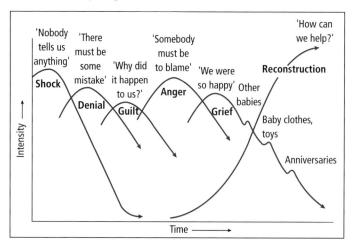

Figure 2.4 Emotional response to bad news.

Summary

We have described how the paediatric history and consultation differs from adult medicine. There are different elements (such as birth, immunizations, development), but more importantly there is a different approach. This includes involving the child according to age, understanding the constraints of working through a third party (the parent), and being aware of the possibility of child abuse. There is no substitute for practice, and we hope you will enjoy taking and presenting many paediatric histories, and reviewing them with your teachers.

 OSCE TIP

- History of any common presenting symptom or problem.
- Counselling and explaining common and important paediatric problems, e.g. constipation, weaning, immunization, gastro-oesophageal reflux, asthma, febrile convulsions, epilepsy, enuresis.

 FOR YOUR LOG

Summarizing a history is key clinical skill. Write a brief (2–3 sentence) summary for every history you take. The process clarifies what is important in your mind, makes your verbal presentation clearer, and means you finish neatly. OSCE stations involving history taking or presentation will often ask for a summary.

OSCE station 2.1: Counselling

Clinical approach:

- Read any facts given to you
- Have mental/written list of main points
- Ask open questions at beginning and end (e.g. is there anything else you would like me to talk about?)
- Note reasons for special concern (e.g. other member of family with same problem)
- Deal with common concerns
- Remember body language — yours and the mother's
- Listen
- It may help to write down the diagnosis, or draw a diagram.

Information to give

- Diagnosis, description of problem
- What do we know?
- The cause
- Explain the child's symptoms
- What can be done?
- How will it affect the child?
- What treatment?
- What investigations?
- Follow up

Please talk to this mother. Her 3-year-old son had a febrile convulsion 2 days ago and is now well. She would like to discuss this with you before going home

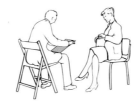

- Listen to what she knows
- Explain diagnosis
  - ◇ Fit caused by fever in healthy child
  - ◇ 6 months — 5 years of age
- Common (3% of all children)
- Fits are frightening but seldom dangerous
  - ◇ How did parents feel during child's fit?
  - ◇ Many parents think that their child is dying
- Prognosis good
  - ◇ Most have no more febrile fits
  - ◇ One third will have a second episode
  - ◇ Epilepsy rare
- Prevention
  - ◇ Recognition of fever
  - ◇ Light clothing, antipyretic, tepid sponging
- Further fits
  - ◇ First aid
  - ◇ When to seek help

Member of staff is likely to play role of mother
The child is not present

Never forget:

- Say hello and introduce yourself
- General health — is the child ill?
- Empathic enquiry: how is Sally today?
- Are you and the child's parent comfortable?

Look around for:

- Hospital records
- Information leaflets

Special points

- In some exams, you will be given a history first
- Listen for hints to unexpressed worries
- 'Parent' may be a trained actor or a hospital secretary — you usually do not need to put your arm round them

3

Examination of children

Chapter map

Examining children, especially the very young, seems daunting at first, but most children are cooperative, and clinical examination should be a happy experience for them. Children are usually accompanied by a parent, who will help you and appreciate being involved. This chapter assumes you are already competent to do systems examinations in adult patients. We will show you how to adjust your examination according to the child's age, show you how to approach any clinical examination of a child, and emphasize key differences in paediatric examination, including attention to growth, nutrition and pubertal status.

The obvious reason for examination is to find abnormal signs that help make the diagnosis. In acute illness, symptoms are often non-specific. The general impression of a child's health is all important. You will miss essential signs (e.g. infected throat, stiff neck or infected urine) if you do not look for them systematically. In chronic illness, subtle signs can be clues to the diagnosis. For example, minor congenital abnormalities or dysmorphic features can point to a syndrome, or chronic chest deformity or clubbing may indicate chronic respiratory disease. Assessment of growth is always helpful.

Parents and children often come to the paediatrician concerned about severe disease. A 'thorough examination' is a powerful therapeutic weapon in the face of parental anxiety. Parents do not readily accept reassurance from the doctor who has not examined the child – and quite right too!

PRACTICE POINT Chaperones

As a student, think carefully before performing sensitive or intimate examinations that might cause a child or adolescent embarrassment. It will rarely be appropriate for you to proceed. As a doctor, consider requesting a chaperone at these times.

Paediatrics Lecture Notes, Ninth edition. Simon J. Newell and Jonathan C. Darling. © 2014 John Wiley & Sons, Ltd. Published 2014 by John Wiley & Sons, Ltd.

PRACTICE POINT Age-specific approach to examining children

- *Newborn infants*: in the early weeks of life, patience, warm hands and a quiet voice are needed. Bedside manner contributes little (but is important to parents).
- *2–10 months*: infants respond to the friendly doctor, and examination is often easy if the child is generally comfortable. A smiling face can evoke rapport, and even cooperation.
- *10 months–5 years*: toddlers present the biggest challenge. The toddler is generally suspicious of strangers. Their confidence must be won, perhaps by giving them something to hold, or taking interest in their toy. An unhurried, confident approach is most likely to lead to success. Young children do not like to be separated from their parents, rapidly undressed or made to lie flat. Examine the child on their parent's knee rather than an examination couch. Be patient and adapt the pace and the order of the examination to the child's level of comfort and confidence.
- *5–10 years*: school-age children are used to being without their parents, but still want them close by in unfamiliar surroundings. They are generally cooperative. They enjoy neurological examination and like to listen to their heart through a stethoscope. A worried child can be diverted by chatting to them.
- *10 years to teenage*: the process of examining the older child and teenager is usually straightforward. Cooperation is almost guaranteed if the doctor respects their independence, maturity and modesty. Ask them whether they would prefer their parents to be present, and seek their permission to examine them. Often the history-taking will be dominated by a parent, and most teenagers cannot tell you their birthweight! The time of the examination is an opportunity to talk to the older child about their perspective and concerns.

3.1 A system of examination

In acute paediatrics, outpatients and in undergraduate exams, clinical examination begins with general assessment and then moves on to look at specific systems. All who are new to paediatrics must begin by learning these skills.

 PRACTICE POINT

Watch paediatricians closely to pick up ideas to add to your own repertoire of ways to help children feel at ease.

A good history will raise specific questions, e.g. this history could be pneumonia. Is this child unwell? Is she tachypnoeic or febrile?

3.1.1 Initial assessment

Clinical examination has certain essential elements; these are made during the first approach to the child and should be carefully recorded. The most striking finding in a young child with pneumonia, for example, is that they appear ill. The positive clinical findings of lobar consolidation are difficult to elicit, and may be absent.

3.1.2 HIGHCOST

This acronym emphasizes the importance of the first clinical impression and simple observation, which

are central to good paediatric clinical assessment. It might also remind you that good clinical assessment is expensive of time, but highly cost effective! It is a useful approach to systems examination in the OSCE (Chapter 28).

Hello

Introduce yourself

General inspection

Health and hands

Centiles

Obvious

Systems examination

Thank you

3.1.3 Hello

Children are quick to assess adults, and often very accurate. Approach the child with courtesy, a smile and a friendly greeting. There are two essential reasons that every undergraduate should remember this: it is an important clinical skill, and in almost every OSCE you will get marks for it!

3.1.4 Introduce yourself

Introduce yourself and find out to whom you are speaking. What does the child like to be called? Matt may only be called Matthew when his parents are annoyed with him.

3.1.5 General inspection

During the general introduction, and often while taking the clinical history, you will learn a lot about the child, her parents and the relationships between them. You should also note if the child has an unusual appearance or abnormal features which fit into a recognized pattern (e.g. Down syndrome, achondroplasia).

PRACTICE POINT

Do not tower over the child, or lean over them during examination, but get down to their level.

Note the following:

- Does the child look well cared for? (Be careful – some clean, well-behaved children are unloved, while some caring parents may not see hygiene and clothing as a priority.)
- Is there a loving relationship between the child and the parents? Do the parents talk as if the child were not there, or as if she is an inanimate object? Are the parents showing an appropriate level of concern whilst sharing the problem with you?
- Is the child confident or clinging to the parent? Is he crying? When he seeks reassurance from his parent, does he get it? These are difficult assessments, particularly when a child is unwell.
- Does the child have any unusual features? Are the body proportions appropriate? Look at the child's face. Before you decide a child is dysmorphic, look at the parents' faces.

3.1.6 Health and hands

- Is the child ill or well? Ask yourself this question every time you examine a child.
  - In the young child, this is often the most important clinical sign. In the acutely unwell, 6-month-old infant, a pale, listless unresponsive appearance with glazed eyes has essential implications for diagnosis and immediate management. The experienced parent who simply reports that their child is ill should be listened to carefully.

🔑 Children can change very quickly. A child who was satisfactory at triage may be moribund an hour later. If in doubt, don't press on with your assessment but call a member of staff.

Facial appearance may be helpful. Look for swelling, pallor, jaundice, or cyanosis and assess hydration (see Figure 21.4). Jaundice may be difficult to detect in artificial light. Examine the palprebral conjunctiva for signs of anaemia (evert the lower eyelid).

PRACTICE POINT

A hospital doctor who receives a phone call from a GP stating that the diagnosis is not clear, but that the child looks ill, should appreciate the urgency and importance of this statement.

- Features that raise concern:
  - A child who is inattentive, limp or intermittently distressed
  - pallor, mottled skin or the infant who appears grey
  - hypoxia may make a child sleepy or agitated
  - cyanosis may be hard to see
  - dehydration (Section 21.1.4.1)
  - increased work of breathing (Section 3.5.3)
  - fever, particularly if there is no clear cause.

It is often helpful to start the examination by holding the child's hand. It is not only a friendly gesture, but is often informative.

- Quickly assess the pulse. The radial pulse is commonly used, but in infants the brachial may be easier to feel.
- Assess perfusion. Are the hands well perfused or cold and clammy?
- Capillary refill is assessed by gently squeezing the nail so that the nail bed becomes pale. Upon release, the nail bed should again become pink within 2 seconds. Pale hands may indicate anaemia, which is better assessed from the conjunctiva.
- Look for clubbing. Although uncommon in children, when present it is an important physical sign.

3.1.7 Centiles

Assessment of growth is a fundamental part of paediatric examination (see below). Although with experience you can make some assessment visually, you should always plot measurements on a centile chart. In an exam, saying that you would like to do this may be all that is necessary. If possible, compare with previous measurements in the parent-held record or the hospital notes. The trend of the plots is more important than their absolute positions.

3.1.8 Obvious

It is surprisingly easy to omit or even not notice the obvious, especially when you are focusing on a particular system, so include this as a deliberate step in your assessment. Often these observations give important clues to the diagnosis. Record or comment on the leg in plaster, the central venous line, the nasogastric tube, ankle/foot orthoses (splints) or a pile of inhalers. Record any injuries.

3.1.9 Systems examination

In paediatrics, each system does not need to be examined in a fixed order. Often examination of the body systems must be opportunistic. If the toddler is undressed and lying peacefully in his mother's arms, you might begin by listening to the heart. Leave potentially upsetting procedures (inspection of the throat) until last. Many children prefer not to be undressed completely, although by the end of examination all parts of the body should have been inspected. In undergraduate examination, genitalia should not be examined, except in young infants, and rectal examination should never be performed. During systems examination, put the child at ease by asking about their family, friends, pets, hobbies or favourite TV programmes. Keep any instruments (tendon hammer, auroscope, etc.) out of sight until you need them, then show them to the child and explain how they work.

3.1.10 Thank you

Gratitude for the privilege of examining a child is never misplaced. The family will all appreciate praise for a child's good behaviour and cooperation.

> **OSCE TIP**
>
> In an exam, never do anything that is painful, likely to cause discomfort, or which is emabarassing. Some tasks are not practical in the OSCE settting. If you are going to omit part of the examination for these reasons, explain this to the examiner (e.g. in the cardiac examination, say that you would want to: plot growth centiles, measure BP with correct cuff, and examine femoral pulses).

3.2 Growth and nutrition

The characteristics of children which most clearly distinguish them from adults are growth (increase in size) and development (organ maturation, sexual development and the acquisition of new skills) (Figure 3.1).

> **PRACTICE POINT**
>
> Plot with a single dot as accurately as you can – crosses and circles obscure subsequent plots. Use the chart already in the notes. If you have to start a new one, label it.

3.2.1 Centile charts (Figure 3.2)

To assess growth, plot weight and height (and head circumference in infants, Figure 3.3) on centile charts. These are constructed from measurements of many children who are free from recognized

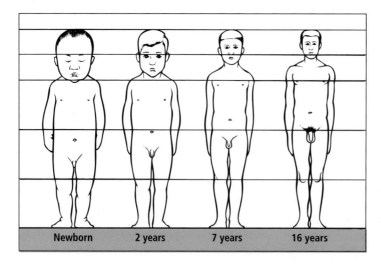

| Newborn | 2 years | 7 years | 16 years |

Figure 3.1 Body proportions from birth to adulthood. The ratio of the parts above and below the symphysis pubis falls from 1.7 : 1 in the newborn to 0.9 : 1 in the adult.

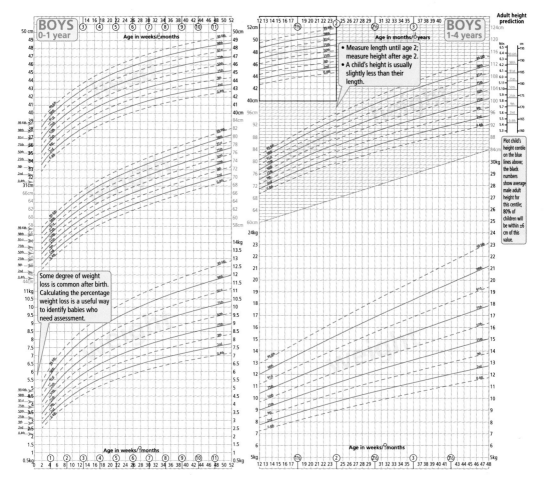

Figure 3.2 Growth centile charts for boys aged 0-4 years. Separate charts are available for girls and older children at www.rcpch.ac.uk/child-health. These charts are developed and maintained by RCPCH/WHO/Department of Health. © 2009 Department of Health.

problems which affect their growth. Children should be weighed either in underclothes (babies in nappies) or naked, but always the same way because changes in weight are more important than absolute values. Height is measured with a wall-mounted stadiometer, and you need tuition and practice to be able to do this accurately. For a child who is not yet walking, measure length supine on a horizontal stadiometer with a moveable foot board. Two people are needed to do this accurately. If children are upset at

the prospect of being weighed and measured, postpone until the clinical examination is over: tears are more easily prevented than stopped.

3.2.2 Normal growth

Growth rates are good indicators of general health and nutrition. Children who are growing normally usually have height and weight measurements that progress parallel to the centile lines, are in proportion (i.e. not more than 2 centile lines difference between height and weight). 95% of healthy children are between the 2nd and 98th centiles.

3.2.3 Growth velocity and puberty

Growth velocity refers to gain in weight or height over time. Height velocity is measured in cm/year. It is

> **PRACTICE POINT**
>
> Remember to adjust plots for prematurity (i.e. less than 37 weeks gestation) for the first year of life. A dotted horizontal arrow from the plot for the actual age to the one for the adjusted age makes the adjustment clear.

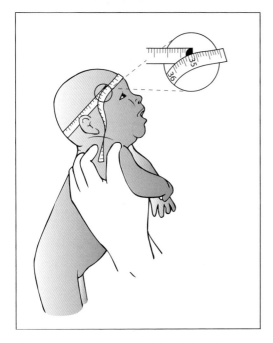

Figure 3.3 Measuring an infant's head circumference:
• *head circumference* is an important measurement, and reflects the volume of the cranial contents with surprising accuracy;
• a good quality, inelastic tape is used;
• the tape passes over the occiput, above the ears, and the prominence of the brow;
• two or three measurements are taken in slightly different planes, and the largest is recorded as the head circumference.

highest in the first year and then gradually falls until the pubertal growth spurt when there is a second smaller peak. Depending on whether puberty starts early or late, a child's height and weight may move away from their 'normal' centile around this time. If puberty is early, growth will accelerate towards a higher centile, and then gradually level off as the rate of the pubertal growth spurt slows. Full assessment of height may require information about pubertal status (Figures 3.5 and 3.6) and bone age (see Section 3.2.5).

3.2.4 Nutritional assessment

Accurate nutritional assessment is difficult and complex. The initial clinical impression is usually valuable. An undernourished child is 'all skin and bone'; the limbs are slender, the bony prominences are conspicuous and loss of muscle bulk may be observed. In the younger child, this is seen as wasting

of the buttocks. Mid-upper arm circumference is measured simply with a tape measure around the arm at the mid-point between the elbow and the shoulder. Centile charts provide reference data but, in the child aged 1–5 years, a circumference less than 14 cm suggests poor nutrition and needs further assessment. If weight loss has been recent, folds of skin on the lower abdomen and inner aspects of the thighs may be seen. Excess fat is most evident on the trunk. Weight for height can be assessed by looking at the relative centiles for the two measurements.

> **PRACTICE POINT**
>
> Body mass index {BMI = weight (kg) ÷ height (m)^2} varies with age, and charts are available. A BMI >20 kg/m^2 in a child of 1–10 years indicates obesity. Calculators are available on the internet which chart and help to interpret BMI (e.g. apps.nccd.cdc.gov/dnpabmi).

Other useful measurements include sitting height (which reflects body proportions), and arm span (which is usually similar to height).

3.2.5 Bone age

Bone age (or skeletal age) is a useful index of growth and maturation. A plain X-ray of the hand and wrist is taken. Calcification of the epiphyses, and later their fusion, is noted for each of the bones around the wrist, and compared with standard pictures. The method is complex and requires special skills. In healthy children, bone age relates more closely to height than to age, short children tending to have 'delayed', and tall children 'advanced' bone ages. Significant advance or delay in bone age merits investigation.

3.3 Dental development

The average ages of eruption of the teeth are shown below, but there is a wide normal range. There are 20 deciduous and 32 permanent teeth; permanent teeth appear from the sixth year. The first molars and central incisors appear first. All teeth have appeared by the age of 14 except the third molars. Teeth appear a few months earlier in girls (Table 3.1).

3.4 Sexual development

Human sexual development is concentrated into two brief periods of time: primary sexual development in the embryo and the appearance of secondary

Deciduous		Appearance (months)
Central incisor	Lower	6–10
	Upper	7–10
Lateral incisor	Upper	8–10
	Lower	12–18
First molar		12–18
Canine		16–20
Second molar		20–30

Table 3.1 **Dental development.**

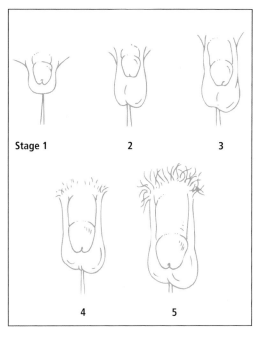

Stage 1   2   3

4   5

Figure 3.5 Stages of male genital development. (1) Pre-adolescent. (2) Enlargement of scrotum and testes. (3) Increases of breadth of penis and development of glans. (4) Testes continue to enlarge. Scrotum darkens. (5) Adult: by this time, pubic hair has spread to the medial surface of the thighs.

sex characteristics during puberty (Figure 3.4). At puberty, changes occur in response to pituitary gonadotrophins. The trigger for release of these hormones is still unknown. The age of onset of puberty is very variable and is influenced by racial, hereditary and nutritional factors.

In girls in the UK today, breast development begins at 11 years of age on average, and pubic hair a little later. Early breast development may be asymmetrical. Mean age of menarche is 13 years, but is commonly between 11 and 15 years. The first signs of puberty are breast development in girls and growth of the testes in boys. In both sexes, puberty is accompanied by an impressive growth spurt, which occurs early in puberty in girls (maximal at age 12 years) and late in puberty in boys (maximal at 14 years) – see Figure 13.5. The progress of puberty is recorded in stages of pubic hair (both sexes), external genitalia (male) and breast development (female) (Figures 3.5 and 3.6). Epiphyseal fusion, with cessation of growth, marks the end of puberty.

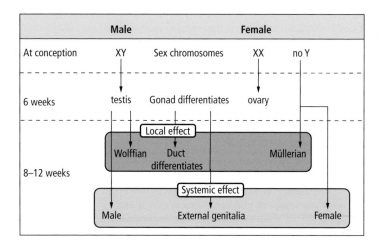

Figure 3.4 Embryonic and fetal sex differentiation.

Breast development

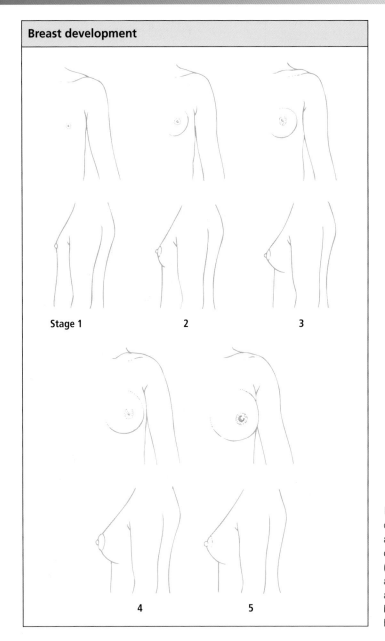

Stage 1   2   3

4   5

Figure 3.6 Stages of breast development. (1) Pre-adolescent – elevation of papilla only. (2) Breast bud stage. (3) Further enlargement of breast and areola. (4) Projection of areola and papilla above level of breast. (5) Mature stage – areola has recessed, papilla projects.

3.5   Systems examination

3.5.1   Head and neck

3.5.1.1   Lymph glands

Superficial lymph glands are always palpable in the neck and groins of children. Normal glands are soft, mobile, non-tender and usually not larger than 1–2 cm. Enlarged tonsillar glands, just behind the

 PRACTICE POINT

Benign lymph nodes are smooth, mobile, non-tender, usually not larger than 1–2 cm, may vary in size and persist for many months. Most don't need any investigation. They are common in the neck, less so in the groins, and rare in the axillae. Hard, craggy, fixed nodes are unlikely to be benign and need urgent referral.

angle of the jaw, indicate past or present throat infections and may persist for months. Generalized lymphadenopathy suggests systemic illness unless it is due to widespread skin disease (e.g. eczema).

3.5.1.2 Fontanelles

Anterior fontanelle – is widely open at birth, but varies considerably in size. It closes between 9 and 18 months. Gentle pressure over the fontanelle gives an indication of its tension. The normal fontanelle is relaxed when the infant is resting. It pulsates with the heartbeat. Tension increases when the infant cries or strains.

Changes may provide important clues if supported by other clinical signs:

- Large fontanelle→hydrocephalus
- Small fontanelle→slow brain growth
- Sunken fontanelle→dehydration
- Bulging fontanelle→raised intracranial pressure.

Posterior fontanelle – far back where the sagittal and lambdoid sutures meet. It closes soon after birth.
Third fontanelle – sometimes present in the sagittal suture just in front of the posterior fontanelle. It may be a marker for other congenital abnormality.

3.5.2 Ear, nose and throat

This is an important part of the general examination of any child, especially an ill child. It is difficult in babies, and young children may dislike having their ears examined. Practice makes perfect. Take time to ensure the young child is securely held – this makes for a much easier examination (Figures 3.7 and 3.8).

 OSCE TIP

You will probably not be asked to do ENT examination in a real child in the OSCE, but it is an essential skill in acute paediatrics. Make sure you can do it.

3.5.2.1 Ears

- Brace with your fingers against the child's cheek to prevent accidental damage to the meatus with the speculum.
- Draw the pinna gently upwards and backwards to allow a clear view of the eardrums.

3.5.2.2 Nose

Note nasal discharge or bleeding. Although not routine, the nasal mucosa may be examined with the auroscope. Note the colour of the mucosa, the presence of oedema, secretions, polyps or foreign bodies.

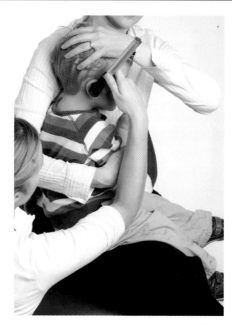

Figure 3.7 Ear examination. Examination of the ear is easier and safer if the infant is held correctly. Note the child is held sideways-on against the parent in a firm 'cuddle'. The rear arm should be behind the parent's back. Hold the auroscope between the thumb and index finger, using the remaining fingers to brace against the child's cheek (this protects against damage caused by sudden movement).

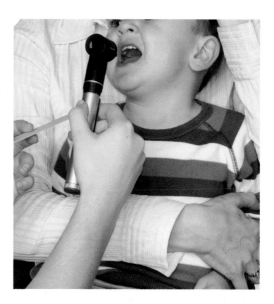

Figure 3.8 Examination of the mouth and throat. Take time to position the child correctly facing towards you on the parent's lap. One of the parent's arms should encircle the child's chest and arms, while the other hand presses on the child's forehead.

3.5.2.3   Mouth and throat

- Note the state of the gums, teeth, tongue and buccal mucosa.
- If children will put their tongue out and say 'ah', the posterior pharynx may be viewed without a tongue depressor. A wooden tongue depressor is well tolerated by most children. It must be used gently, and not placed so far back as to cause gagging. It is difficult to get a good view of the throat in babies.

> **PRACTICE POINT**
>
> Never examine the throat of a young child with stridor: it may precipitate respiratory obstruction.

3.5.3   Chest and lungs

3.5.3.1   Inspect the chest

- *Hyperinflation* is caused by chronic obstructive airways disease as in bad asthma, or seen acutely in conditions such as bronchiolitis.
- *Pectus carinatum*: the sternum is displaced forward, relative to the ribs. Children do not like to hear themselves referred to as pigeon-chested.
- *Pectus excavatum*: a depression in the anterior chest wall above the epigastrium due to a short central tendon of the diaphragm which tethers the lower end of the sternum.
- *Harrison's sulcus*. A bony rib deformity, which is a linear indentation, parallel to and just above the costal margin (Figure 3.9). Its position corresponds to the insertion of the diaphragm and it is due to either increased diaphragmatic pull (chronic respiratory conditions such as poorly controlled asthma) or bone disease such as rickets, where the bones are more easily deformed by normal diaphragmatic action.

> **?   OSCE TIP**
>
> In the OSCE, it does not matter if you forget the latin terms: Pectus carinatum is just increased AP diameter with prominent sternum.

3.5.3.2   Assess respiratory effort

- Respiratory rate. Tachypnoea is important. Breathing should be measured at rest over a full 30s. Normal respiratory rate falls with age: in infants, it should be less than 60/min, in children it should be less than 40/min. Rates less than 20 or intermittent apnoea should always raise immediate and urgent concern.

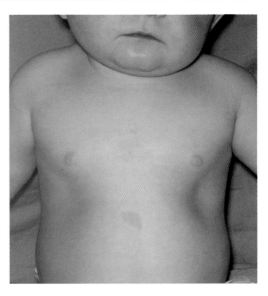

Figure 3.9 Harrison's sulcus. Note the indentation or 'guttering' of the lower ribcage, which is a chronic deformity.

- Pattern of breathing. Prolonged expiration occurs with wheeze. Deep, sighing (acidotic) breathing occurs in diabetic ketoacidosis.
- Recession in the intercostal spaces, epigastrium and suprasternal notch may be seen with increased respiratory effort and obstruction of air flow into the lungs.

> **Signs of respiratory distress**
>
> - Tachypnoea
> - Recession (intercostal, subcostal, suprasternal)
> - Nasal flaring
> - Use of accessory muscles (appears as head bobbing in babies who cannot fix the shoulder girdle)
> - Grunting on expiration (in infants)
> - Cyanosis
> - Difficulty in walking, talking, drinking or speaking.

3.5.3.3   Detect added noises

- Wheeze: a predominantly expiratory sound, due to obstruction in the lower airways. Typical of asthma and bronchiolitis.
- Stridor: a predominantly inspiratory sound, indicating upper airway obstruction and typical of croup or laryngeal oedema.
- Cough: most often arises in the upper respiratory tract. Children tend to swallow sputum rather than spit it out. A barking cough is typical of croup. Paroxysms of coughing occur in whooping cough.

3.5.3.4 Percussion

Place finger firmly, but gently, in contact with the anterior chest wall, and parallel to the ribs. Percuss your own finger lightly. Percuss over the clavicle and the front of the chest and in three positions on each side of the chest posteriorly. In children under 2y, percussion yields limited information, but is important where auscultation is abnormal or asymmetrical.

3.5.3.5 Auscultation

- Use an appropriate sized stethoscope. An adult-sized stethoscope placed on a newborn baby will pick up heart, breath and bowel sounds all at once! Compare air entry on both sides. In small children, it is normal for breath sounds to be bronchial.
- Coarse crepitations are often transmitted from the throat or upper airways. These may clear if the child coughs first.

 PRACTICE POINT Auscultation

If a young child finds it hard to take a deep breath, ask them to blow out, and listen when they breathe in afterwards.

3.5.4 Cardiovascular system

3.5.4.1 Inspection

- Look for increased respiratory rate or other signs of increased work of breathing.
- Watch a baby feeding. The infant sucks well at first, but then has to stop for a rest.

 Poor feeding is a cardinal sign of heart failure.

- Is there cyanosis on rest or on exertion?
- Precordial bulge: the right ventricle pushes the sternum forward.
- Ventricular heave: the right ventricle causes the lower sternum to move forward with each cardiac impulse.

3.5.4.2 Pulse

- The minimum requirement is to count the pulse and to examine its character in both brachials. Check that the femoral pulses are present and that there is no brachio-femoral delay (coarctation of the aorta).
- Rate. Normal rate falls with age.
- Rhythm.
- Character. Small volume in shock; bounding pulse in patent ductus arteriosis.

3.5.4.3 Palpation

- Find the apex beat. It should be in the fourth or fifth intercostal space, just lateral to the nipple.
- Check the apex is on the left.
- Thrills are the vibration of a loud murmur. If you do not hear a murmur, you have not felt a thrill.

3.5.4.4 Auscultation

- Listen for two heart sounds.
- Splitting of the second sound is easily heard in children and is usually normal. The gap between the aortic and pulmonary second sounds increases in inspiration.

3.5.4.5 Murmurs

- Timing: pansystolic, ejection systolic, continuous or, rarely, diastolic.
- Quality: describe the sound or character.
- Site of maximum intensity: where?
- Intensity: how loud is it?
- Radiation: can the murmur be heard in the neck or back?

Intensity grading of heart murmur

1 Barely audible
2 Soft
3 Easy to hear, no thrill
4 Loud, easily audible, thrill
5 Very loud, with easily palpable thrill
6 Audible with the stethoscope held off the chest

3.5.4.6 Blood pressure

The cuff should be wide enough to cover two-thirds of the distance between the tip of the elbow and shoulder. In practice, this is the largest cuff that will comfortably fit around the upper arm. Too small a cuff yields a falsely high blood pressure. Check the systolic pressure by palpation first, then determine systolic and diastolic pressures by auscultation. Automated methods (e.g. Dinamap) are commonly used in paediatrics. Blood pressure should be judged against centile charts. In the neonatal period, mean systolic blood pressure is 70 mmHg. From 6 weeks to 10 years of age, mean systolic blood pressure remains around 95 mmHg, and most children will have a systolic blood pressure less than 115 mmHg. Mean systolic blood pressure is 125 mmHg by 16 years of age.

3.5.5 Abdomen and gastrointestinal tract

3.5.5.1 Mouth

The oral cavity should be examined thoroughly. Note cracking and soreness around the lips.

3.5.5.2 Inspection

- Abdominal distension. Normal toddlers are rather pot bellied. The mother will be able to say whether the abdomen is swollen.
- Visible peristalsis.
- Hernia.
- The acutely painful abdomen does not move normally with respiration.

3.5.5.3 Palpation

Is the abdomen soft or tender with guarding? Palpate gently and then more deeply whilst talking to the child and carefully observing their face for signs of tenderness.

3.5.5.4 Hernia

An umbilical hernia is easily seen (Section 21.2.3.1). Inguinal hernias may not be immediately evident; femoral hernias are hard to find.

3.5.5.5 Hepatomegaly

- The liver is normally palpable 1–2 cm below the costal margin in infants and young children.
- Palpate from the right iliac fossa upwards. The liver edge moves down with respiration.
- Percussion may be helpful.
- The size of the liver is measured below the costal margin in the mid-clavicular line.

3.5.5.6 Splenomegaly

- The spleen tip may be felt in young infants. Palpate from the right iliac fossa, across the abdomen.
- Spleen moves downwards or diagonally on respiration. The notch is palpable. One cannot get above it, and it is felt anteriorly.

3.5.5.7 Renal swelling

- Normal kidneys may be palpable in the newborn period.
- Kidneys felt bimanually.
- Kidneys move down with respiration.

3.5.5.8 Faecal masses

- Frequently felt in the line of the colon and in the left iliac fossa, especially if the child is constipated.

3.5.5.9 Percussion

The liver and large spleen are dull to percussion.

Ascites

- Diffuse swelling, protuberant umbilicus.
- Shifting dullness: gas-filled bowel produces resonant percussion note on the uppermost point of the abdomen. If ascites is present, then when the child lies on his back the abdomen is resonant around the umbilicus and dull in the flanks. Turn the child so that one side is uppermost. The upper flank should now be resonant and the umbilical area dull (Figure 3.10).

3.5.5.10 Auscultation

- Increased bowel sounds: intestinal hurry, e.g. gastroenteritis and early intestinal obstruction.
- Decreased bowel sounds: paralytic ileus.

3.5.5.11 Rectal examination

Rectal examination is rarely indicated in children. It should only be performed by a skilled doctor who can interpret the findings.

Examine stool for colour, consistency and the presence of blood or mucus.

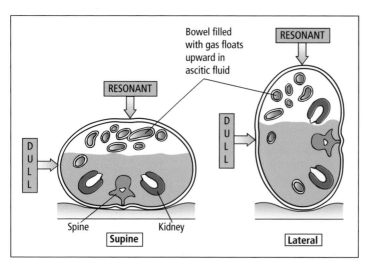

Figure 3.10 Schematic diagram of shifting dullness. Dullness to percussion shifts as the fluid moves and the bowel floats.

3.5.5.12 Urinalysis

Urine should be examined and tested with a multi-reagent stick (OCSE station 22.1).

3.5.5.13 Genitalia

Boys

- Is the penis a normal shape? Is the urethral meatus at the tip of the penis or displaced (hypospadias, epispadias)?
- Scrotum and testes. The retractile testis is drawn back up into the scrotum in response to cutaneous stimulation: this is normal in small boys. Gently sweep down the inguinal region (with a warm hand) from lateral to medial to see if you can bring each testis into the scrotum. If the testis cannot be brought into the scrotum it isundescended or ectopic.
- Scrotal swelling may be fluid (hydrocoele) or hernia. Hydrocoeles transilluminate.

Girls

- Examine vulva and external genitalia.
- Look for soreness, injury, discharge or abnormalities.

3.5.6 Neurology

> **PRACTICE POINT**
>
> All that is needed is space and time: space for the child to run around and time to watch him (Dr Stuart Green).

3.5.6.1 Motor function

Activity

- Formal examination of tone, power and coordination should be used to help confirm or explain the findings made on simple observation (Table 3.2).
- Does the infant show appropriate head control for age? Is the small child floppy when picked up? Are there symmetry and normal patterns of movement? Can the older child walk or run? Ask the child to sit on the floor and rise quickly (Figure 3.11). Can the child walk on tip toe or on his heels?
- These observations should be made before reaching for the tendon hammer. Check with the mother first, and encourage a child gently. If a child is unable to walk, asking him to do so is not kind.

3.5.6.2 Muscle tone

- The normal infant and young child can touch his ears with his toes. Observe head control and look for hypotonia when the infant is picked up.

Table 3.2 Characteristics of upper and lower motor neurone lesions

	Upper motor neurone	Lower motor neurone
Example	Cerebral palsy	Spina bifida
Strength	Decreased	Decreased
Tone	Increased	Decreased
Reflexes	Increased	Absent/ decreased
Clonus	Present	Absent

- Muscle tone is generally assessed on passive movement. Ensure the child is relaxed.
- The most common abnormality of tone is *spasticity* (increased tone around a joint in one direction of movement). The most common groups of muscles affected are the hip adductors (test by abducting the hips) and the plantar flexors (tested by dorsiflexing the foot). When both groups are affected, scissoring and toe pointing is seen.

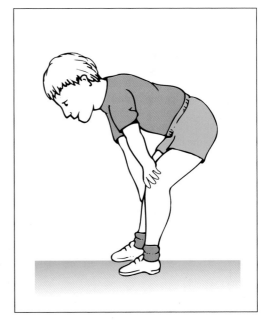

Figure 3.11 Gower's sign. If asked to rise from sitting on the floor, the child turns prone and climbs up his own legs. This indicates limb girdle weakness and is typical of Duchenne dystrophy.

3.5.6.3   Muscle power

This is best tested in children old enough to cooperate by giving simple commands, e.g. 'squeeze my fingers', 'push me away'. Formal grading of muscle power is seldom used in young children. It is best to describe effects of abnormal power on movement and activity.

3.5.6.4   Muscle wasting

Loss of muscle bulk may be seen in a wide variety of disorders. Hypertrophy of the calf muscles is seen in Duchenne muscular dystrophy (Figure 3.10).

3.5.6.5   Tendon reflexes and clonus

- Reflexes are often easier to elicit in a child than in an adult. The child must be relaxed. Reinforcement may be helpful: ask the child to squeeze his hands together.
- Brisk reflexes in association with spasticity suggest an upper motor neurone (pyramidal) lesion.
- Plantar response may be extensor in the normal child until around the age of walking. In older children, a normal flexor response should be seen.
- *Ankle clonus*, if sustained, is suggestive of an upper motor neurone lesion. It is best tested for with the knee semi-flexed. Dorsiflex the ankle sharply, trying different degrees of pressure. Pressing too lightly or too hard may mask clonus.

3.5.6.6   Coordination

This may be tested in children more than 2 years old by the finger–nose and heel–shin manoeuvres. In younger children, it is more helpful to watch for any unsteadiness when playing. A healthy 3-year-old child can stand on one leg briefly, and make a good attempt to walk heel-to-toe along a straight line on the floor.

To test for *dysdiadochokinesis*, ask the child to copy you patting the back of one hand as fast as possible, and then the other. Even 10 year olds cannot do it as quickly as an adult can.

3.5.6.7   Sensation and proprioception

A child who has significant abnormalities in this area is likely to show problems when observed in general activities. Full testing of sensation is rarely performed. It is very difficult in infants and toddlers, but enjoyed by older children. Painful stimuli should not be used.

3.5.6.8   Cranial nerves

- Examination often includes inspection of the eyes, external ocular movement and observation for manifest squint (Section 10.4.4).

Table 3.3 Tests for cranial nerve function.

Nerve	Function	Test
I	Smell	Not often tested
II	Acuity	Simple tests of vision appropriate for age
	Pupils	Direct and consensual light reflex
	Fields	Facing child, who is fixing on your face, test peripheral vision horizontally and vertically
III, IV, VI	Squint, External ocular movements	See Section 10.4.4. Facing child, watch following of bright object in H pattern. In infants and toddlers, head may be held
V	Motor Masseter	Clench jaw
	Sensation	Light touch on face (avoid corneal reflex)
VII	Facial muscles	Observe smiling or crying. Ask child to show teeth, close eyes tight, and watch eyebrows during upward gaze
VIII	Hearing	8 months: distraction testing. Pre-school: cooperation testing. Over 5 years: audiometry. All ages: tympanometry, auditory evoked responses. Ask parents: is she deaf?
IX, X	Swallowing, palate, larynx	Observe swallowing, listen to voice, inspect palatal movement
XI	Trapezius	Ask child to shrug
XII	Tongue	Ask child to stick out tongue and move it from side to side

- Facial nerve function and hearing should be observed. Other tests are only performed if there is indication (Table 3.3).
- Ophthalmoscopy and examination of the fundi is difficult. Looking at the optic disk has been described as 'trying to identify a friend on a passing train'. Ask the child to fix on an object in a dimly lit room, and make sure the ophthalmoscope light is not too bright. Do not worry if you fail – you are in good company!

 PRACTICE POINT

To examine the fundi in a young child, ask her to look at an interesting picture, and ask about it while examining. With patience, the disk can often be seen.

- The eye should also be inspected for corneal opacity, abnormality or cataract. If good visualization of the retina is essential in young children, consider referral to the ophthalmologist.

> **Red reflexes**
>
> This describes the reflection of light from the retina, making the pupil appear red (as in the 'red-eye' seen in flash photography). Anything blocking transmission of light through the eye (e.g. cataract), or changing the colour and character of the retina (e.g. retinoblastoma) will prevent the red reflex. To elicit it, view through the ophthalmoscope in the normal way (focused for infinity), but with the child's face about 0.5–1.0 m away, and with the light shining directly at the pupil.

3.5.7 Examination of bones and joints

Fractures are common in childhood and will cause local pain, tenderness and sometimes swelling. Joint disease is not so common, but arthritis and synovitis do occur. Each joint must be examined carefully:

- *Inspection*: Is there swelling or deformity? Does the skin look red? Compare the two sides. Is there wasting of adjacent muscles? If in doubt, measure. If a joint is painful, ask the child to show you how far it will move without pain before you touch it.
- *Palpation*: Does the skin feel hot? Is there tenderness? Is there fluid in the joint? Is there crepitus when the joint moves? Put the joint through the full range of movement in every direction, watching the child's face to be sure you do not hurt him. Compare the two sides.
- *Measurement*: comparison of muscle bulk can be made by measuring the greatest circumference of the calves, upper arm or forearm muscles. Thighs should be measured about their middle, marking the same distance above the patella on the two sides. Leg lengths are measured with the legs in line with the trunk, from the anterior superior iliac spine or the umbilicus to the medial malleolus at the ankle, taking the tape medial to the patella.

3.5.7.1 Joint movements

Joint movement should be tested gently if pain may be present. Active and passive range of movement should be noted. The *hip* movements are internal and external rotation, adduction, abduction, flexion and extension. Hip disease may be associated with buttock wasting and/or leg shortening. All newborns are tested for stability of the hip joint (Section 23.1.7).

The *knee* normally extends beyond 180° and flexes until the heel touches the buttock. Knee disease is often associated with quadriceps wasting.

The *spine* should be examined for abnormal curvature and for mobility.

> **RESOURCE pGALS (Paediatric Gait, Arms, Legs, Spine)**
>
> Go to **www.arthritisresearchuk.org** and search for 'pGALS' for a video on how to do a musculoskeletal screening examination in a child, and other useful resources.

 # Summary

Examining children is a key skill. You can only learn it by doing it! But we hope this chapter will be a useful starting point, and we encourage you to take every opportunity to hone your skills.

> **FOR YOUR LOG**
>
> - Make sure you have mastered every system examination adapted for children. Don't forget child development and squints (see Section 9.2 and Section 10.4.4).
> - Measure child growth (height, weight and head circumference) and be able to plot and interpret a centile chart (including BMI).
> - Assessing respiratory distress.
> - Know normal and common features e.g. benign cervical lymph nodes and the normal fontanelle.

> **OSCE TIP**
>
> - Any systems examination in a child
> - Development assessment in a young child.
> - Assessment through video of clinical examination findings (e.g. respiratory distress).
> - Before a paediatric OSCE, go back to the wards and do a history, a complete examination, and a developmental assessment.

4

Emergency paediatrics

Chapter map

The European Resuscitation Council (ERC) provides clear guidelines for emergency care and paediatric life support. They also publish the scientific evidence on which, wherever possible, these guidelines are based.

 Early and skilled resuscitation saves lives. It is essential that all who work in health care are trained to recognize emergencies and to act appropriately. Training needs to be kept up to date.

RESOURCE

- Visit **www.erc.edu**, European Resuscitation Council Guidelines for Resuscitation 2010, section 6, Paediatric Life Support (**www.cprguidelines.eu/2010/**).
- iResus is a free mobile phone app published by the Resuscitation Council UK (but not yet available on all platforms) – provides the key algorithms in an easy-to-access format (**www.resus.org.uk/pages/iresusdt.htm**).
- *Spotting the sick child* (**www.spottingthesickchild.com**) is an excellent UK interactive resource (requires registration) that will help you to improve your skills of assessing ill children. It is worth working through it early in your course. It includes videos and self-testing.

Basic life support (BLS) for children over the age of 1 year is now similar to adult life support. The ERC have stated that if someone is trained only in adult life support, the basic life support techniques should be used in the child. If you are training in paediatrics, you will need to learn paediatric life support and the important differences between the child and adult.

KEY POINTS

- Children's lives are saved by recognizing impending or imminent danger, and intervening before terminal collapse
- Cardiac arrest usually occurs at the end of a long sequence of deterioration
- Children seldom collapse because of a primary cardiac event
- The outlook for the child who has a cardiac arrest is very poor

The aim of resuscitation training is to give you a clear systematic approach to treatment of the collapsed child. It is helpful to understand the science and evidence underlying these guidelines. It is equally important to

---

Paediatrics Lecture Notes, Ninth edition. Simon J. Newell and Jonathan C. Darling. © 2014 John Wiley & Sons, Ltd. Published 2014 by John Wiley & Sons, Ltd.

be trained and practise them so that they become automatic if you are faced with such an emergency.

4.1 Basic life support

Paediatric BLS is similar to the adult scheme, and follows the 'ABC approach'. The main difference is that the algorithm starts with five rescue breaths (after determining that the child is unresponsive and calling for help) (Figure 4.1). This is because respiratory arrest is much more common in children than a primary cardiac event.

It is always important to ensure safety for the child, for you and anyone assisting the resuscitation.

Is the child unresponsive? Gently stimulate the child and see if there is a response. If the child responds, attend to other first-aid measures (e.g. pressure on bleeding points), and reassess while help is obtained.

Call for help by asking someone present to call an ambulance, or dial the crash call number when in hospital. Intense anxiety for the child may prevent someone carrying out this simple task. If you are in charge, make sure that it is done. The arrival of skilled help is extremely welcome when someone collapses and you are one of the first people to arrive.

PRACTICE POINT

- Ensure you know the telephone numbers for crash calls in your hospital.
- If the child may have suffered trauma, particularly a road traffic accident, stability of the cervical spine must be maintained. Try to avoid moving the child. Do not shake them. If an airway manoeuvre is required, use chin lift or jaw thrust.

4.1.1 Airway

If the child does not respond, open the airway. This is achieved using head tilt and chin lift. Lift the chin with your finger on the mandible. Do not place your fingers in the soft tissue under the chin as this will compress the airway.

4.1.2 Breathing

Look, listen and feel for breathing. Do not take longer than 10 s doing this. Lean down with your face near to the child and look down their chest. You may be able to hear or feel breathing. If the child is not breathing or if they are breathing irregularly and infrequently, commence resuscitation. Give five rescue breaths.

4.1.2.1 Child (Figure 4.2)

With an open airway pinch the nose. Take a deep breath, place your mouth over the child's mouth and gently but firmly inflate the chest for around 1 s. You will see the chest rise. Then allow the child's chest to fall as the lungs deflate. Give five breaths.

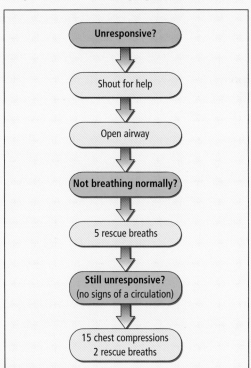

Figure 4.1 Paediatric basic life support algorithm.

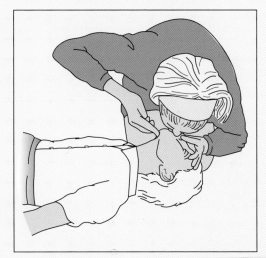

Figure 4.2 Mouth-to-mouth ventilation for a child.

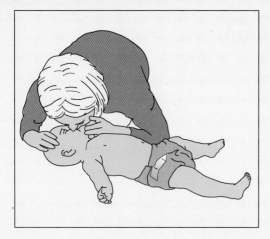

Figure 4.3 Mouth-to-mouth and nose ventilation for an infant.

4.1.2.2   Infant (under 1 year) (Figure 4.3)

Ensure the airway is open. Take a deep breath. Cover the baby's nose and mouth with your mouth. Inflate the chest for 1 s. Allow deflation. Repeat this five times.

If the child or infant's chest does not rise with inspiration, assess the position of the airway. Consider the possibility of a foreign body (see below).

4.1.3   Circulation

If the child is not recovering, assess circulation. Checking the pulse in an emergency, especially in young children, is quite difficult. In children, use the carotid pulse. In infants the brachial pulse is recommended. Do this quickly in up to 10s. You are also looking for some response to the rescue breaths: if regular breathing or spontaneous movements occur, it is likely that adequate circulation is established.

Commence cardiac massage with chest compression if:

- there are no signs of circulation
- OR a slow pulse of less than 60 with poor perfusion
- OR you are not sure.

 PRACTICE POINT

The aim of cardiac massage is to compress the heart, ejecting its contents. Compression should be provided over the lower sternum but at least 1 cm above the xiphisternum. The aim is to compress the chest one-third of its depth at a rate of around 100/min.

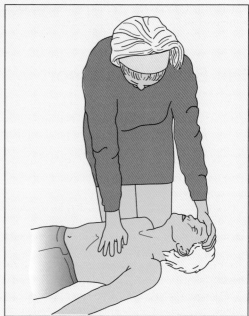

Figure 4.4 Chest compression with one hand.

Give 15 compressions and then two breaths and continue with this pattern.

4.1.3.1   Child (Figure 4.4)

The heel of the hand is placed over the lower one-third of the sternum. In bigger children, both hands may be used as in adults.

4.1.3.2   Infant (Figure 4.5)

If you are on your own, two fingers are placed over the lower sternum to provide compressions. If there is more than one person, use both hands. The two thumbs are placed on the lower sternum pointing

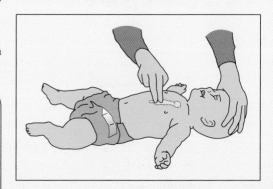

Figure 4.5 Chest compression for an infant.

towards the infant's head. The fingers of the hands encircle the chest.

Continue resuscitation until the child recovers or a more experienced person arrives and is able to decide what is best. If you are on your own, it is recommended to give 1 min of CPR and then go for help.

4.2 Recognition of impending or imminent collapse

There are two main mechanisms of collapse in children and infants. These are respiratory failure and shock. Each has many causes. Early recognition of a child's worsening condition will allow the team to intervene before collapse occurs. The younger the child, the more quickly he will deteriorate. It can be very difficult to predict these problems in young infants.

This section describes the progress from respiratory distress to failure and the evolution of shock. In many conditions, both occur together.

4.2.1 Respiratory distress and failure

Respiratory distress is common – it means increased work of breathing.

Respiratory failure is uncommon – it means that the child's breathing is insufficient to ensure adequate oxygenation and ventilation.

> **PRACTICE POINT Signs of respiratory distress**
>
> - Increased respiratory rate
> - Intercostal or subcostal recession
> - Use of accessory muscles and head-bobbing
> - Grunting
> - Cyanosis.

In the presence of respiratory distress, a child should be monitored carefully and given oxygen. Full clinical assessment (history, examination and investigations) will provide a diagnosis and guide specific treatment (e.g. antibiotics for pneumonia).

If there is known or suspected respiratory failure, it is essential to seek urgent help. Do the following:

- Support, comfort and assess
- Ensure there is a patent airway

> **PRACTICE POINT Signs of respiratory failure**
>
> The following raise concern that respiratory distress is leading to respiratory failure. Here the child or infant's breathing is not enough to ensure oxygenation and the removal of carbon dioxide. Any of the following should raise concern:
>
> - The respiratory rate is very rapid, irregular or is becoming slow in the absence of recovery
> - Cyanosis
> - Poor oxygen saturation readings
> - Poor response to facial oxygen
> - Increasing tachycardia
> - Apnoea or respiratory arrest
> - Altered level of consciousness (agitation or decreased consciousness).
>
> This list provides the features of respiratory failure. Those lower on the list mark a more severe and worrying picture.

- Give oxygen
- Consider oxygen saturation monitoring and seek help.

The child should be transferred to a place that can provide high dependency or intensive care.

4.2.2 Shock

The word shock is used widely. In some medical use it refers to extreme illness often requiring full intensive care. Circulatory shock may progress to this stage but also means the situation where the child is poorly perfused and where there is danger of progression to life-threatening or damaging circulatory failure or even arrest.

> Shock occurs when the circulation is not adequate to maintain organ perfusion.

Shock is common particularly in young children and infants. The most common reason is hypovolaemia due to dehydration. Any other cause of loss of circulating volume will lead to shock. This may include blood loss, or sepsis (when fluids leaks out of the vascular space). Occasionally there is a primary cardiac problem so that the heart is not pumping adequately. The diagnosis of shock depends upon clinical examination.

PRACTICE POINT Features indicating shock

- Poor peripheral circulation with cool hands and feet
- Prolonged capillary refill time (>2 s) (Chapter 3)
- Increased heart rate
- Weak or thready peripheral pulses
- Direct evidence of poor organ perfusion (poor urine output, metabolic acidosis)
- Decreased blood pressure
- Altered level of consciousness.

worsening severity

As the cause of shock, e.g. dehydration (hypovolaemia), worsens, the child will initially show compensation. The compensatory features include the rising pulse and diminished perfusion of the peripheries. Intervention at this stage is highly successful. A child will maintain normal blood pressure by these compensatory methods until decompensation begins to occur. This is followed rapidly by life-threatening deterioration.

Recognition of compensated shock or early signs of decompensation is vitally important. The administration of volume to an infant with dehydration or hypovolaemia of any cause is life saving. The usual treatment is intravenous fluid using a bolus of normal saline (20 ml/kg).

PRACTICE POINT

So much of acute paediatric care and resuscitation is helped by knowing a child's weight. Practise making an estimate of children's weight when you meet them and then check in their notes. The formula Weight = 2 × (Age in years+4) is approximate but useful.

4.3 Paediatric advanced life support

If you pursue a career looking after children, you will need to learn these skills and remain updated. There are four main areas:

- Management of the airway
- Vascular access
- Drugs
- Management of cardiopulmonary arrest.

4.3.1 Airway management

Support and maintenance of the airway is a key clinical skill. The simplest and most important aspect is position. In children, an oral airway may be used if the tongue is obstructing ventilation in the child with diminished conscious level. The correct size of oral airway is inserted gently under direct vision using a tongue depressor and torch, or the laryngoscope.

If a child is not breathing, ventilations can usually be achieved with a bag and mask. Mask ventilation is important at all ages but it is a skill that must be learned by practical instruction.

An airway may be achieved with a laryngeal mask or tracheal intubation. These specialist techniques require the selection of the correct equipment, specific training and continuing practice.

4.3.2 Vascular access

PRACTICE POINT

In an emergency this is achieved with:

- Peripheral intravenous line (usually limiting yourself to 2–3 attempts).
- Intraosseous access – used in life-threatening situations in the unconscious child. If peripheral access cannot be obtained, a specially-designed needle is inserted into the upper tibia avoiding the growth plates. Samples may be taken for investigations. Fluids and drugs may be given through the line.

If vascular access has not been obtained, some drugs can be given through the tracheal tube. These include adrenaline.

4.3.3 Drugs

A number of drugs are used during resuscitation. The two most commonly used are oxygen and adrenaline.

TREATMENT Adrenaline

- Catecholamine (alpha and beta stimulant)
- Vasoconstriction
- Raises blood pressure
- Increased myocardial contractility
- Cardiac arrest

Adrenaline is also called epinephrine.

Oxygen should be given to any infant or child who has collapsed or who is in danger of collapse. It is given to the child in respiratory distress during assessment. Oxygen may be given by face mask or used with bag/mask ventilation or tracheal intubation.

Adrenaline may be given intravenously or through an intraosseous line. It can be given through the endotracheal tube. It is also helpful in the management of anaphylaxis (acute allergic collapse).

 TREATMENT

Adrenaline is a dose that all doctors in paediatrics should know: 10 micrograms/kg (0.1mL/kg of 1:10,000) initial dose

4.3.4 Cardiopulmonary arrest

The initial management of cardiopulmonary arrest is as described for basic life support.

 PRACTICE POINT

If there is no cardiac output, the problem falls into one of two groups:

- Asystole or pulseless electrical activity. The heart has stopped or is showing electrical activity without contractions. This will not respond to an electric shock. The airway is secured, the child is ventilated, cardiopulmonary resuscitation and adrenaline are given. Any cause is treated.
- Ventricular fibrillation or pulseless ventricular tachycardia. These conditions are shockable. Defibrillation is used and other drugs may be helpful.

4.3.5 Foreign body airway obstruction (FBAO)

Choking with airway obstruction is not uncommon in young children. Death is rare. Simple measures are very effective. Most children who choke do so while they are playing or eating. The result is that most episodes are observed and intervention is successful while the child is still conscious.

 PRACTICE POINT **General signs of FBAO**

- Witnessed episode
- Coughing/choking
- Sudden onset
- Recent history of playing with/eating small objects

Obstructed airway	Airway clear
Unable to vocalize	Crying or verbal response
Quiet or silent cough	Loud cough
Unable to breathe	Able to take a breath
Cyanosis	Pink
Decreased consciousness	Fully responsive

First assess whether the child has an effective cough or not (Figure 4.6). If the child is able to cough and respond, simply encourage them to do so and continue to assess. If you have any concerns seek help.

If coughing is becoming ineffective, call for help immediately and perform one of the procedures that gives an artificial cough. The artificial cough in the conscious child is provided by back blows or abdominal/chest thrusts.

To give back blows it is best to have the child head downwards and in a prone position with the lower

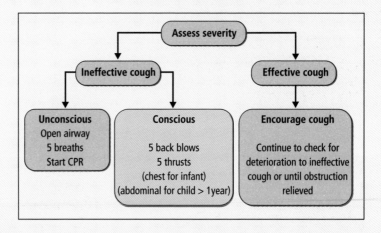

Figure 4.6 Foreign body airway obstruction algorithm.

jaw supported to open the airway. The infant can be picked up. A small child can be placed across the lap whilst older children will need to be supported.

Five back blows are given. The heel of the hand is used to provide a firm blow between the shoulder blades. They work best if the child is head down because the manouevre is then assisted by gravity.

Chest thrusts are used in children under 1 year of age. These are like cardiac compressions but sharper and given at a slower rate. Five chest thrusts are given. Abdominal thrusts are used in children over 1 year. This is the Heimlich manoeuvre. Your clenched fist is placed between the umbilicus and the xiphisternum while standing behind the child. The other hand grasps the fist. A sharp upwards pull is given.

Once the airway obstruction is relieved, a child will usually recover if they are conscious at the time.

If the child becomes unconscious, place him supine. Examine the mouth. If there is a foreign body visible, then remove it. Do not simply place a finger in the mouth in the hope of finding something. Give mouth-to-mouth resuscitation. After five breaths, give cardiac compressions. Repeat artificial respiration, again examining the mouth for the presence of a foreign body which has become dislodged.

4.4 Recognition of the ill child

It's far better to recognize signs of serious illness early and prevent deterioration, than to perform a perfect resuscitation once a child has collapsed. Paediatric advanced warning scores are increasingly used to help spot the sick child. Here abnormal observations such as heart rate, respiratory rate and fever are used to give a score – high scores require early review. NICE guidelines use a 'traffic light system' to help identify serious illness (see Table 4.1).

 ## Summary

Emergencies in children are different from in adults and often there is a period of deterioration before collapse. Recognition and early intervention in respiratory distress and failure, and in shock can prevent life-threatening collapse. In the child who has stopped breathing, simple things done well, promptly, save lives.

 OSCE TIP

- Basic life support.
- Choking/foreign body.
- Mannikin: recognition of dehydration – ask for the signs.
- Video of severe respiratory distress.

 FOR YOUR LOG

- If you are present at a resuscitation, reflect on what you have seen with a member of the team.
- Do a paediatric basic life support course, or when you do an adult course, find out what is different for children.

See EMQ 4.1, EMQ 4.2 and EMQ 4.3 at the end of the book.

Table 4.1 Traffic light system for identifying likelihood of serious illness

	Green — low risk	Amber — intermediate risk	Red— righ risk
Colour	• Normal colour of skin, lips and tongue	• Pallor reported by parent/carer	• Pale/motted/ashen/blue
Activity	• Responds normally to social cues • Content/Smile • Stays awake of awakens quickly • Strong nornal cry/not crying	• Not responding normally to social cues • Wakes only with prolonged stimulation • Decreased activity • No smile	• No response to social cues • Appears ill to a healthcare professional • Unable to rouse or if roused does not stay awake • Weak, high-pitched or continous cry
Respiratory		• Nasal flaring • Tachypnoea: • RR > 50 breaths/minute age 6-12 months • RR > 40 breaths/minute age > 12 months • Oxygen saturation ≤ 95% in air • Crackles	• Grunting • Tachypnoea: • RR > 60 breaths/minute • Moderate or servere chest indrawing
Hydration	• Normal skin and eyes • Moist mucous membranes	• Tachycardia • >160 beats/min, age <12m • >150 beats/min, age 12-24 m • >140 beats/min, age 2-5y • Dry mucous membrane • Poor feeding in infants • CRT ≥ 3 seconds • Reduced urine output	• Reduce skin turgor
Other	• None of the amber or red symptoms or signs	• Fever for ≥ 5 days • Rigors • Swelling of a limb or joint • None-weight bearing/not using an extermity	• Age 0–3 months, temperature ≥ 38°C • Age 3–6 months, temperature ≥ 39°C • Non-blanching rash • Bulging fontanelle • Neck stiffness • Status epilepticus • Focal neurological signs • Focal seizures

CRT: capillary refill time
RR: respiratory rate

Source: National Institute for Health and Clinical Excellence (2013) CG 160 Feverish illness in children: assessment and initial management in children younger than 5 years. London: NICE. Available from http://guidance.nice.org.uk/CG160. Reproduced with permission.

OSCE station 4.1: Shock

Task: Jamie is 21 months of age. Two days ago, he developed diarrhoea and then vomiting. This has become more frequent, and Jamie is reluctant to feed. His 5-year-old brother recently had a similar illness and is now well. He had been brought to A&E because his parents are more worried. Jamie has become quiet, but is crying intermittently. He is pink and blood glucose is 5 mmol/L.

Take a brief history from Jamie's mother (4 min). Then discuss his assessment with the examiner (4 min).
Don't forget:

Brief history

How ill is he?	Is he feeding, hungry, alert? Does he recognize parents? Is he talking?
History of acute problem?	How long has he been ill? How severe is diarrhoea? How often is he vomiting? Is he febrile? Are there any other symptoms?
Feed and fluids?	How much milk is he taking? Is he drinking anything else? Have the parents been given any special drinks (glucose/electrolyte mixture)?

Assessment and management

A B C	Jamie is crying and pink.
Is Jamie in shock?	The examiner will ask you how you will assess hydration, peripheral perfusion and shock.
Early detection of shock is important to prevent progression	Early signs such as dry mouth and eyes, cool hands and feet and prolonged capillary refill time can be treated with rehydration and restoration of circulating volume. Progression to loss of peripheral perfusion, poor urine output, hypotension and decreased level of consciousness is dangerous.
Management	If signs of early shock, give intravenous fluid, with a bolus of saline. Then, maintain good hydration with IV fluids and later oral rehydration if possible.

Jamie is moderately dehydrated and has a capillary refill time of 4 s. He is given a bolus of saline (20 mL/kg) IV, and looks better. IV fluids are given and he is regraded to oral rehydration fluid and then milk. Gastroenteritis leads to dehydration by increased losses (diarrhoea, vomiting, fever) and intake (poor feeding, vomiting).

Part 2

Normal and abnormal in childhood: growth, development, behaviour and prevention

This section follows the child's journey from the very earliest beginnings (genetics) to adolescence, and covers some of the key things that happen along the way (normal and abnormal).

Many conditions in paediatrics have a genetic basis, and it is helpful to be able to record a clear family tree, and know the principles of genetic mechanisms, investigation and counselling. These are summarized in Chapter 5.

Chapters 6–8 cover the transition from fetal life to newborn infant, including prenatal diagnosis, and minor and major problems of the newborn (including prematurity).

You cannot work effectively in paediatrics without understanding development, learning, and the emotional and behavioural aspects of child health and disease. These are covered in Chapters 9–11.

Chapters 12 and 13 are about nutrition and growth, which are foundational to paediatric practice. Knowing the range of normal underpins much advice given to parents.

In Chapter 14, we review childhood infections, immunity and the key public health intervention of immunization.

Chapter 15 covers accidents and child abuse: the former one of the commonest causes of death in childhood, the latter one of the most challenging areas in the specialty – but one that everyone in paediatrics needs to know about.

We reach adolescence in Chapter 15, with its unique problems and challenges. These include consent, chronic illness management, self-harm and the transition to adult services.

5

Genetics

Chapter map

Childhood and fetal life is when many genetic problems present. It is important to understand the principles of inheritance, and the wide variety of genetic disease. The clinician needs to know about the range of investigations in suspected genetic disease and have an approach to genetic counselling. This chapter does not deal with the individual conditions, many of which can be found elsewhere in this book.

5.1   The human genome

Successful sequencing of the genome was announced on 26 June 2000. Understanding of structure has preceded explanation of function. Current knowledge offers a wealth of new diagnostic tests, increasing therapeutic benefits and the future possibility of gene therapy.

The diploid human cell contains DNA extending to around 6 billion base pairs in 23 chromosome pairs. Only 2% of DNA codes for protein expression in some 20 000 genes. Some of the remaining DNA offers

> 'It has not escaped our notice that the specific pairing we have postulated immediately suggests a possible copying mechanism for the genetic material.' Watson, J.D. and Crick, F.H.C. (1953) Molecular structure of nucleic acids: a structure for deoxyribose nucleic acid. *Nature*, 4356, 25 April, 171: 737–8; see also Figure 5.1)

regulation and control of gene expression, genetic replication and chromosomal architecture, while the function of other non-coding DNA is not yet known.

The base pair structure of DNA allows replication. During cell division, chromosomes align, replicate and divide. In *mitosis*, identical diploid daughter cells result. In *meiosis*, haploid gametes are produced: eggs and sperm containing half the genetic material, with just one of each of the pairs of chromosomes. In meiosis, genetic material may be swapped between chromosomes, while all cell division carries potential for mutation.

Genes code for polypeptide sequences and these may constitute or may be built into proteins. Post-translational changes modify structure and function and result in functional proteins.

The potential for errors is massive, but most do not result in disease. It is important to understand the principles underlying genetic disease for diagnosis, prognosis, treatment and genetic counselling.

Paediatrics Lecture Notes, Ninth edition. Simon J. Newell and Jonathan C. Darling. © 2014 John Wiley & Sons, Ltd. Published 2014 by John Wiley & Sons, Ltd.

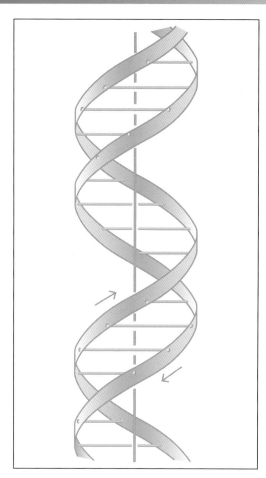

Figure 5.1 DNA – the Nobel Prize winning description of the double helix.
Source: Watson and Crick (1953).

For any characteristic (height, blood pressure, etc.), our phenotype (the way we are) is the result of complex interaction between our genotype (genetic material related to that characteristic) and our environment (Figure 5.2).

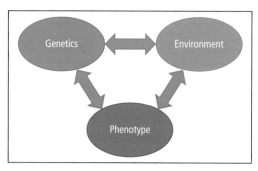

Figure 5.2 There is a complex interaction between genotype, environment and phenotype.

RESOURCE

Useful refresher videos and animations on DNA and the human genome can be found at:
- **www.hhmi.org**
- **www.dnalc.org/resources**
- **www.dnatube.com**

5.2 Genetic mechanisms of disease

- Chromosomal
  - Abnormal number (aneuploidy)
  - Translocation (balanced or unbalanced)
  - Duplication
  - Deletion
  - Copy number variation (abnormal numbers of copies of section of DNA)
- Single gene disorders
  - Mutations
    - Missense (protein product is abnormal, e.g. amino acid substitution)
    - Nonsense (protein product is not complete)
- Triplet repeat (base pair triplets)
- Gene imprinting (e.g. modification of gene expression by gender of parent)
- Mitochondrial DNA abnormalities
- Multifactorial inheritance

5.2.1 Chromosomal abnormalities

Aneuploidy means that there is an extra chromosome (e.g. Trisomy 21, Down syndrome; 47XXY, Klinefelter syndrome) or one missing (e.g. 45XO, Turner syndrome). Most aneuploidy arises because of non-disjunction (failure of the pair of chromosomes to separate), and often it results in spontaneous miscarriage. Down syndrome (trisomy 21), Edward syndrome (trisomy 18), Patau syndrome (trisomy 13) and the sex chromosome aneuploidies account for most infants with abnormal chromosome number. Risk of Down syndrome aneuploidy rises with maternal age.

Down syndrome is most commonly due to non-disjunction. In around 5% of affected children, other patterns are seen: unbalanced translocation (see Figure 5.3), and mosaicism (the phenotype varies with the balance in number between 2 cell lines, one of which is trisomy 21).

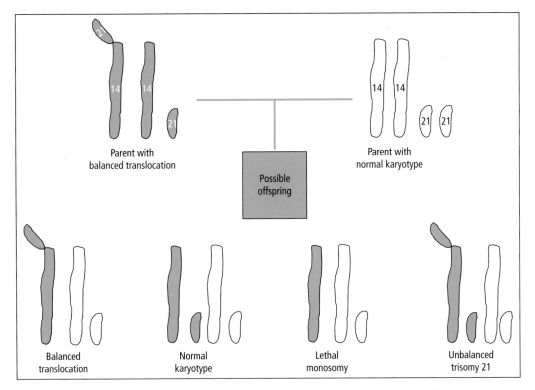

Figure 5.3 A balanced 21 translocation in a healthy parent can result in Down syndrome in the child.

Translocations occur when a part of one chromosome is stuck to another. If the total chromosome content is normal or near normal (a balanced translocation), the phenotype may be normal. The risk for this person is that their offspring may inherit an unbalanced karyotype.

The other chromosomal abnormalities are associated with a wide variety of phenotypes. Some deletions or duplications may be a chance finding in a healthy child or their family. On the other hand, some are small and not visible on microscopy, yet may result in a variety of important syndromic abnormalities (e.g. 22q deletions: Di George syndrome spectrum with hypocalcaemia, T-cell deficiency, cardiac defects).

> 🔑 A syndrome is a phenotype with a recognizable pattern of various abnormalities or problems.

5.2.2 Single gene disorders

These may adopt the classical Mendelian patterns of inheritance.

Symbols for a genetic pedigree are shown in Figure 5.4.

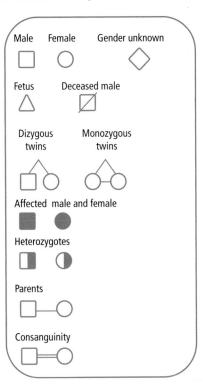

Figure 5.4 Symbols for genetic pedigree.

The features of each pattern in a family is described. You do not need to learn lists of inheritance patterns but should know some of the commoner ones. Discussion of individual conditions here is to illustrate patterns of inheritance. Please see other chapters for discussion of conditions that are more common or important in paediatrics.

One phenotype may be the result of a number of different mutations.

Phenotype may vary between family members who share a genetic abnormality, reflecting variation in expression and penetrance.

5.2.2.1   Autosomal dominant (Figure 5.5)

- Parents affected
- Females and males affected
- Female and male transmission
- 50% recurrence risk
- High new mutation rates
- Variable penetrance in some conditions

Autosomal dominant conditions

- Achondroplasia
- Huntington's chorea
- Polyposis coli
- Marfan syndrome
- Tuberous sclerosis
- Mytonic dystrophy
- von Willebrand disease

Trinucleotide repeat disorders

- Trinucleotide repeats (triplet repeat) are normal up to a certain number in some genes. The area is unstable, may expand on transmission to the next generation and cause disease.
- *Anticipation is seen* – earlier presentation and greater severity with successive generations.
- Most are autosomal dominant (e.g. myotonic dystrophy – chromosome 19).
- Fragile X is X-linked recessive (see below).

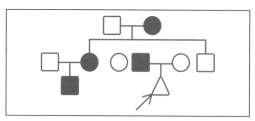

Figure 5.5 Autosomal dominant: parents seek advice on risk to the fetus.

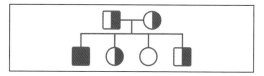

Figure 5.6 Cystic fibrosis: a 1 in 4 risk of affected offspring.

In some dominant conditions, phenotype varies even in the same family. In achondroplasia, the new mutation rate is 50%. Huntingdon's chorea and polyposis do not present until after childhood.

5.2.2.2   Autosomal recessive (Figure 5.6)

- Parents not affected
- Parents heterozygote carriers
- 1 in 4 risk of condition if carrier parents
- 2 in 3 risk of unaffected sibling being carrier
- More common with consanguinity (Section 1.3.3)

Autosomal recessive conditions

- Cystic fibrosis
- Phenylketonuria
- Sickle cell disease
- Thalassaemia
- Various inborn errors of metabolism (e.g. congenital adrenal hyperplasia)

Rates of gene carriage vary greatly between ethnic groups (e.g. cystic fibrosis carriage in Europe is around 1 in 25, while considerably lower across Asia). Most parents will not know that they carry the rare gene until they have a child with another carrier.

5.2.2.3   X linked recessive (Figure 5.7)

- Affects males
- Carrier female usually unaffected
- 50% of boys of carrier mother affected
- 50% of daughters of carrier mother are carriers
- 100% of daughters of affected men are carriers
- No transmission from father to son
- New mutations not uncommon

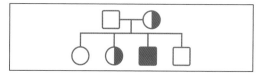

Figure 5.7 Haemophilia A: there is a 1 in 2 chance that girls will be carriers and boys will be affected.

X linked recessive conditions

- Fragile X
- Duchenne muscular dystrophy
- Haemophilia A and B
- G6PD deficiency
- Red green colour blindness

The abnormality on one X chromosome is not usually sufficient to lead to disease in the carrier woman. In some women, the Lyon phenomenon (random inactivation of one of the X chromosomes) may result in disease. In fragile X (an important cause of language and developmental problems) women may have mild learning difficulties (Section 10.3.2).

5.2.3 Gene imprinting

Certain genes express differently depending on whether they are inherited from the mother or the father. Current understanding suggests that this is rare in clinical disease.

Affected individuals have the unopposed effect of maternally or paternally inherited genes. This occurs because of a mutation in the gene on one chromosome, or because of inheritance of two copies of the gene from the same parent (uniparental disomy).

Example of imprinting (part of chromosome 15q)

Two different disorders result (both rare), depending on whether the maternal or paternal contribution of this imprinted gene is lacking:

- No *paternal* contribution
  - Mutation of the paternally inherited gene, *or*
  - Maternal uniparental disomy
- No *maternal* contribution
  - Mutation of the maternally inherited gene, *or*
  - Paternal uniparental disomy

- *Prader Willi syndrome* (short stature, obesity, eating and behaviour problems, hypogonadism)
- *Angelman's syndrome* (ataxia, motor problems, abnormal behaviour apparently happy, epilepsy)

5.2.4 Mitochondrial DNA abnormalities

- Maternal inheritance (mitochondria are acquired in the cytosol of the ovum)

- Rare conditions affecting tissues with high energy needs
- Tissues affected: eyes, brain, liver, muscle

5.2.5 Polygenic or multifactorial conditions

The characteristics of our phenotypes have many origins. Some are genetic. Growth has genetic and environmental drivers. Complex features like intelligence are clearly multifactorial.

> 🔑 Polygenic conditions are much more common than single gene disorders.

Patterns of inheritance are not well defined and calculation of risk for polygenic disease is based upon studies of populations. If a family has such a condition (e.g. atopy, diabetes), risk increases with the number of close relatives who are affected.

It is increasingly evident that the health of the fetus and young child has long-term implications for adult health. *Programming* refers to the ability of the early environment during a critical period of development to influence long-term outcome (e.g. the small fetus is more likely to suffer coronary artery disease or diabetes at the age of 60 years).

This makes fetal and childhood well-being the birthplace of adult health.

Polygenic or multifactorial conditions

- Atopy (e.g. asthma, eczema)
- Spina bifida
- Cleft lip and palate
- Congenital heart disease
- Adult coronary heart disease
- Adult hypertension
- Diabetes
- Epilepsy

5.3 Investigations

5.3.1 Karyotype

Chromosomes are separated during cell division, allowing counting and examination for defects (Figure 10.1). Banding studies (staining) allows definition of chromosomes or parts of chromosomes in duplication or deletion. Resolution is limited by microscopy.

5.3.2 FISH (Fluorescence in situ hybridization)

A fluorescent labelled specific DNA probe sequence binds to complementary DNA on the chromosome. The probe can be seen because it is fluorescent. This can be used to count chromosomes without waiting for a full karyotype. Searching for part of chromosome 21 will show 3 areas of fluorescence in Down syndrome. FISH can also look for specific genes or abnormalities, or localize a known DNA sequence.

5.3.3 DNA analysis

Specific gene probes are increasingly available. Clearly they require that the practitioner suspects the condition being tested for.

DNA microarray comprises multiple DNA probes applied simultaneously. This allows more rapid and accurate detection of a wide variety of abnormalities, and the search for duplications and deletions.

Polymerase chain reaction (PCR) uses a DNA replication enzyme to achieve exponential increases in the number of copies of a specific section of DNA. PCR amplification makes it much easier to study the DNA. PCR is used to detect small amounts of specific DNA (e.g. detection of Herpes virus in CSF).

5.4 Approach to suspected genetic disease

> **PRACTICE POINT**
>
> Constant vigilance is necessary to detect inherited disease.

> **Benefits of early diagnosis of genetic disease**
>
> - Families are often helped by having a diagnosis
> - Prognosis
> - Early intervention during or before disease
> - Genetic counseling

It is important to approach a potential genetic diagnosis with some caution. Accuracy is key, usually demanding a multiprofessional team including Clinical Genetics. The implications for the child and her

family may be massive. Premature mention of a possible genetic diagnosis may lead a family to deep and unnecessary anxiety – access to detailed and full, and occasionally inaccurate, information is easy for anyone who can find Google.

> **RESOURCE**
>
> The Online Mendelian Inheritance in Man database (OMIM) at **www.ncbi.nlm.nih.gov/omim** is a useful compendium of human genes and genetic phenotypes.

5.4.1 Genetic counselling (Figure 5.8)

An accurate diagnosis is ideal for all. Not uncommonly, a firm diagnosis may be difficult, and often syndromic diagnoses are made on probability rather than certainty.

Risks for the child and family require careful and complex assessment. Many genetic conditions vary greatly in how much they affect individuals even within one family. Naturally, families will be drawn to expect the same problems with the same diagnosis. The number and gravity of possible outcomes in some conditions (e.g. neurofibromatosis) can be bewildering and cause great worry.

> **Complex issues in genetic counselling**
>
> - Recurrence risk in a family
> - Carrier detection in healthy parents, siblings, and extended family
> - Paternity
> - Predictive testing of children who may be pre-symptomatic
> - Reproductive choices including fetal intervention

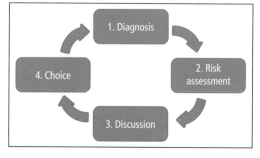

Figure 5.8 Genetic counselling – key steps.

The complexity and ethical difficulties that arise in this area of medicine are many. Families may seek testing for a genetic disorder in the hope of a reassuring result. This should not take place without careful counselling about the implications of an abnormal test result. Testing of children for diseases that will only affect them as adults, and where early intervention does not bring clear benefit (e.g. Huntingdon's chorea, Adult polycystic kidney disease) is not generally accepted.

PRACTICE POINT

Clinical Genetics services have great expertise in this area and work closely with paediatrics.

Careful, clear and honest explanation of these complex issues to a concerned family is very challenging. Often families will need to be seen on a number of occasions.

 Good information given with care and compassion will enable families to make the right choices.

 # Summary

You should now understand the main mechanisms of inherited disease, the variety of patterns of inheritance, and something of the clinical approach to investigation, diagnosis and counselling. The immediately obvious complexity is the reason why the child and family are usually best helped by a combined team of paediatrics, community services and clinical genetics.

FOR YOUR LOG

- Include a family tree in your paediatric histories, and extend when concerned about inherited disorders.
- Be able to recognize different genetic mechanisms of inheritance.
- If there is an opportunity during paediatrics, or elsewhere in your course, observe genetic counselling.

 OSCE TIP

- Questions about a pedigree.
- Counselling about simple problems related to inherited or multifactorial conditions.

6

Fetal medicine

Chapter map

Multidisciplinary collaboration is the key to fetal medicine. Good contraceptive advice is important for the young person, while assisted conception allows more couples the joy of parenthood. Primarily an obstetric specialty, advice to the expectant couple often provides diagnostic and ethical problems, demanding input from paediatrics, genetics and surgery. You should understand that ultrasound, amniocentesis, chorionic villus sampling, fetal blood sampling, DNA analysis and fetoscopy allow assessment of fetal health, early detection of many anomalies and sometimes treatment of the fetus, taking Down syndrome and spina bifida as important examples.

6.1   Control of fertility

6.1.1   Contraception

In developing countries, high birth rates and high child mortality tend to go hand in hand. Medical care reduces mortality from disease, but large family size threatens good nutrition, education, and socioeconomic growth. Safe, effective, cheap contraception coupled with education is key.

In Europe, the challenge of providing good, supportive advice to teenagers is widely acknowledged. The UK is now seeing a fall in the teenage pregnancy rate (around 40/1000 15–17 year olds), although it remains high compared with the rest of Europe.

6.1.2   Infertility treatment

Methods of helping infertile couples continue to advance. Techniques of ovulation control, in vitro fertilization, prolonged storage of gametes and the embryo, and surrogacy permit the separation of functions previously regarded as inseparable:

- Production of ova and sperm
- Place of fertilization
- The uterus in which the fetus develops
- The adult(s) responsible for rearing the child.

The ovum could come from Ms A, be fertilized in the laboratory by sperm from Mr B, be implanted in the uterus of Ms C and be reared by Mr and Ms D. This may raise psychosocial and ethical issues. Limiting the number of embryos implanted has reduced multiple pregnancies. Some studies raise concern that congenital abnormality may be more common after induced pregnancy.

PRACTICE POINT

Gillick competency: this important ethical concept arose when the courts decided that a teenager could obtain contraception without parental knowledge. The principle is that a competent teenager may seek treatment or advice as long as the treating doctor is convinced that the child understands the implications of their choice.

Paediatrics Lecture Notes, Ninth edition. Simon J. Newell and Jonathan C. Darling. © 2014 John Wiley & Sons, Ltd. Published 2014 by John Wiley & Sons, Ltd.

6.2 Antenatal and pre-pregnancy care

Preparation for a baby is aided by good physical and emotional health in both parents. Hereditary conditions should be discussed.

> **PRACTICE POINT**
>
> Women should be immunized against rubella before conception. All but the most essential drugs should be stopped before pregnancy. Smoking and alcohol should be avoided.

Some social and behavioural factors increase risk of problems:

- Socioeconomic deprivation: ↑ low birthweight; ↑ prematurity; ↑ perinatal mortality
- Young mothers: ↑ fetal growth problems; ↑ perinatal morbidity and mortality
- Older mothers: Down syndrome
- Obesity: ↑ gestational diabetes, ↑ perinatal mortality, ↑ difficult delivery
- Drug-abuse: effects of drugs on fetus and newborn
- Viral infection; HIV; hepatitis B and C.

Ideally, women should be in good health and prepared for pregnancy at the time of conception. The fetus may suffer long-term effects from early adverse influences (Figure 6.1).

6.3 Congenital malformations

About 2% of all babies are born with serious congenital defects, sufficient to threaten life, to cause permanent handicap or to require surgical correction.

Distressingly little is known of the causes of congenital abnormalities. Single-gene defects and chromosome anomalies account for 10–20% of the total. A small number are attributable to intrauterine infections (e.g. cytomegalovirus, rubella), fewer to teratogenic drugs and even fewer to ionizing radiation. The ideal is prevention.

> **TREATMENT Folate in spina bifida: a paradigm of prevention**
>
> Laboratory and epidemiological studies showed the importance of folate. Increased folate intake reduces the incidence and prevents recurrence.

Nature protects against birth of children with serious anomalies. The incidence of serious defects and chromosomal anomalies amongst early spontaneous abortuses is very high (Table 6.1). It can be shown, for example, that at least 90% of embryos/fetuses with trisomy 21, and a much higher proportion of embryos with sex chromosome anomalies, are aborted. Liveborn, malformed infants therefore represent the small minority of abnormal conceptuses.

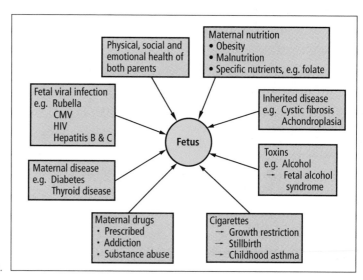

Figure 6.1 Factors affecting fetal nutrition, growth and development.

Table 6.1 Incidence of some congenital problems

Down syndrome	1 : 600
Club foot	1 : 700
Polydactyly/syndactyly	1 : 700
Cleft lip/palate	1 : 800
Congenital heart disease	1 : 1000
Spina bifida/anencephaly	1 : 2000
Oesophageal atresia	1 : 3000
Diaphragmatic hernia	1 : 3500

6.3.1 Prenatal diagnosis (Table 6.2)

Choice of technique for prenatal diagnosis is difficult. More invasive tests may provide more definitive information, but may risk precipitation of miscarriage. Amniocentesis has a 1% risk of miscarriage. Some fetal intervention is highly successful (e.g. fetal blood sampling, or transfusion for anaemia or thrombocytopenia) while fetal surgery (e.g. relief of urinary obstruction, or diaphragmatic hernia) remains experimental.

 Reasons for prenatal diagnosis

- Reassurance of parents
- Management of pregnancy and delivery
- Selective termination of pregnancy
- Planned neonatal management
- Intrauterine treatment.

 PRACTICE POINT Screening for Down syndrome

- Ultrasound (increased nuchal thickness – the depth of the skin fold over the back of the neck)
- Triple test (maternal blood: ↓ α-fetoprotein, ↑ gonadotrophin and ↓ oestriol)
- Karyotyping for trisomy 21 (chorionic villus sampling/amniocentesis).

6.4 Embryonic and fetal growth and development

In early pregnancy the embryological timetable determines teratogenic hazards. Infective, chemical or physical agents that cause birth defects may only be teratogenic at certain times in pregnancy. Rubella, for example, has devastating effects in the first trimester, and almost none in the third trimester.

In the second and third trimesters, fetal growth, estimated clinically or by ultrasound, is an important indicator of fetal health. Ultrasound can also be used for fuller assessment of well-being (fetal biophysical profile). The healthy fetus shows normal growth, fetal breathing movements, good volume of amniotic fluid and has normal blood flow velocities measured in the fetal arteries by Doppler. Loss of these features implies fetal compromise and is useful in timing delivery.

Table 6.2 Modes of prenatal diagnosis

Mode	Type of investigation	Example
Ultrasound	Fetal measurement	IUGR
	Fetal anomaly	
	• Missing structures	Anencephaly, renal agenesis
	• Enlarged organs	Polycystic kidneys
	• Abnormalities	Cardiac
		Oligohydramnios: IUGR
		Polyhydramnios: oesophageal atresia
Amniocentesis	Fluid analysis	↑ Alphafetoprotein in spina bifida
		↑ Bilirubin in haemolysis
	Fetal cells	Karyotyping/DNA analysis
Maternal blood	Biochemistry	Triple test for Down syndrome
Chorionic villus sampling	Genetic testing/Karyotyping/DNA analysis	Down syndrome or cystic fibrosis
Fetoscopy, cordocentesis (fetal blood sampling)	Fetal blood and tissue	Wide variety of investigations

The increase in size from conception to birth is phenomenal. At 8 weeks, all major organs have been formed. All serious congenital malformations have their origins in these early weeks. More serious malformations often result in early fetal death and spontaneous abortion.

At 8 weeks the embryo, who only weighs 1 g, becomes a fetus. Weight gain accelerates, and at 24 weeks (the lower limit of viability) the fetus weighs just around 600 g. Weight gain increases through the final trimester to 100–250 g/week.

 ## Summary

Multidisciplinary care, supported by innovations in technology have led to dramatic changes in our knowledge of fetal well-being, and detection of abnormality. A healthy child with healthy, loving parents is the best outcome in every pregnancy. In your attachment to paediatrics or obstetrics, ask to attend fetal ultrasound, and consider going to a fetal medicine clinic.

 FOR YOUR LOG

(Note that some items in this section may be more easily carried out in a clinical placement in Obstetrics and Gynaecology.)

- Understand the principle of Gillick competency and observe/reflect on scenarios where this applies.
- Observe a consultation where pre-natal screening is discussed.
- Observe antenatal ultrasound.

See EMQ 6.1 at the end of the book.

7

Birth and the newborn infant

Chapter map

The delivery of a baby is a wonder. In moments, the fetus, crumpled and wet, is transformed into a free-living baby. This transition from intrauterine to extrauterine life is vital. The fetus must escape potential damage during birth, adapt physiologically to a new environment and, after birth, evade environmental hazards such as hypothermia and infection. Understanding the physiology helps understand logical management.

Perinatal hypoxic ischaemic brain injury is potentially preventable but may have lifelong consequences. Most newborn infants are healthy and you should understand the routine examination of the newborn and some of the more common findings.

> 🔑 There is a greater risk of dying on the first day of life than on any other day (except the last).

For most fetuses these events occur without problems; a minority suffer potentially damaging asphyxia along the way.

7.1 The effects of birth on the fetus

7.1.1 Normal physiology (Table 7.1)

The most dramatic events are the switch from placenta to lung as the organ of gas exchange, and the change from fetal to adult circulation (Figure 7.1).

7.2 Perinatal asphyxia and its prevention

In the healthy fetus the Po_2 is only about 4 kPa, which is the arterial Po_2 at the summit of Mount Everest (normal child 12–15 kPa). The needs of the fetus are fully met thanks to fetal adaptation, but oxygenation around the time of birth is in a state of delicate balance which depends critically on many factors.

Paediatrics Lecture Notes, Ninth edition. Simon J. Newell and Jonathan C. Darling. © 2014 John Wiley & Sons, Ltd. Published 2014 by John Wiley & Sons, Ltd.

Table 7.1 Normal physiological events at birth

Phenomena	Effects
Stress of labour $\Rightarrow$ catecholamine and steroid	$\downarrow$ Lung liquid and $\uparrow$ surfactant release
Compression of thorax in birth canal	Expulsion of lung liquid
Sensory stimuli and clamping of umbilical cord	Initiation of breathing
Air enters lungs $\Rightarrow$ $\uparrow$ lung tissue oxygen	Pulmonary vascular resistance $\downarrow$ $\Rightarrow$ $\uparrow$ pulmonary blood flow $\uparrow$ arterial Po_2
Systemic pressure > pulmonary pressure	Foramen ovale closes
Ductus arteriosus fills with oxygen-rich blood	Ductus arteriosus closes

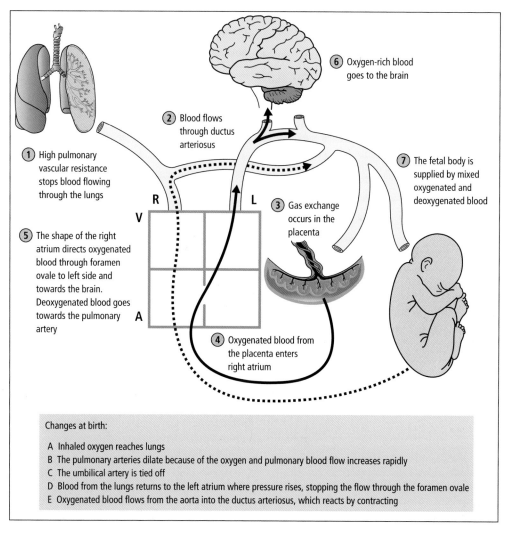

1. High pulmonary vascular resistance stops blood flowing through the lungs
2. Blood flows through ductus arteriosus
3. Gas exchange occurs in the placenta
4. Oxygenated blood from the placenta enters right atrium
5. The shape of the right atrium directs oxygenated blood through foramen ovale to left side and towards the brain. Deoxygenated blood goes towards the pulmonary artery
6. Oxygen-rich blood goes to the brain
7. The fetal body is supplied by mixed oxygenated and deoxygenated blood

Changes at birth:

A Inhaled oxygen reaches lungs
B The pulmonary arteries dilate because of the oxygen and pulmonary blood flow increases rapidly
C The umbilical artery is tied off
D Blood from the lungs returns to the left atrium where pressure rises, stopping the flow through the foramen ovale
E Oxygenated blood flows from the aorta into the ductus arteriosus, which reacts by contracting

Figure 7.1 Fetal circulation. Follow the circulation in the fetus 1 to 7. Then review the changes which occur at birth, which are listed A to E at the bottom of the figure.

Fetal adaptations to hypoxia

- High haemoglobin (18 g/dL)
- Fetal haemoglobin with left shifted dissociation curve (Chapter 25)
- High cardiac output.

It is not surprising that the fetus has good defences against acute hypoxia. These include redistribution of blood flow in favour of vital tissues, and a myocardium and nervous system more resistant to hypoxic damage than those of the adult. Despite this, a small minority of fetuses suffer perinatal brain damage. Fetal hypoxia calls for prompt obstetric action and resuscitation at birth in order to prevent permanent damage.

7.2.1 Resuscitation (Figure 7.2)

Rapid assessment and action is needed for any baby who does not breathe within 30 s of birth, or who exhibits slow or irregular gasping. Bradycardia indicates hypoxia (Tables 7.2 and 7.3).

Avoid hypothermia by drying, and use the radiant heater (Figure 7.3). If needed, clear secretions from the mouth and then the nose with a soft suction catheter. In the correct position, the neck is extended,

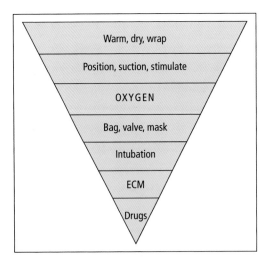

Figure 7.2 Resuscitation of the newborn. If you are at a delivery, rapidly assess pulse, respiration and colour. All babies are cleaned, dried and wrapped. If assessment is not satisfactory, move down the steps of the triangle, re-assess frequently, and go back up the triangle as the baby improves. External cardiac massage (ECM) and drugs are not used very often. You will need special training when you work with newborns.

Table 7.2 Apgar score, usually recorded at 1, 5 and 10 min after birth

Score	0	1	2
Heart rate	Absent	<100/min	>100/min
Respiratory effort	None	Slow, irregular	Regular, with cry
Muscle tone	Limp	Some tone in limbs	Active movements
Reflex irritability	None	Grimace only	Cry
Colour	Pallor	Body blue	Pink body

Table 7.3 Pointers to fetal hypoxia

Obstetric	Fetal
Antepartum	
Placental disease (pre-eclampsia, diabetes)	Intrauterine growth retardation
Placental abruption	Reduced fetal movements
Severe maternal illness	Abnormal fetal blood flow (Doppler's)
Intrapartum	
Umbilical cord prolapse/ compression	Meconium-stained liquor
Obstructed labour/ shoulder dystocia	Abnormal fetal heart rate (cardiotocograph)
Placenta praevia/ placental abruption	Metabolic acidosis (fetal blood sample)
	Postpartum
	• Bradycardia/apnoea
	• Low Apgar score
	• Delayed onset of respiration
	• Metabolic acidosis (cord blood)

 PRACTICE POINT

In almost all infants, an airway and adequate ventilation is all that is needed for effective resuscitation. Simple actions done well prevent mortality and morbidity.

allowing for the infant's large occiput. If hypoxia is not far advanced, breathing can usually be started by stimulation: gentle rubbing with a towel dries and stimulates! Some asphyxiated infants are pale, limp, apnoeic and bradycardic, and intermittent positive

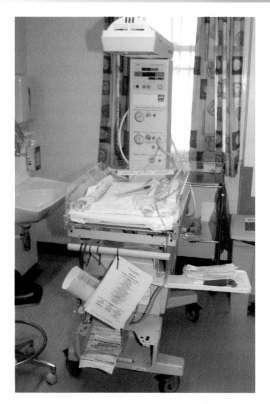

Figure 7.3 The resuscitaire comprises a heater, source of oxygen and suction, and an equipped platform for neonatal resuscitation.

pressure ventilation is begun by either bag and mask or tracheal tube.

Infants who recover rapidly should be given to their mothers as soon as possible. Some babies with severe asphyxia need to be admitted to the neonatal unit.

7.2.2 Birth asphyxia

Birth asphyxia is the consequence of intrapartum fetal hypoxia/ischaemia. Most infants will recover rapidly with prompt resuscitation. More severe asphyxia may lead to hypoxic ischaemic encephalopathy (HIE), the acute neurological illness due to the effects of asphyxia on the fetal brain. HIE occurs in 1–2 per 1000 deliveries.

 TREATMENT

Perinatal asphyxia induces a sequence of events over the first days, leading to neuronal death by apoptosis. Therapeutic hypothermia (cooling to 34 °C for 3 days), increases the chance of recovery without brain injury, and reduces the risk of cerebral palsy.

Table 7.4 Hypoxic ischaemic encephalopathy (HIE) grading

HIE grade	Prognosis
Mild: irritable with a high-pitched cry and poor feeding	Normal
Moderate: lethargic and hypotonic, poor feeding and occasional fits	40% risk of cerebral palsy
Severe: diminished conscious level, no spontaneous movement, multiple seizures and multi-organ failure	30% mortality 90% cerebral palsy

HIE is graded by clinical severity in the first days. The grade is important for prognosis (Table 7.4).

HIE requires intensive care. Some 20% of cerebral palsy is due to intrapartum hypoxic-ischaemic damage.

7.3 Routine care of the normal baby

Labelling. All newborn babies should have name bands attached to wrist and ankle in the delivery room and in the presence of the mother.

Vitamin K. Newborn babies have low levels of vitamin K and its dependent clotting factors. Untreated, in less than 1%, this causes haemorrhagic disease of the newborn with bleeding from the gastrointestinal tract, into the skin or mucous membranes, or rarely into the brain. Haemorrhagic disease is prevented by prophylaxis.

 TREATMENT

Vitamin K is given to all newborns as an oral supplement or as a single IM injection. Oral vitamin K is repeated over the first month in breast-fed infants.

The umbilical cord has two arteries and one vein. A single artery may be associated with congenital malformation. The cord is clamped about 1 cm from the skin surface and cut close to the clamp. The cord stump should be observed carefully for signs of infection. Staphylococcal infection is important but unusual.

Bathing. It is tempting to wash the newborn clean after birth, but bathing risks hypothermia and can be deferred for a few days. Vernix, a natural layer of grease which is present *in utero*, is absorbed naturally.

Passage of meconium and urine. It is important to note the time of first passing meconium and urine, and often this occurs at or soon after delivery. Both are usually passed within 24 h of birth, and delay should prompt a search for underlying pathology.

Feeding. This topic is dealt with fully in Section 12.1 and Section 12.3. The ideal is to put the baby to the breast shortly after birth. The first feed, of either breast milk or a formula, should be offered within 6 h of birth.

7.4 Examination of the newborn

All newborn babies should have a clinical examination in the first 24 h. The mother should be present, and in the vast majority, it will be possible to reassure parents that all is well.

PRACTICE POINT

The aims of newborn examinations are to:

- Detect conditions that:
  - Will benefit from early treatment
  - Need long-term supervision
  - Have genetic implications
  - Indicate systemic illness.
- Discuss parental anxieties, and take a brief medical, genetic and social history, seeking information that may be relevant to the future health and development of the baby.
- Provide advice on matters such as infant feeding, attendance at baby clinics, and immunization.
- Advise on minor abnormalities which may lead to worry.

7.4.1 Suggested scheme for routine clinical examination

General observation. Does the infant look well? Is she pink and responsive? Is she tachypnoeic or pale? Check for the normal flexed posture and symmetrical limb movements. Are there dysmorphic features? Look for cyanosis, jaundice, skin rashes and birthmarks.

Measurements. Check weight, length and occipito-frontal head circumference for gestational age on a centile chart.

Head. Check head shape. Moulding (change of head shape during delivery) is common and resolves in

days. Assess the tension of the anterior fontanelle and the width of the sutures. These vary greatly between babies, but a full fontanelle with wide sutures may indicate hydrocephalus.

Face. Has the baby got a normal face, or any dysmorphic features? Is there a facial nerve palsy?

Eyes. Simply look carefully at the eyes and make sure there is a red reflex (excluding cataract) (Section 3.5.6, p. 39). Asymmetry of eye size is abnormal: small eyes may occur in congenital viral infection or developmental defect, or one eye may be large (congenital glaucoma). The eye should be checked for signs of infection.

Common conditions of little clinical importance

Skin lesions

- Strawberry naevi (Figure 24.3)
- 'Stork' marks (Figure 24.1)
- Milia (small collections in the sebaceous glands which disappear soon after birth) (Figure 7.4)
- Erythema toxicum (a blotchy red rash; each spot has a yellow centre which is full of eosinophils. Spots come and go. It is benign and should be distinguished from skin sepsis)
- Mongolian blue spots (Section 24.1.2.2)
- Epithelial 'pearls' (small white cysts near the midline on the palate)

Subconjunctival haemorrhage

Cephalhaematoma (Figure 7.5) – see 'Soft tissue injuries' later in this chapter

Positional talipes (you need to distinguish from structural talipes that needs surgery (Section 23.1.6)

Peripheral and traumatic cyanosis (blue hands and feet are normal in the first days. Facial congestion looks like cyanosis)

Breast enlargement (due to maternal oestrogen; this resolves with time)

Oral and vulval mucosal tags

Sacral dimple (extremely rarely connects with spinal cord but make sure you can see the bottom of the dimple)

Skin tags and diminutive accessory digits.

Mouth. The palate should be inspected for clefts and palpated for submucosal clefts (Figure 7.6). The oral cavity should be checked for the presence of teeth, cysts or thrush (candida infection).

Jaw. A small or recessed mandible (retrognathia) can lead to feeding difficulty or respiratory obstruction.

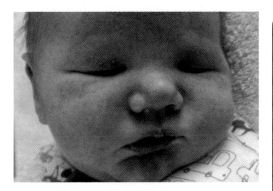

Figure 7.4 Milia. Small raised, white spots over the nose and cheeks. This baby also has two erythema toxicum spots on the right eyelid.

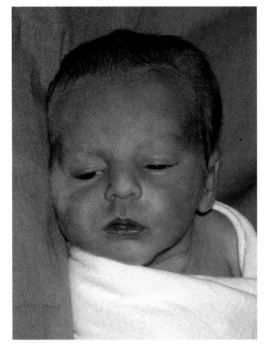

Figure 7.5 Unilateral cephalhaematoma.

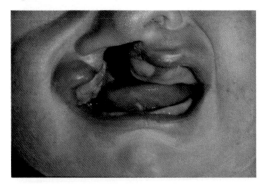

Figure 7.6 Unilateral cleft lip and palate.

Primitive reflexes

Grasp - birth to 4 months The infant grasps an object placed in palm or under toes.

Moro (startle) reflex - birth to 4 months
- Hold the infant supporting the head, and allow the head to drop gently a few centimetres. The infant will look surprised or even cry, throw its arms outwards and then bring them back to the midline. Explain what you are doing to the mother.

Asymmetric tonic neck reflex (ATNR) - birth to 7 months
- On turning the head to one side, the ipsilateral arm and leg are extended.

Rooting reflex - from birth
- On touching the infant's face, he turns, opening his mouth as if to suck on the finger.

Persistence of the Moro and ATNR is abnormal and may indicate cerebral palsy.

Chest. Check the baby is pink and not breathless.

Heart. Which side is the heart best heard on? Where is the apex beat? Heart murmurs are very common in babies and most relate to the transition from fetal to adult circulatory pattern and disappear in the first days. It is difficult to tell which murmurs are significant and it is important not to worry parents unnecessarily. Pansystolic, diastolic or very loud murmurs are likely to be important.

Abdomen. The liver edge is usually palpable 1–2 cm below the right costal margin, and the spleen can be tipped in at least 20% of normal babies. The lower poles of both kidneys may be palpable.

Groin. Absent femoral pulses may denote coarctation of the aorta. Check for hernias.

Genitalia. Check that the genitalia are clearly either male or female. If there is doubt, do not ascribe sex. In boys, check that the testes are in the scrotum and that the urethral meatus is where it should be. In girls, inspect the genitalia and remember that a little vaginal bleeding or discharge of clear mucus is normal secondary to the influence of maternal and placental hormones.

Anus. Ask if the baby has passed meconium, and check that the anus is present, patent and normally located.

Spine. Turn the baby prone. Inspect the entire spine for lumps, naevi, hairy patches, pits or sinuses which may indicate spinal cord abnormality.

Hips. Examination of the hips is very important (Section 23.1.7). It is best left to the end of the examination as it may upset the baby.

Central nervous system. Is the baby moving spontaneously? Is there symmetry of movement? Are limbs held in the usual flexed position? Ask about feeding behaviour. Assess tone by picking the baby up and holding her in ventral suspension. Elicit the Moro reflex (see above, this chapter, 'Primitive reflexes').

Biochemical screening. Routine screening on blood spot tests is carried out on day 5–7 for phenylketonuria (Section 27.7.1) (Guthrie test), hypothyroidism (Section 27.3), cystic fibrosis (Section 19.8), haemoglobinopathy (Section 25.2.2.1) and MCADD (Section 27.7.2).

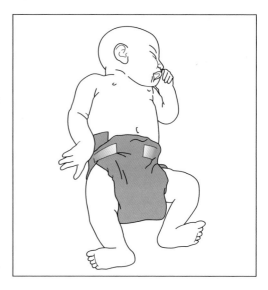

Figure 7.7 Erb's palsy.

7.5 Birth injury (physical trauma)

Serious birth injury is rare. Tentorial tears (injury to the fold of dura between the cerebrum and cerebellum) can be fatal or lead to permanent cerebral damage, but are hardly ever seen now. Minor trauma is quite commonly discovered on routine examination. Trauma is more common after obstructed labour (due to a small pelvis or a large baby), precipitate labour, malpresentation and heroic instrumental delivery.

7.5.1 Nerve palsies

Most lesions recover as traumatic swelling subsides, but minor disability persists in about 15%, and a few are left handicapped.

7.5.1.1 Brachial plexus palsies

These usually follow the difficult delivery of a big baby.

 PRACTICE POINT

Erb's palsy (Figure 7.7) affects C5/6 roots, resulting in weakness or paralysis. The affected arm lies straight and limp beside the trunk. The forearm is internally rotated and with the fingers flexed (waiter's tip position). When the Moro reflex is elicited, the affected arm does not respond.

Rarely, the lower roots C8/T1 are injured, resulting in weakness of wrist extensors and intrinsic muscles of the hand (*Klumpke's palsy*).

7.5.1.2 Facial nerve palsy

The facial nerve may be injured by pressure from the maternal pelvic bones or by forceps blades. It is a lower motor neurone defect, usually unilateral.

7.5.1.3 Phrenic nerve palsy

Rarely, the cervical roots of the phrenic nerve are damaged, causing diaphragmatic paralysis and respiratory difficulty.

7.5.2 Skeletal injury

7.5.2.1 Clavicle fracture

This commonly follows shoulder dystocia. Complete breaks are painful and limit the baby's arm movements. Clavicle fractures heal well, but often with considerable callus formation.

7.5.2.2 Humerus and femur

Fractures and epiphyseal injury may rarely occur during difficult births. They heal well.

7.5.2.3 Skull fractures

The compliant skull of the newborn is remarkably resistant to fracture. Asymptomatic linear fractures of the parietal bone are most common. Depressed fractures require surgical elevation.

7.5.3 Soft tissue injuries

7.5.3.1 Cephalhaematoma

 PRACTICE POINT

Subperiosteal bleeding is common, occurring in 1–2%. The swelling and the amount of blood loss are limited by the periosteum attached to the margins of the skull bone so a cephalhaematoma does not cross the midline (Figure 7.5).

It may make jaundice worse as the blood in it is reabsorbed. Infection may occur if the skin is broken. The vast majority resolve spontaneously, although the edge may calcify.

7.5.3.2 Subaponeurotic haemorrhage

Haemorrhage between the periosteum and galea aponeurotica (a thick membrane going from the eyebrows to the occiput) is potentially lethal. The space is not limited like a cephalhaematoma, and serious blood loss can occur. It is more common after Ventouse delivery. The baby appears pale with a raised fluctuant swelling of the scalp.

7.5.3.3 Sternomastoid tumour

This is a fusiform fibrous mass in the middle of the sternomastoid muscle. It may follow trauma. It usually disappears over about 6 months. Gentle physiotherapy to prevent shortening of the muscle is required.

7.5.3.4 Bruising and abrasions

Difficult births are often accompanied by bruising. Usually there is little serious harm. Breakdown of extravasated blood may contribute to neonatal jaundice. Skin abrasions are portals of entry for microorganisms and should be observed for signs of infection.

7.6 Congenital malformations

Congenital abnormalities are an important cause of perinatal mortality and short- and long-term morbidity (Figure 7.8). Most of the common

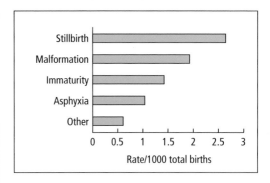

Figure 7.8 Causes of perinatal death (the stillbirth rate is for fetuses without abnormality).

defects are described in the relevant chapter. Causation and prenatal diagnosis are discussed in Section 6.3 and 6.3.1.

Most congenital defects can be detected at birth or by the routine clinical examination. Some will present with symptoms such as vomiting, cyanosis, jaundice or failure to pass urine or meconium. Some abnormalities, especially in the cardiovascular system or renal tract, may escape detection. It is important to remember that multiple defects are quite common.

 PRACTICE POINT

Finding of any congenital anomaly should always lead to a careful search for others.

Some constellations of defects may fit into recognized syndromes. Some syndromes are well known (e.g. Down syndrome) but most are rare. A diagnosis often gives a reasonably accurate prognosis and genetic risk of recurrence.

The problems of helping parents to cope with the bad news that there is something wrong with their baby are discussed in Section 2.2.3.1.

Summary

This chapter has reviewed the changes in the fetus at birth. Routine examination of the newborn is important; usually leading to reassurance of the parents but also detection of important congenital abnormality.

Good obstetrics usually avoids significant birth trauma or asphyxia but both can happen with the best of care.

FOR YOUR LOG

Note common neonatal variations. You will see milia, storkmarks and erythema toxicum in examining the healthy newborn.

OSCE TIP

- Manikin: first day examination of newborn.
- Illustrated station with congenital abnormality.
- Examination of the hips – model (OSCE Station 23.1).
- Video of primitive reflexes, e.g. Moro, asymmetric tonic neck reflex.
- Recognition of common congenital abnormalities.

See EMQ 7.1 and EMQ 7.2 at the end of the book.

8

Disorders of the newborn

Chapter map

Most newborns are healthy and need warmth, love and milk. The cost of illness can be great and the newborn is prone to severe problems that may have long-lasting consequences. In the term infant, early detection of illness such as infection is key. In the preterm infant, expert perinatal and neonatal care has transformed and improved outcome. When considering a newborn, think of three main groups: preterm, small for gestational age, and term.

8.1   Birth weight and gestation

Careful classification of a baby by weight and gestation is important (Figure 8.1). Abnormalities of weight for gestation may indicate maternal diabetes, intrauterine infection or chromosome abnormality. The preterm infant's problems are due to immaturity. SGA babies are at risk of hypoglycaemia (see Section 8.4.3).

> **Definitions**
>
> - Low birthweight (LBW): <2500 g (7% of UK births)
> - Very low birthweight (VLBW): <1500 g (1% of UK births)
> - Extremely low birthweight: <1000 g
> - Preterm: <37 weeks gestation (6% of UK births)
> - Term: 37–41 weeks gestation
> - Post-term: ≥42 weeks gestation
> - Small for gestational age (SGA): birthweight <2nd centile for gestation
> - Large for gestational age: birthweight >98th centile for gestation
> - Appropriate for gestational age (AGA): birthweight 2nd to 98th centile for gestation.

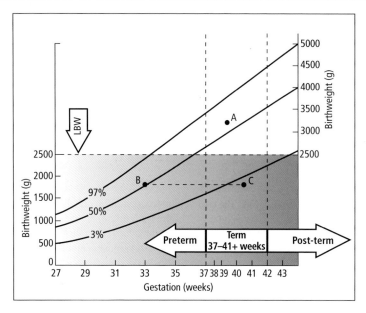

Figure 8.1 Growth chart with 50th, 3rd and 97th centiles. Three babies are marked: A is term and appropriate for gestation; B and C both have the same birthweight and both are LBW but they will have very different clinical problems; B is LBW and preterm – he is appropriate for gestation; C is LBW and term – he is small for gestation.

 Different problems occur when low birth weight is due to prematurity or intrauterine growth restriction.

The best guide to gestation is the menstrual history and ultrasound estimate of fetal size made before 20 weeks' gestation. Physical and neurological features of the newborn change with gestation. As gestation increases, skin becomes keratinized, thicker, and has less lanugo (fine hair). Ear cartilage and the breast nodule develop during the third trimester. In boys, the testes descend into the scrotum at around 36 weeks. In girls, the labia majora cover the labia minora towards term. As gestation increases, muscle tone and ligamentous laxity increase.

8.2   The preterm baby

Preterm infant: problems are due to immaturity

- Respiratory distress syndrome (surfactant deficiency)
- Recurrent apnoea
- Poor thermoregulation
- Renal function, fluid and electrolyte balance
- Nutrition
- Patent ductus arteriosus
- Intraventricular haemorrhage and other brain damage
- Anaemia
- Necrotizing enterocolitis
- Jaundice.

8.2.1   Respiratory distress syndrome (RDS)

RDS, also known as hyaline membrane disease, is virtually confined to preterm babies and is common below 32 weeks.

PRACTICE POINT

Antenatal maternal steroids lead to a 60% reduction in the likelihood of RDS, and should be used whenever possible.

Surfactant lowers surface tension in the liquid that lines the respiratory tract. Without surfactant, the alveoli cannot be inflated and tend to collapse. The result is atelectasis (poor aeration) and the appearance on X-ray (Figure 8.2). Increased work of breathing (respiratory distress) occurs, leading to poor oxygenation and carbon dioxide retention (respiratory failure), and often to apnoeic spells.

 Respiratory distress

- Tachypnoea (>60 bpm)
- Intercostal recession
- Subcostal recession
- Grunting
- Nasal flare
- Cyanosis.

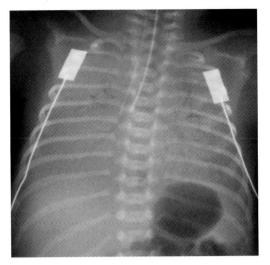

Figure 8.2 Respiratory distress syndrome: note the characteristic ground glass appearance in all lung fields. In this picture, the tracheal tube is too far down, and was pulled back afterwards.

Surfactant replacement therapy can be given through the endotracheal tube soon after birth, and leads to reduced mortality, less risk of pneumothorax and reduced lung damage. RDS resolves over a period of 3–7 days as surfactant production increases. The key to management is to keep the baby alive and undamaged during this period. Infants with significant RDS need assisted ventilation (mechanical ventilation or continuous positive airway pressure). Careful monitoring is crucial.

8.2.2 Bronchopulmonary dysplasia (BPD)

This chronic lung disease occurs in some preterm babies who have been ventilated for severe RDS. It is due to lung damage by high oxygen concentration and high positive pressures. Steroid therapy is helpful in ventilator-dependent infants, but has side effects. Some babies with BPD require prolonged oxygen therapy for months.

 PRACTICE POINT **Blood gas stability is essential**

	Blood oxygen	Blood carbon dioxide
Low	Tissue or brain damage	Brain ischaemia and PVL
High	Retinopathy of prematurity	Intracranial haemorrhage

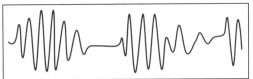

Figure 8.3 Irregular breathing in a preterm infant with periods of apnoea or shallow breathing.

8.2.3 Recurrent apnoea

Preterm infants do not breathe regularly (Figure 8.3). If periods of shallow breathing or apnoea exceed 10–20s, they are associated with bradycardia and cyanosis. Apnoeas may be the first sign of neonatal illness but commonly are due to immaturity. Caffeine is given to stimulate regular breathing. Apnoea monitors are in regular use on neonatal units! (see Figure 28.2f).

8.2.3.1 Temperature control

Hypothermia increases oxygen consumption and predisposes to RDS and infection. It must be avoided. Incubators and radiant heaters are used so that the baby uses little energy keeping warm or cooling down.

 PRACTICE POINT

Tiny preterm infants are placed in a polythene bag at birth to prevent evaporative loss of fluid and heat.

Risks for hypothermia

- Large surface area relative to body mass
- Little subcutaneous fat
- Large insensible water and heat loss.

8.2.4 Fluid and electrolyte balance

Renal function is relatively poor in the preterm baby. Coupled with a high (but largely unmeasurable) water-loss through the very permeable skin, this can lead rapidly to dehydration and electrolyte disturbance.

8.2.5 Nutrition

If the preterm newborn is to equal the fetal growth rate, requirements are high. If the baby is not ill, milk is given. Frequent, small volume nasogastric feeds are used. The best milk is the mother's expressed breast milk – it is better tolerated, induces gut maturation and reduces risk of necrotizing enterocolitis. In VLBW infants, protein and calories are added to breast milk. Nutritive sucking and swallowing develops at about 34 weeks. For tiny sick babies, parenteral nutrition is often used.

> **Nutrition requirements**
>
> Energy 120 kcal/kg/day in 150–180 mL/kg/day
> Protein and energy needs are four times those of the adult (per kg!).

8.2.6 Patent ductus arteriosus (PDA)

The ductus arteriosus (Figure 8.4) of the preterm infant often fails to close, especially when RDS is present. Left-to-right shunting may lead to heart failure. Most close with time. The PDA can be closed by giving a prostaglandin synthetase inhibitor (e.g. ibuprofen), but sometimes surgical closure is required.

8.2.7 Intraventricular haemorrhage and other forms of brain damage

In the walls of the lateral ventricles of the preterm baby's brain are fragile capillaries (the germinal matrix), where bleeding may occur. Haemorrhage,

easily seen on cranial ultrasound through the fontanelle, may be local or extend into the ventricles or brain tissue. The more extensive the haemorrhage, the more likely are brain damage and hydrocephalus. It is estimated that some degree of haemorrhage occurs in 40% of very small babies, although it causes serious damage in only a small minority.

Periventricular leukomalacia (PVL) is the most important pattern of brain damage in the preterm. It is seen in 5–10% under 32 weeks. White matter beside the ventricle is damaged by hypoxia/ischaemia and also inflammation and low carbon dioxide levels. It characteristically leads to spastic diplegia.

8.2.8 Anaemia

Anaemia is common because of red cell breakdown, and 'bleeding into the laboratory'. Transfusion is often used. Extra iron is given with breast feeding when the preterm infant is 6 weeks old. Preterm formula milk is supplemented with iron.

8.2.9 Necrotizing enterocolitis (NEC)

NEC is the most common surgical emergency in neonatal medicine. Surgery is often needed. Mortality is 20%. The infant becomes sick and acidotic with a distended abdomen due to gut necrosis. NEC is almost restricted to the preterm. Aetiology is unknown, but immaturity, infection, gut ischaemia

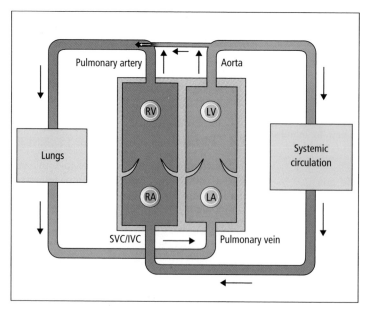

Figure 8.4 Patent ductus arteriosus.

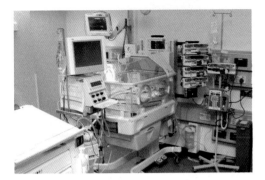

Figure 8.5 Neonatal intensive care. The hi-tech set-up is daunting for the parents.

and enteral milk feeding all contribute to pathogenesis. Breast milk feeds reduce the risk of NEC considerably.

8.2.10 Management of the preterm infant

Preterm infants who are unwell are looked after in neonatal units or special care baby units (SCBUs) (Figure 8.5).

Only babies who need to be should be separated from their mothers. Parents must be allowed free access to the unit, involved in their baby's care and kept up to date regularly. Hospitals that cannot provide intensive care often transfer infants to a regional unit. Babies travel well in expert hands.

Improved obstetric and neonatal care means that the mortality rate among preterm infants has fallen considerably and continues to do so. The very preterm infant is at risk of disability (Figure 8.6). The survival rate for VLBW infants (<1500 g) who are free of lethal malformation is currently better than 90%, and serious handicap occurs in no more than 6–10%. Survival rates fall off rapidly at gestations below 28 weeks and are virtually zero below 24 weeks. Resuscitation of babies at the extremes of viability is an area of ethical and scientific dilemma.

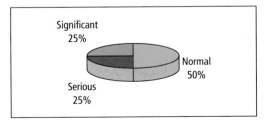

Figure 8.6 Disability at 2 years in preterm infants <26 weeks.

8.3 The small-for-gestational age (SGA) baby

> **Risks for the SGA baby**
>
> Perinatal asphyxia
>
> - Poor placental function
> - Risk of meconium aspiration
>
> Hypoglycaemia
> Hypothermia
> Congenital malformation or chromosome abnormality
> Poor postnatal growth.

Paediatric management begins by preparing for delivery. SGA infants are more likely to need resuscitation, and the paediatrician must be there if meconium is present in the liquor to prevent aspiration. Small size and little insulation from body fat increase the risk of hypothermia (Figure 8.7). The most important, common problem is hypoglycaemia. Initiate early, frequent feeds and routine testing of blood glucose. Any symptom could be hypoglycaemia, and demands a blood glucose check.

Most SGA infants have asymmetric intrauterine growth restriction (relatively large head compared with birthweight) due to placental insufficiency, and have a good prognosis. Look carefully for congenital abnormalities or a cause in symmetrical SGA infants (Table 8.1). More severe SGA babies may have poor

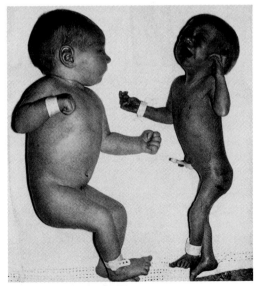

Figure 8.7 Two babies born at term. The baby on the right shows severe growth restriction.

Table 8.1 Types of SGA babies

Type	Growth pattern	Cause
Asymmetrical	Head circumference significantly higher on centiles than weight	Late fetal malnutrition Pre-eclampsia Smoking
Symmetrical	Head circumference and weight equally reduced	Genetic Normal small Fetal abnormality Early fetal malnutrition Congenital viral infection Drug effect

fetal brain growth with future neurodevelopmental problems, and these babies often fail to show 'catch up' growth postnatally.

8.4 The newborn term infant

8.4.1 Respiratory problems

Respiratory distress has many causes in the term infant. Infection, congenital heart disease, metabolic acidosis and diaphragmatic hernia can all lead to respiratory distress.

PRACTICE POINT

Any baby with tachypnoea (rate >60 bpm) must be seen. It is vital not to miss the early signs of infection. GBS can kill an infant in hours. Early infection screen and antibiotics give a good prognosis.

The following lung disorders are common:

Transient tachypnoea. Tachypnoea for a few hours after birth due to delayed clearance of lung fluid. It is more common after caesarean section.

Meconium aspiration. Intrapartum asphyxia in full-term babies may cause passage of meconium into the liquor. If inhaled, it can cause severe illness with pneumonitis and persistent pulmonary hypertension, with persistence of the fetal pattern of circulation. Clearing the upper airway and trachea of meconium at birth reduces the risk, but do not delay bag and mask ventilation of an apnoeic infant if intubation expertise is not available.

Congenital pneumonia. When microorganisms invade the amniotic cavity before delivery, the baby may be born infected. This is particularly likely when there has been prolonged rupture of the membranes (longer than 18 h). Group B streptococci (GBS) and Gram-negative organisms such as *Escherichia coli* are most commonly incriminated.

Pneumothorax. Tiny, spontaneous pneumothoraces are not uncommon after birth and they are usually asymptomatic. Occasionally a chest drain is needed, and the prognosis is good.

8.4.2 Jaundice

Around 50% of infants are visibly jaundiced during the first week of life. The most common mechanism is 'physiological' and reflects slow conjugation. In the fetus, bilirubin is not conjugated which enables it to be excreted by placental transfer, but after birth conjugation and hepatic excretion of bilirubin must take over. Some jaundiced infants need investigation or therapy.

PRACTICE POINT Golden rules of physiological jaundice

- Jaundice is not apparent in first 24 h.
- The infant remains well.
- The serum bilirubin does not reach treatment level.
- The jaundice has faded by 14 days.

These infants do not need investigation or intervention, other than to measure the bilirubin level if jaundice appears marked.

Jaundice apparent within the first 24 h is never physiological and strongly suggests excessive haemolysis or sepsis.

8.4.2.1 Kernicterus

Unconjugated bilirubin (but not conjugated) can enter the brain and cause neuronal damage. High serum bilirubin, preterm birth, acidosis or hypoxia increase the risk. The rare clinical syndrome of bilirubin encephalopathy (kernicterus) may result in death or serious handicap.

When serum bilirubin is high, treatment with phototherapy is started. Light of a wavelength that converts unconjugated bilirubin to non-toxic isomers allows bilirubin excretion without conjugation. The infant is nursed naked wearing an eye shield under a phototherapy unit, or on an illuminated fibreoptic mat. In

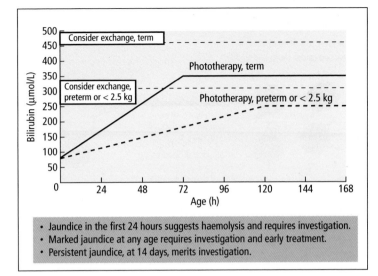

- Jaundice in the first 24 hours suggests haemolysis and requires investigation.
- Marked jaundice at any age requires investigation and early treatment.
- Persistent jaundice, at 14 days, merits investigation.

Figure 8.8 Serum bilirubin is plotted against age to decide upon therapy.

severe or rapidly worsening jaundice, exchange transfusion is performed (Figure 8.8). An umbilical vessel is catheterized, and fresh donor blood obtained. A small volume of blood is removed from the infant and discarded, and then replaced with donor blood. This is repeated many times.

Causes of neonatal jaundice

Physiological (obeys golden rules)

Haemolytic (often begins <24 h)
- ABO incompatibility
- Rhesus or other isoimmunization
- Red cell defects (e.g. G6PD deficiency)

Physiological plus
- Prematurity
- Bruising
- Polycythaemia
- Dehydration
- Sepsis

Prolonged
- Physiological (normal variation)
- Breast milk
- Biliary atresia
- Neonatal hepatitis
- Hypothyroidism
- Inborn errors of metabolism (e.g. galactosaemia).

🔪 **TREATMENT Exchange tranfusion**

- Removes bilirubin
- Removes haemolysing red cells
- Corrects anaemia
- Removes antibody

8.4.2.2 Pathological jaundice

Jaundice in the first day is characteristically due to haemolysis. Look for maternal antibodies on antenatal blood tests and check the baby's bilirubin, haemoglobin and Coombs' test (Figure 8.9).

ABO incompatibility is the most common cause of haemolytic jaundice: usually the mOther is group O, the bAby group A and the problem is maternal anti-A. ABO occasionally requires an exchange transfusion. Anti-A occurs naturally in people who are group O.

In Rhesus (Rh) haemolytic disease, the Rh-negative mother is sensitized by exposure to Rhesus-positive red cells and produces anti-D in her next pregnancy. Rh alloimmunization causes serious haemolysis, leading to jaundice and anaemia. The affected fetus may need in utero transfusion, and exchange transfusion is often needed in the infant. Rh disease is now rare because anti-D immunoglobulin is given to women.

Alloimmunization

- STEP 1 Mother meets foreign antigen
  - Miscarriage, amniocentesis, delivery
  - Blood transfusion
- STEP 2 Mother expresses antibody
- STEP 3 IgG crosses placenta.

Breast milk jaundice is quite common and harmless. It presents as delayed resolution of physiological jaundice. Breast milk interferes with conjugation. Stools remain pigmented, and clinical and biochemical investigation is satisfactory. Breast feeding can continue.

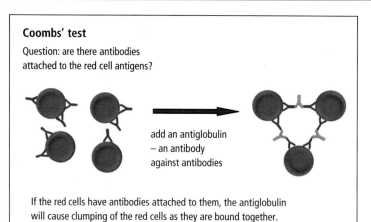

Coombs' test

Question: are there antibodies attached to the red cell antigens?

add an antiglobulin
– an antibody
against antibodies

If the red cells have antibodies attached to them, the antiglobulin will cause clumping of the red cells as they are bound together.

Figure 8.9 Coombs' test.

 PRACTICE POINT

Biliary atresia is rare, but early recognition is essential for successful surgery. It leads to prolonged conjugated jaundice and pale stools. Biliary atresia must be considered in all babies who are still jaundiced at 14 days.

 Hypoglycaemic symptoms

- Jitters, irritability
- Poor feeding
- Pallor, sweating
- Hypotonia
- Seizures.

8.4.3 Hypoglycaemia

High risk for hypoglycaemia

- Small for gestational age
- Preterm
- Infants of diabetic mothers
- Any perinatal illness

At birth, continuous supplies of glucose that cross the placenta are cut off and the baby must maintain her own blood glucose from stored glycogen and fat until feeding is established. Glucose is an essential fuel for the nervous system. Early symptoms of hypoglycaemia are non-specific, and late signs are associated with risk of cerebral damage. Levels of glucose as low as 1–1.5 mmol/L may be seen in asymptomatic healthy term infants but the brain is protected by its ability to use other fuels. Symptomatic hypoglycaemia is an emergency and must be corrected urgently. This also applies in the infant at high risk of hypoglycaemia, where it is essential to keep blood glucose at or above 2.5 mmol/L, by early and frequent milk feeds and, if necessary, by IV infusion of dextrose. In these infants, blood sugar is checked 4–6 hourly for the first 1-2 days.

8.4.3.1 Infant of a diabetic mother

If a mother has diabetes or gestational diabetes, the altered metabolic climate of the fetus can cause the following problems after birth:

- Hypoglycaemia
- Large size and obesity
- Increased risk of RDS
- Polycythaemia
- Congenital malformation.

Good diabetic control before conception and during pregnancy has vastly reduced these problems.

8.4.4 Infection

8.4.4.1 Fetal infection

Micro-organisms rarely succeed in crossing the placenta or penetrating the intact amnion. The effect of fetal infection depends on the nature of the organism, and the stage of gestation. Very early infections may cause fetal death, abortion or major malformation.

Rubella. The rubella virus causes malformation if infection occurs early in pregnancy. An infected baby may also be born with evidence of active viraemia: jaundice, hepatosplenomegaly, purpura and sometimes lesions of the bones and lungs (Figure 8.10).

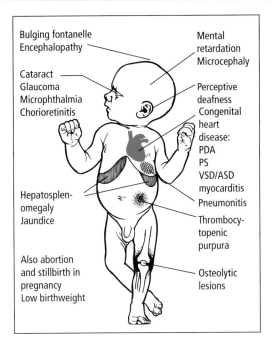

Bulging fontanelle
Encephalopathy

Mental retardation
Microcephaly

Cataract
Glaucoma
Microphthalmia
Chorioretinitis

Perceptive deafness
Congenital heart disease:
PDA
PS
VSD/ASD
myocarditis

Hepatosplen-
omegaly
Jaundice

Pneumonitis

Thrombocy-
topenic
purpura

Also abortion
and stillbirth in
pregnancy
Low birthweight

Osteolytic
lesions

Figure 8.10 Features of congenital rubella syndrome.

Congenital rubella is prevented by herd immunity through immunization.

Cytomegalovirus (CMV). The incidence of congenital CMV infection is in the region of 3 or 4 cases per 1000 births. The brain and auditory pathway are the major targets for damage, which occurs in about 15% of infected fetuses. It is an important cause of deafness.

Toxoplasmosis. This rare disease is caused by a protozoon whose usual host is the cat. CNS involvement with hydrocephalus and retinitis may occur.

Human immunodeficiency virus (HIV) (Chapter 14). In Europe, measures taken (see box) reduce risk of perinatal, vertical transmission from mother to infant to 1–2%. Without these strategies, approximately 10–20% of infants of HIV seropositive mothers are prenatally or perinatally infected with HIV. This vertical transmission accounts for the majority of AIDS in childhood. Symptoms of AIDS may begin at any time from birth, and usually within 2 years. More common symptoms are failure to thrive, diarrhoea, recurrent infections and severe candida infection. The number of AIDS cases in babies and young children in the UK is small. Worldwide it is rapidly becoming the major cause of infant mortality.

 TREATMENT

Vertical transmission of HIV is reduced by:

- Antenatal, maternal antiviral therapy
- Delivery by caesarean section
- Avoidance of breast feeding
- Neonatal antiviral therapy.

Hepatitis B infection. Risk of vertical transmission varies, but is high if mothers have the e antigen. Protection is by combination of passive immunity with hepatitis B immunoglobulin, and active immunity with hepatitis B vaccine. Lower risk babies should receive hepatitis B vaccine.

Syphilis, tuberculosis and malaria can cause fetal infection; they are rare in Europe, although TB is now seen more often.

8.4.4.2 Intrapartum infection

When the membranes rupture, the uterus may be invaded by organisms from the birth canal. Some infections are particularly likely to be acquired in this way:

- Pneumonia and/or meningitis due to group B streptococci
- *E. coli* septicaemia and/or meningitis
- Gonoccocal and chlamydia eye infection
- Herpes simplex.

8.4.4.3 Infection acquired after birth

Once born, the baby rapidly becomes colonized by bacteria and usually this occurs without harm. Infection is especially likely if colonization is heavy or if the organisms are of high pathogenicity. Organisms in the blood stream may give rise to septicaemia, meningitis or pneumonia.

 PRACTICE POINT Common early signs of infection

- Lethargy and hypotonia
- Poor feeding, abdominal distension or vomiting
- Pallor and mottling of the skin
- Disturbed temperature regulation
- Tachypnoea or recurrent apnoea.

Any baby with suspected infection should be examined carefully. Perform an infection screen: full blood count, blood culture, chest X-ray, microscopy and culture of urine and CSF. Immediate investigation and antibiotic may be life saving. GBS (see above) is the commonest and most important infection while other common organisms are *E. coli, Staphylococcus aureus* and *Listeria*. Coagulase-negative staphylococcus is the most common pathogen in the preterm infant.

TREATMENT

Do not wait for results – if infection is suspected give broad-spectrum antibiotics, typically amoxycillin and gentamicin.

8.4.4.4 Sticky eye

The cause of most sticky eyes is poor drainage down the nasolacrimal duct. Often all that is necessary is to bathe the eye with warm saline. More serious eye infections may be due to staphylococci and coliforms.

PRACTICE POINT

If a baby has severe purulent eye infection in the first 10 days, this is typical of gonococcus and *Chlamydia trachomatis* infection. Urgent diagnosis and treatment is needed.

8.4.4.5 Skin infection

Septic spots and paronychia, usually due to staphylococcal infection, are relatively common and responsive to local treatment, but may need systemic antibiotics.

8.4.4.6 Candida infection

Infection of the mouth and nappy area by yeasts is common. It responds well to nystatin or miconazole. Therapy should be continued for a few days longer than it takes to clear the signs of infection. Hygiene of bottles and dummies must be scrupulous.

8.4.5 Convulsions

Convulsions occurring in the first days of life have many causes. Perinatal brain injury is important. Severe seizures are a poor prognostic sign.

Seizures always require immediate and thorough investigation and treatment of any underlying disorder. If the cause cannot be remedied, anticonvulsant medication is given.

Causes of seizures

- Intrapartum asphyxia
- Intracranial bleeds
- Hypoglycaemia
- Meningitis
- Low Ca or Mg
- Inborn error of metabolism
- Brain malformation or abnormality

 Summary

Most problems in the preterm infant are due to organ immaturity, and are closely linked to gestation. Each week below 32 weeks increases the chance of serious problems. The outlook for the preterm infant has improved massively in the last 2 decades. In the infant who is small for gestational age, problems relate to the cause of the low birthweight and to poor fetal nutrition. In the term infant who becomes unwell, always consider infection and hypoglycaemia, especially in high-risk infants. Every baby that is successfully treated acquires over 70 quality adjusted life years.

 FOR YOUR LOG

- Visit the neonatal intensive care ward. Ask to join the ward round. Go there when you are on call.
- Look at the chest X-ray of a baby with respiratory distress syndrome.
- Make sure you have seen an apnoea monitor and know how to set it.
- See a baby having phototherapy.

See EMQ 8.1, EMQ 8.2, EMQ 8.3 and EMQ 8.4 at the end of the book.

9

Child development and how to assess it

Chapter map

Child development is the gradual acquisition of new skills and behaviours through childhood. Knowledge of development helps you to understand the presentation and impact of illness in children, and will help you to adapt your history and examination for age. In this chapter we describe normal development and a practical approach to assessment.

 Healthy development has a wide range of 'normal'.

9.1   Normal development

Development is normally divided into several separate areas; learn these for a systematic approach, but be flexible.

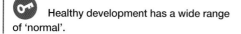
PRACTICE POINT **Four areas of development**

- Posture and movement (gross motor)
- Vision and manipulation (fine motor/adaptive)
- Hearing and speech (language)
- Social and play (personal/social).

9.1.1   Range of normal

The age at which a normal child achieves a particular physical or developmental goal is extremely variable; 50% of children can walk 10 steps unaided at 13 months, but a few can do this at 8 months, and others not until 18 months. It is best to talk to parents of the 'usual' age for developing a skill rather than the 'normal', since abnormal implies problems. Quite commonly one field of activity appears delayed in a normal child, but it is rare for all four fields of development to be delayed if the child is normal. In the preterm infant, correct age for gestation before assessing development.

Delayed development that is following a normal sequence is likely to be normal unless the delay is severe. Bizarre and unusual patterns of development are more worrying.

Paediatrics Lecture Notes, Ninth edition. Simon J. Newell and Jonathan C. Darling. © 2014 John Wiley & Sons, Ltd. Published 2014 by John Wiley & Sons, Ltd.

9.1.2 Milestones are stepping stones

Parents tend to think of certain developmental skills as essential milestones. It is truer to regard them as stepping stones. In general, one cannot reach a particular stepping stone without using the previous ones – and a child does not run until she can walk, or walk until she can stand. However, different people may use different stepping stones, and occasionally miss one out. Most children crawl before they stand, but some shuffle on their bottoms, never crawl, yet stand and walk normally in the end. *Bottom shuffling* is a typical example of the sort of variation in development that can cause parents unnecessary worry, particularly as bottom shufflers tend to walk later than other children.

Using stepping stones, we may go in sudden bounds rather than at an even rate – children often develop that way, appearing static for a few weeks then suddenly mastering a new skill. If the next stepping stone is a particularly hard one, all the child's energy may appear to be devoted to just one of the four areas of development, whilst the other three seem static; posture and movement skills may advance rapidly about the age of 1 year as walking is mastered, whilst hearing and speech development appear static.

> Whether we like it or not, many parents view their child's developmental assessment in the same way as an undergraduate examination, and all parents want their child to 'pass'. Therefore:
>
> - When we 'test' beyond expected skills – reassure that we do not expect the 9- to 12-month-old child to walk.
> - Announce 'results' early – if development is normal, say so.
> - Handle 'failure' carefully – be sure before you diagnose developmental delay.

9.2 Developmental assessment

There are two purposes of developmental assessment:

- Early detection of significant delay so that help (advice, physiotherapy, spectacles, hearing aid) can be provided early.
- To provide reassurance to parents.

There are two parts to developmental assessment:

- History
- Observation

The history is usually reliable and augments the clinical examination. Parents may exaggerate their child's abilities or misinterpret involuntary movements.

9.2.1 History

- Ask in detail about present skills.
- Cover the four main categories.
- How do these compare with those of older siblings at that age? (This may influence parents' perceptions.)
- School performance (if at school) – a significant developmental problem is unlikely if the child is coping well in a normal class.
- Past history – especially dates of early milestones.
- Some parents recall milestones well, others not at all. Many have documented them in the parent-held record. If an experienced parent says 'she was very quick', it may not be necessary to obtain exact detail of past achievements.

9.2.2 Observation

- Play with the child in the presence of the parent.
- Demonstrate each skill where possible.
- Define the limit of achievement by noting both the skills the child has and those he has not.

You can easily carry out the following simple tests in any surgery or clinic. No special equipment or expertise is needed. They are screening tests which identify children who need more detailed expert assessment. The ages given are the average ages at which the skill is seen.

> **PRACTICE POINT The first 6 months**
>
> This is the most difficult time to assess the baby, because it is not until about 6 months that many of the easier developmental tests can be used. Therefore, developmental testing before the age of 6 months is less reliable than at any other time.

9.2.3 Posture and movement

Body control is acquired from the top downwards:

- Head on trunk – the newborn baby held upright can balance his head briefly but laid on his back and pulled up by arms or shoulders, there is complete head lag. By 4 months the head comes up in line with the trunk. By 6 months the head comes up in advance of the trunk.
- Trunk on pelvis – by 6 months a baby can sit supported on a firm, flat surface, but left will topple over (do not let this happen). By 9 months he sits without arm support and can turn without falling.

- Pelvis on legs – by 9 months he will weight bear and helps to stand up. At 12 months he is pulling himself up to stand and cruising (walking holding on) round the furniture. By 15 months he can walk unaided.

9.2.4 Vision and manipulation

9.2.4.1 Visual attention

- At 8 weeks a baby observes with a convergent gaze a dangling toy or bright object held 20–30 cm (9–12 inches) from his face, and moves his head and neck in order to follow it.
- From 2 months a baby prefers to watch a face rather than anything else. The ability to fix and follow improves and can be tested by watching the baby follow a rolling ball, the toddler matching toys (Figure 9.1) or the 5-year-old matching letters.

PRACTICE POINT

Babies may squint transiently in the first 3 months, but a persisting true squint (as distinct from a pseudo-squint as seen with epicanthic folds) is always abnormal and requires referral to a specialist (see Chapter 10).

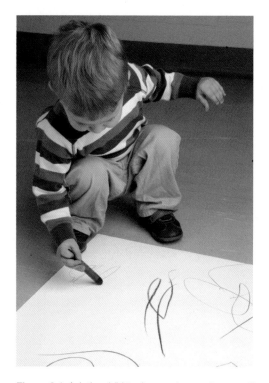

Figure 9.1 Ask the child to draw and copy shapes with a crayon.

9.2.4.2 Grasp and pincer grip

Palmar grasp

- Offer a large object
  - A wooden tongue depressor
  - A 2.5 cm cube
- Observe how it is grasped
  - At 6 months there is a clumsy palmar grasp, object approached with the ulnar border of the hand.
  - At 9 months he approaches it with the radial border and takes it in a scissor grasp between the sides of thumb and index finger before transferring it to the other hand and putting in his mouth.
  - At 12 months he approaches it with the index finger and picks it up precisely between the ends of the thumb and index finger in a pincer grasp.

Pincer grip

- Offer a small object, e.g. a sultana (check with parents first). Observe for an index finger approach (9 months) and a pincer grasp (9–12 months).
- Once this is developed, parents notice that their child can pick up the tiniest bits of fluff on the carpet (Figure 9.2).

PRACTICE POINT

Do not expose the child to danger during developmental assessment. Children may choke on small objects. Scissors are perilous.

9.2.5 Hearing and speech

9.2.5.1 Localization of sounds (distraction test)

The baby is sat on the parent's knee facing another adult about 3 m (10 feet) away whose function is to keep the baby's visual attention straight ahead (but

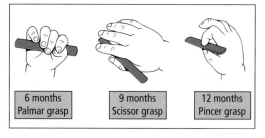

| 6 months Palmar grasp | 9 months Scissor grasp | 12 months Pincer grasp |

Figure 9.2 Development of grasp.

without being so fascinating that the baby ignores the test sounds).

A variety of quiet, soft sounds are made lateral to either ear and out of the line of vision. Rustling tissue provides a high-frequency sound; a spoon gently scraped round a cup, or a high-pitched rattle are other suitable sounds. Provided the baby has reasonable hearing, she will turn to locate the source. At 7 months the baby turns to sounds 0.5 m from either ear. At 9 months he turns promptly to sounds 1 m away. The optimal age at which to test an infant's hearing is 7 months.

The distraction test used to be a child's first screening hearing test, but there have been concerns about how well it performs. Neonatal screening of hearing is now used in the UK, and routine distraction testing is not necessary.

9.2.5.2 Speech

3 months – open vowel sounds (ooh, eeh) – cooing

6 months – consonants (goo, gah) – gurgling

9 months – varied and tuneful babbling

1 year – single word labels used for familiar objects and people – 'Mum', 'Dog'

2 years – words joined to convey ideas – 'Dadad gone' – child follows simple instructions, e.g. 'Put the spoon in the cup'

3 years – sentences used to describe present and past happenings.

Throughout this period, the child's understanding of language is far ahead of his ability to utter it.

9.2.6 Social behaviour

9.2.6.1 Smiling

Seen at 4–8 weeks in response to mother's face.

9.2.6.2 Reacting to strangers

Up to 9 months most babies will be handled happily by anyone; from 9 months they begin to cry or fret if handled by a stranger.

9.2.6.3 Feeding

At 9 months, lumpy food is chewed. At 18 months, the child cooperates with feeding, and drinks from an ordinary cup using two hands. At 3 years, he can feed himself efficiently with a spoon and fork (Table 9.1).

Table 9.1 Developmental milestones (average age of achievements)

Age	Posture and movement	Vision and manipulation	Hearing and speech	Social behaviour
3 months	Prone: rests on forearms, lifts up head and chest Pulled to sit: head bobs forwards, then held erect Held standing: sags at knees	Vision: alert, watches movement of adult Follows dangling toy held 15 cm from face Hands: loosely open	Chuckles and coos when pleased Quietens to interesting sounds	Shows pleasure appropriately
6 months	Sits erect with support Prone: lifts up on extended arms Held standing: takes weight on legs	Reaches out for toy and takes in palmar grasp, puts to mouth Transfers object from hand to hand Watches rolling ball 2 m away	Makes double syllable sounds and tuneful noises (gurgles) Localizes soft sounds 45 cm (15 inches) lateral to either ear	Alert, interested Still friendly with strangers
9 months	Sits unsupported for 10 min Prone: wriggles or crawls Held standing: bounces or stamps	Scissor grasp Looks for toys that are dropped	Babbles tunefully Brisk localization of soft sounds 1 m lateral to either ear	Distinguishes strangers and shows apprehension Chews solids
12 months	Walks round furniture stepping sideways (cruising) Crawls on all fours; walks with hands held	Index finger approach to tiny objects then pincer grasp Drops toys deliberately and watches where they go	Babbles incessantly A few words Understands simple commands	Cooperates with dressing, e.g. holding up arms Waves bye bye
18 months	Walks alone and can pick up a toy from floor without falling	Builds tower of three cubes Scribbles	Uses many words, sound labels Occasionally two words togethe	Drinks from cup using two hands Demands constant mothering
2 years	Runs Walks up and down stairs two feet to a step	Builds tower of six cubes	Joins words together in simple phrases, as sound ideas	Uses spoon Indicates toilet needs, dry by day Play imitates adult activities
3 years	Walks upstairs one foot per step, and down two feet per step Stands on one foot momentarily	Builds tower of nine cubes Copies O	Speaks in sentences Gives full name	Eats with spoon and fork Can undress with assistance Dry by night
4 years	Walks up and down stairs one foot per step Stands on one foot for 5 s	Builds three steps from six cubes (after demonstration) Copies O and +	Talks a lot Speech contains many infantile substitutions	Dresses and undresses with assistance
5 years	Skips, hops Stands on one foot with arms folded for 5 s	Draws a man Copies O, + and □	Fluent speech with few infantile substitutions	Dresses and undresses alone Washes and dries face and hands

9.3   Notes and memory aids

 PRACTICE POINT Notes and memory aids (Figure 9.3)

Small wooden 2.5 cm (1 inch) cubes are best.

The tower of bricks is roughly three times the age in years (between 1.5 and 3 years) (Figure 9.4).

A cross is part of the figure '4' and is copied at 4 years.

Age 3 is the age of '3's and circles:

- The bridge at age 3 has 3 bricks, the tower 3 × 3 bricks.
- A 3-year-old kicks a ball, draws a circle, rides a trike (three wheels), knows (at least) three body parts and three colours, and speaks in (at least) three-word sentences.

Age (yr)	Tower of bricks (number of bricks in a tower)	Shape with bricks	Copying shapes
1.5	3		
2	6		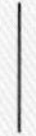 |
2.5		Train 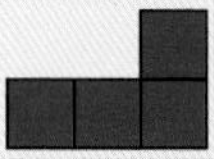	
3	9	Bridge 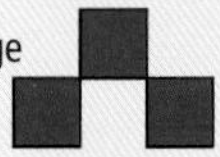	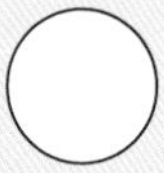 ◯
4	–	Steps 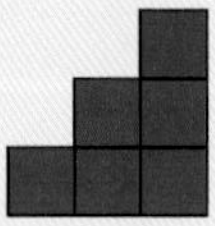	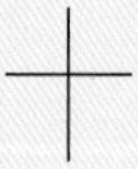 +
5	–		□

Figure 9.3 Assessing fine motor development. Small wooden 2.5 cm (1 inch) cubes are best for tower building and brick shapes. Ask the child to copy the shapes.

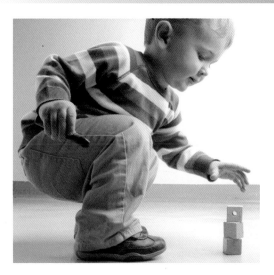

Figure 9.4 Small bricks (for tower-building and shapes) are used to assess fine motor skills.

9.4 Limitations of developmental assessment

The range of normal means assessment cannot be too precise. Aim to give a range of a few months for each area. Practice improves reliability of assessment, but simply listening to the parents and observing the child will provide useful information in the four main fields of development. If the parents' account differs greatly from what is observed, it may be that the child is having an 'off day', in which case observing on another occasion will be more reliable.

 PRACTICE POINT

Remember that all 'candidates' can have an off day – interpretation is difficult during illness.

 Summary

Developmental assessment is a key skill in paediatrics. Use the 'four areas' to help you, and build up an understanding of normal sequences that run through each.

 FOR YOUR LOG

- Do developmental assessments on children aged about 6 months, 12 months and 18 months.
- Observe normal child development and behaviour in a pre-school or nursery setting.

 OSCE TIP

- A child of up to 2 years with normal development (see OSCE Station 9.1).
- A video of a child with developmental delay.
- A child with Down syndrome with global developmental delay.
- A child who is deaf with speech and language delay.

See EMQ 9.1 and EMQ 9.2 at the end of the book.

OSCE station 9.1: Developmental assessment

Clinical approach:

- Combine history, observation and clinical testing
  ◇ Watch the child playing
  ◇ Think of four areas of development
- Assessment of four areas:
  ◇ **Gross motor/posture and movement**
  ◇ **Fine motor/vision and manipulation**
  ◇ **Hearing and speech**
  ◇ **Social/personal**
- Think in 3-month intervals
- In each area of development:
  ◇ Find a skill that the child can do
  ◇ Find a more advanced skill that the child cannot do
  ◇ Developmental age is between the two
- Use any set of recognized milestones
- Present findings for each area of development
- Summarize your findings

This is Rachel and her mother. Please perform a developmental assessment and tell me how old she is

Posture and movement

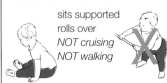

sits supported
rolls over
NOT cruising
NOT walking

Vision and manipulation

index approach
scissor grip
transfers
NOT pincer grip

Hearing and Speech

passed health visitor test
turns to sound
babbles— lots of sounds
NO words

Social/personal

waves bye holds, bites, chews biscuit holds bottle when feeding
NOT handing things back
STILL mouthing

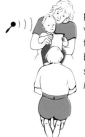

Rachel is a healthy child of 10 months

Never forget:

- Say hello and introduce yourself
- General health — is the child ill?
- Quickly assess growth, nutrition and development
- Mention the obvious (e.g. bandage on arm)

Look around for:

- Walking aids
- Hearing aids, evidence of feeding problems
- Glasses
- Adapted buggy

Special points

- Praise the things a child can do and reassure them when they cannot perform
- Developmental age may not be the same in each of the four areas — this can be normal
- Did the child perform to her ability?
- Children in the developmental OSCE are usually normal healthy children
- As soon as development is considered, start observing the child — they may perform brilliantly until you begin formal assessment, and then go on strike!

10

Learning problems

Chapter map

School attendance and education is second only to the family in influencing a child's life. Doing well at school is part of a child's overall health, and we should try to prevent illness disrupting a child's social and academic education as much as possible. For some children who get little support or encouragement at home, school may be a place of sympathy and understanding.

It is therefore of great importance that:

- Children are in the best physical, mental and emotional health to benefit from their education.
- Schools encourage learning in a broad perspective, supporting each child in achieving their individual potential.
- Children leave school self-confident, healthy and self-directed in their aspirations.

10.1 Medical causes of educational difficulty

In the UK, over 90% of children are educated in the public sector, while state and private schools run side by side. Around 20% of children will have special educational needs at some stage, that vary from minor to major. Most will simply need some extra support within mainstream schools. Some, if the problems are more severe, will receive education in a special school designed, staffed and organized to meet their needs.

The main medical problems which can affect children's education may be considered in groups, and not infrequently children have problems in more than one group.

Paediatrics Lecture Notes, Ninth edition. Simon J. Newell and Jonathan C. Darling. © 2014 John Wiley & Sons, Ltd. Published 2014 by John Wiley & Sons, Ltd.

10.1.1 Physical – motor

Disorders such as cerebral palsy (Section 17.8), muscular dystrophy and severe congenital abnormalities clearly are very important. Other children have minor motor problems such as clumsiness, or difficulty with more complex tasks (dyspraxia), which can be difficult to recognize. Motor problems may make games, stairs, corridors or getting round the school difficult. Wheelchair users cannot negotiate stairs and need wide toilets. Problems of manipulation may prevent the use of normal writing implements: special pens or a computer may be needed.

10.1.2 Physical – sensory

Impaired vision or hearing present obvious barriers to education. If they are severe, and especially if they are combined (the deaf/blind), special equipment and specially trained teachers are necessary. Early recognition and support of children with mild or severe problems is very important and changes a child's prognosis.

10.1.3 Intellectual (learning) disability

Intelligence is difficult to define, but it has to do with understanding, reasoning and the association of ideas. It is not closely related to memory or creativity, nor has it much to do with sociability, which may be conspicuous by its absence in the super-intelligent.

Intelligence can be measured by a wide variety of 'intelligence tests', the results of which are often expressed as intelligence quotients (IQ). Quotients are calculated as the child's functioning age as a percentage of their chronological age. A global and detailed assessment of a child's ability is more helpful than a single quotient. This provides a more comprehensive picture of the particular strengths and weaknesses of the individual child, and hence an indication of the particular kinds of help needed.

> If IQ or other learning ability is measured in an unselected population, the median is 100 and the distribution curve is approximately normal (Gaussian), with a longer tail to the left (low IQ) than to the right.

Most children with intellectual disability are between 2 and 3 SDs below the mean of the normal distribution curve, and often there is no obvious cause, although they may have parents of low IQ. Children with skills >3.5 SD below the mean are more likely to have a cause for their leaning problems, congenital or acquired.

Children with moderate learning difficulties are usually best served by the provision of extra help in the classroom (usually non-teaching aides) in mainstream schools. More severe impairment needs the facilities and specially trained staff of a special school.

10.1.4 Emotional

Emotional problems often reflect social problems at home. A few children are difficult to motivate, in sharp contrast to the normally insatiable appetite for information in young children. Others are hyperactive, aggressive, destructive or antisocial. Not only are they difficult to teach, but they disrupt the classroom and make the teacher's task very difficult.

10.1.5 Communication

Communication is receptive and expressive. Receptive problems are usually due to deafness or associated with learning difficulties. Some children with dysarthria and cerebral palsy, or other motor disorders, may understand but not be able to express. There are also a variety of disorders, including autism (Section 11.5.3.1) and dyslexia (see Section 10.4.1) which cause severe difficulties. The detailed diagnosis of these problems, and the devising of a suitable educational programme, call for very special skills.

10.1.6 Chronic illness

Chronic illness can interfere with education in a number of ways. Intractable asthma, for example, may result in frequent absences from school and in tiredness, and may result in poor academic progress. Epilepsy may place some restrictions on physical activities. Diabetes and coeliac disease affect meals taken at school. Juvenile arthritis limits physical activities.

10.2 Early diagnosis and assessment

10.2.1 Developmental delay

One of the main reasons for recommending that all young children should undergo regular developmental assessment (Section 9.2) is to detect significant delay as early as possible. Another reason is to reassure parents who are unnecessarily anxious about their child. Learning disability is likely to present as delayed development, unless there are physical features (e.g. Down syndrome, microcephaly) which permit early prediction of difficulty. Although all children with learning disability are late developers, the reverse is not necessarily true.

> **PRACTICE POINT**
>
> Express a child's achievement in a particular field or ability as appropriate to the *average* child of a particular age (e.g. head control is at the 3-month level).

10.2.2 Assessment

Faced with a child who is reported or found to be late smiling, sitting, walking or talking, a full paediatric history is essential:

- Was the baby very preterm? Has she spent long periods in hospital? Has she had proper care at home?
- Is she delayed in all developmental areas or only in selected aspects? Most children with more severe learning disability have delay in all areas, although gross motor development is often better than social and language development.
- Can a specific cause be found for a specific delay? If speech is delayed, is she deaf? If walking is delayed, does he have muscular dystrophy?
- A single assessment, especially if the child is having an 'off' day, is usually inadequate for decision making. Re-examination, to assess progress is often helpful.
- Progressive (degenerative) brain disease leads to loss of previously achieved skills. It is rare and important.

> **Causes of learning disability**
>
> **Congenital 75%**
> - Chromosome abnormalities (30%), e.g. Down syndrome.
> - Metabolic disease (under 5%), usually recessively inherited, e.g. galactosaemia, phenylketonuria.
> - Neurocutaneous syndromes (under 5%), often dominantly inherited, e.g. tuberous sclerosis, neurofibromatosis.
> - Other genetic causes, e.g. X-linked intellectual disability and some cases of microcephaly.
> - Idiopathic – the cause cannot be identified.
>
> **Acquired 25%**
> - Prenatal, e.g. alcohol, infections (rubella, CMV).
> - Perinatal, e.g. prematurity, haemorrhage, hypoxia, meningitis, septicaemia, hyperbilirubinaemia, hypoglycaemia.
> - Postnatal, e.g. trauma, infection.

10.2.3 Diagnosis

There are three stages in the diagnosis of a 'late developer':

- Is the delay significant? Or does the child fall within the range of normal?
- What is the nature of the problem - learning disability, deafness, social deprivation?
- What is the cause? This may be relevant to treatment and genetic counselling. Clinical assessment may indicate investigation (biochemical screening of blood and urine for metabolic disorders; serological tests for prenatal infections; neuroradiological studies).

10.2.4 Management

Prevention is unfortunately often not possible. Genetic counselling may prevent recurrence of genetic disorders; rubella immunization should be universal; neonates are screened for phenylketonuria and hypothyroidism (Section 27.3.3); and, clearly, avoidance of acquired damage should help.

Support of the child and family is the mainstay of management. For most children with severe disability there is no cure. With modern health care, life expectancy is often normal. These circumstances place great strains on families. Children with disabilities can take up all the time and energies of both parents, leading to physical exhaustion (especially as the children get older and heavier), neglect of siblings and the breakdown of marriages. The problems faced by single parents and families with socioeconomic problems are multiplied.

The principle is to help the child to develop to his full potential, however little this may be, and to offer all possible help and support to the family. Many children with learning disability have additional problems

> **Multidisciplinary team**
>
> This may include:
> - Community paediatrician
> - Physiotherapist
> - Orthopaedic surgeon
> - Audiologist
> - Social worker
> - General practitioner
> - Health visitor
> - Occupational therapist
> - Worker with visually impaired
> - Neurologist
> - Teacher
> - Educational psychologist.

such as cerebral palsy, epilepsy or deafness. Multi-disciplinary assessment is therefore essential before any treatment programme is drawn up. Although the health services have an important role, it is the social and educational services which have the chief respon-sibilities for helping children with learning disability. Many systems have been devised for encouraging maximal progress. Some are variations on traditional methods, which have been properly assessed. Some, which unfortunately attract great media attention, play (to their considerable profit) on the eternal hope of parents that a cure may be found. Doctors must be understanding of parents who decide to try unortho-dox methods, and must be prepared to help pick up the pieces if disappointment follows.

> **Disability Living Allowance (DLA)**
>
> This comprises two parts.
>
> **Care allowance**
> - Actual care needed above other children
>
> **Mobility allowance**
> - Over age of 5 years if severely limited
>
> Make sure the family are claiming DLA. The doctor completes the medical section.

The main forms of family support are:

- Home visits by an individual who can become a friend, offer friendly support and who is at the same time well informed about practicalities
- Provision of equipment for use at home, from incontinence pads to bath hoists, and adaptations to the home such as ramps for wheelchair access, or downstairs toilets
- Respite care for the family, when the child with problems spends time with a foster family or in residential care
- Financial assistance, such as Disability Living Allowance, or help from the Family Fund.

10.3 Conditions

10.3.1 Down syndrome

This affects approximately 1 in 600 pregnancies: it is less frequent for younger women and more frequent for those over 35 years. Most children with Down syndrome have an extra chromosome 21 resulting from non-disjunction at the time of gamete forma-tion (Figure 10.1). A few result from a translocation

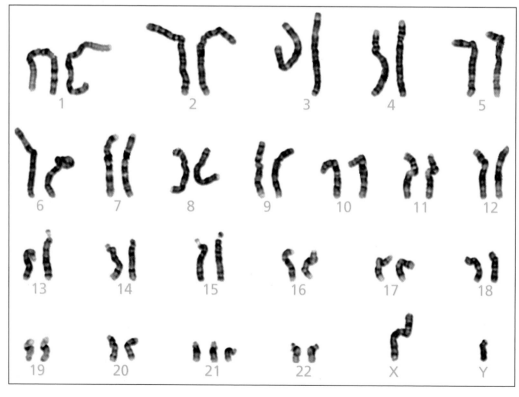

Figure 10.1 Karyotype in Down syndrome, showing trisomy 21.

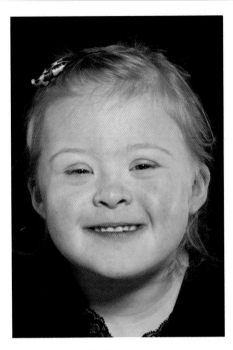

Figure 10.2 A child with Down syndrome.

> **Features**
> - Eyes
>   - *Oblique palpebral fissures*
>   - *Prominent epicanthic folds*
>   - *Brushfield spots* – tiny pale spots on the iris from infancy
> - Head and face
>   - *Brachycephalic skull* – face and occiput are flattened
>   - *3rd fontanelle* – at birth, between the anterior and posterior fontanelles
>   - *Mouth* small and drooping
>   - *Tongue* – becomes large and furrowed, often protrudes after infancy
>   - *Pinna* may be abnormal in shape and low-set
>   - *Neck* – short and broad, with excess skin posteriorly (the nuchal fold used in fetal screening)
> - Hands and feet
>   - *Hands and fingers* short and stubby
>   - Single transverse palmar crease
>   - *Clinodactyly* – short, incurved little finger
>   - *Sandal gap* – wide gap between the first and second toes
> - General
>   - *Short stature* (there are Down centile charts)
>   - *Hypotonicity* (floppiness) is always present
>   - *Delayed development* in all aspects
> - Associated congenital abnormalities:
>   - *Congenital heart disease* in 50% (usually atrioventricular septal defect)
>   - *Duodenal atresia* and *congenital leukaemia* are associated, but much less common
> - Long-term
>   - Increased risk of infections
>   - Increased risk of leukaemia
>   - Increased risk of thyroid problems and diabetes
>   - Presenile dementia

carried by a parent giving a high risk of recurrence (Section 5.2.1).

Prenatal diagnosis (Section 6.3.1) has made little impression on the birth prevalence of the condition. The news of an unexpected diagnosis on the day of birth can be devastating for a family, and demands senior and skilled handling (Section 2.2.3.1).

Although none of the characteristic features of Down syndrome is pathognomonic, and any may be present in a normal child, the association of several features usually enables a clinical diagnosis to be made (Figure 10.2). Recognition in very small pre-term babies is difficult, and the condition is easily overlooked in aborted fetuses.

10.3.1.1 Diagnosis

This can usually be made with confidence on clinical grounds but should be confirmed by chromosome analysis, which is also necessary for genetic counselling.

10.3.1.2 Progress

Apart from any problems arising from associated congenital abnormalities, Down babies may be difficult to feed in the early weeks. Thereafter they tend to be placid and to thrive, although they have an excess of respiratory tract infections. Most have moderately severe learning difficulties and require special educational help, but usually in their local school. As adults they require continuing supervision. Their life expectancy is somewhat shorter than normal because of degenerative disorders of advancing age which develop a decade or two earlier than usual. Libido is diminished. Males have low fertility, females are fertile.

10.3.2 X-linked disability

Fragile X syndrome is the second most common genetic cause of severe learning disability; Down syndrome is the most common. More men than women are affected by non-specific learning disability.

> **Fragile X syndrome**
>
> - Cognitive: moderate to severe learning difficulties
> - Speech and language delay
> - Behaviour: autistic features; aggression
> - Physical: long thin face, big jaw, macro-orchidism.

Fragile X syndrome is due to a triplet repeat on the X chromosome (Section 5.2.2.1, p. 54). The excess genetic material makes the area unstable when grown in special medium in the laboratory, hence the name.

Boys are most affected. Women may carry the condition or are affected less severely due to random inactivation of one of the X chromosomes. A positive family history is an important clue to the diagnosis.

10.3.3 Microcephaly

Primary microcephaly is associated with an inadequately developed brain at birth. The head circumference is small and falls further below the normal centiles. The fontanelles close early. In severe cases, the infant has a characteristic appearance: the face is normal but the skull vault is disproportionately small. Some cases are genetic (autosomal recessive). Others are caused by intrauterine infections (rubella, cytomegalovirus), toxins (alcohol) or (rarely) radiation. If the brain is damaged in the perinatal period, the poor head growth will become evident later.

Microcephaly must not be confused with craniosynostosis (Section 17.10.1). This is a disorder of fusion of sutures which will only result in a small head if it is neglected.

10.3.4 Disorders of speech and language

Normal language development varies considerably (Section 9.1). Children who are late in beginning to talk, or whose speech is thought to be abnormal, need careful assessment. Most will, in fact, go on to normal development. Some children have a sizeable vocabulary before their first birthday while others say little until 3 or 4 years old. A lisp is a common phase of speech development. Many 3- and 4-year-olds trip over their words because their thoughts and questions tumble out of their minds more quickly than they can articulate them. The average 4-year-old asks 26 questions an hour!

Significantly delayed or abnormal speech may be helped by early intervention. It is often helpful to refer any child with a speech problem to a speech therapist so that parents can be advised how best to help. The wrong kind of intervention may make the problem worse. There is a strong link between language delay and later educational difficulties.

If speech development is delayed:

- Is the child being spoken to? Speech is learned by imitation.
- Can the child hear? Deafness is an important cause of speech delay.
- Are other spheres of development delayed? If so, learning disability must be considered.
- Is there evidence of emotional/behavioural disorder? Late speech is usual in autism (Section 11.5.3.1) and fragile X.

The main abnormalities of speech are disorders of fluency (stammer/stutter) and of articulation. *Stammering* is common in young children and is much more common in boys than in girls. It usually goes spontaneously especially if it is ignored. If it persists into school age it becomes a barrier to communication and a social embarrassment. Speech therapy is very effective.

> **Speech problems**
>
> - Consonant substitution (e.g. 'Come' is pronounced 'Tum')
> - Nasality, resulting from cleft palate or nasopharyngeal incompetence
> - True dysarthria, as in some kinds of cerebral palsy (Section 17.8)
> - Faulty enunciation, e.g. normal, orthodontic.

Articulation disorders are common in young children. If they persist or are severe, the child may be unintelligible. Speech therapy is essential for assessment and treatment. Occasionally palatal or oral surgery is helpful.

10.4 School difficulties

If a healthy child of normal intelligence and good vision and hearing has educational difficulties, an emotional problem will often be found. There may be unhappiness at home, or at school (from bullying or fear), or family overexpectation or indifference. Conversely, emotional problems may be the result of learning problems. A report from the school is an important part of the assessment of the schoolchild.

More detailed assessment of intelligence and abilities by an educational psychologist will provide recommendations for remedial help.

> **Reasons for poor performance at school**
>
> **Social/cultural**
> - Absence of family support for child and school
> - Truancy
> - Bullying, problems at school
> - Poor home support for the child's study.
>
> **Neurological/psychological**
> - Major learning disability – usually detected before school
> - Hearing, vision, fine motor, perceptive skills – often not detected.
>
> **Chronic ill health (any condition)**
> - Aim is to minimize effect on education.
>
> **School refusal (school phobia).**

> **Learning problems: information needed**
>
> **Clinical assessment**
> - Chronic illness
> - Neurodevelopment
> - Emotional problems
> - Socioeconomic difficulties.
>
> **School report**
> **Educational psychology**
> **Vision and hearing.**

10.4.1 Reading problems

Some children are much worse at reading, speech and language than at other skills, and remedial therapy is difficult. This is more common in boys and occurs in all social classes. It is not associated with neurological abnormalities. This includes dyslexia, but a broad spectrum of problems is recognized.

10.4.2 Developmental coordination disorder

Also known as developmental dyspraxia or clumsy child syndrome, this is another important cause of school difficulties. Apart from difficulty with dressing or physical activities, some children may have great difficulty with writing and drawing. They may be considered wrongly to be stupid or lazy. Incoordination in clumsy children may sometimes represent a mild form of cerebral palsy. Occupational therapy may enable these children to overcome their problems.

10.4.3 Visual impairment

Severe visual impairment is a terrible handicap at any age. Whether it is congenital or originates in early childhood, it presents a serious threat to development and education.

Local authorities keep a register of children with severe visual problems so that the families can be helped and suitable education planned. Experienced home advisers from the local authority or the RNIB (Royal National Institute for the Blind – a charitable organization) visit the family to provide continuing advice and support. They provide practical advice, e.g. 'Wear noisy shoes and give a running commentary about all your household activities so that she can understand and learn about the things she hears, sometimes smells and feels, but never sees.' Severe visual impairment requires formal education by methods not involving the use of sight; the specialist schools for the blind teach Braille. For children with sufficient sight to use educational material involving large print and type, there are residential schools for the 'partially sighted'. Schools for the visually impaired are few in number and may be some distance from home.

10.4.4 Squint (strabismus)

Nearly 1 in 15 children have a squint when they commence school (Figure 10.3). The incidence is even greater in children with brain damage or learning disability. Most squints in children are non-paralytic (concomitant). In non-paralytic squint, there is a normal range of external ocular movements, and a constant angle of squint between the two eyes in all directions of gaze. In latent squint, there is extraocular muscle imbalance but the eyes do not deviate most of

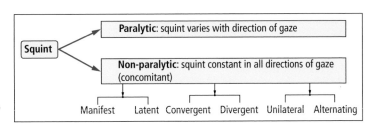

Figure 10.3 Classification of squints. For example, one child may have a manifest, convergent, alternating non-paralytic squint.

the time. A latent squint is not visible on inspection and difficult to diagnose. A decrease in visual acuity in one eye can be the cause, so the eyesight should be tested. Paralytic squints, caused by paralysis of one of the external ocular muscles, are unusual in children.

 New onset paralytic squint may be due to a brain tumour and needs urgent referral.

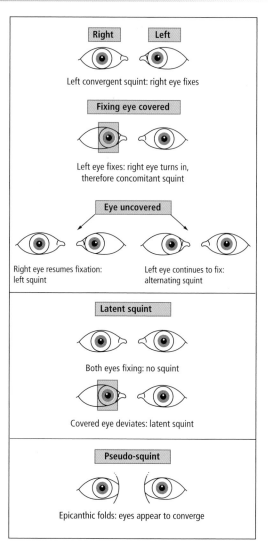

PRACTICE POINT Squint

Most squints are idiopathic
Some are due to decreased acuity
Rare causes include:
- Cataract
- Glaucoma
- Retinal disease
- Retinoblastoma.

Examination for a squint is a special technique and a favourite of undergraduate examinations (Figure 10.4; see also OSCE station 10.1). Babies sometimes falsely give the impression of having a squint because of a low nasal bridge, epicanthic folds or wide-spaced eyes (*hypertelorism*). This is a *pseudosquint* and is unimportant.

Any child with an untreated squint will suppress vision from the squinting eye in order to avoid blurred images and double vision (Figure 10.5). Unused, the eye can develop permanent *amblyopia* (diminished acuity of central vision). Early treatment before school age should prevent this. If left untreated, vision will be lost in the squinting eye, denying the child binocular vision for life.

Refractive errors are common in children with squints. In many, early use of spectacles is sufficient treatment. Occlusion of the non-squinting eye is unpopular with children. The aim is to force the child to use the squinting eye. Patching or occlusion may be needed for several months. Severe squints may require surgery, if only for cosmetic reasons.

Figure 10.4 Examination of the eyes for squint. The white dot on the pupil is the reflection of the examiner's torch.

TREATMENT Non-paralytic squint

- Full ophthalmic examination
- Detection and correction of refractive error
- Patching or occlusion of the squinting eye
- Surgery.

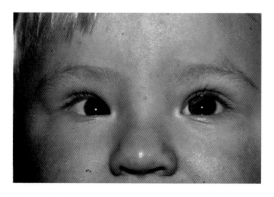

Figure 10.5 This child has a right convergent squint.

10.4.5 Hearing impairment

Hearing exists before birth and can be tested in neonates. They startle to a loud noise, or become quiet in response to a quiet voice. In the UK, all newborns go through neonatal screening for sensorineural deafness (Section 9.2.5). At 7–8 months of age a child's hearing may be tested by distraction testing – does she turn to sound? Pure tone audiometry is not usually possible before 3–4 years.

Congenitally deaf babies are noticed by parents before health professionals. They may have early communication problems or temper tantrums and behavioural problems.

Causes of deafness

Prenatal
- Maternal infection (e.g. rubella)
- Malformation

Perinatal
- Hypoxia
- Prematurity

Postnatal
- Hyperbilirubinaemia
- Infection (meningitis, encephalitis)
- Otitis
- Ototoxic drugs.

Most deaf children have some residual hearing, and so will be helped by a hearing aid, which can be fitted as early as 3 months of age. That is the start of the treatment, not the end. The child requires prolonged exposure to speech and sounds at a level that she can hear with the hearing aid.

Skilled help is needed from a team of otologist, audiologist, hearing aid technician and specially trained teachers. Education for the deaf can be started from early childhood. Most deaf children will enter the partially hearing unit of a nursery school at 3–4 years and then progress to similar units attached to normal schools or to special schools for the deaf.

10.5 Special educational needs

The normal educational provision of mainstream schools meets the needs of over 80% of children. The rest need something more or something different.

In the past, some of these children were labelled according to the nature of their problem (e.g. intellectual disability, physical disability, deaf) and were placed in special schools bearing similar labels. The rest tended to flounder in the bottom layer of mainstream schools, often leaving without any educational qualifications.

More recent policy rests on four principles:

- Early recognition or anticipation of special educational needs
- Detailed assessment through psychological, medical, social, parental and other reports
- Integration into mainstream schools for most, with extra support (the school Special Educational Needs Coordinator – SENCO – is key)
- Special schooling for those who need it.

10.5.1 Statement of special educational needs

This process involves the child, her parents, doctors and health workers in a process led by the education authorities, which aims to define a child's special needs at the earliest opportunity. Education for such children may start as early as 2 years and is particularly important for children with visual or hearing impairment, who need to establish good methods of communication with teachers and other children before formal education is possible.

All children with special needs undergo a comprehensive assessment which results in a report ('Statement') which is discussed with the parents and then forwarded to the education authorities who have the responsibility for the child's educational provisions and any further assessment. The process of assessment is sometimes referred to as *statementing*.

- 3% of school children have statements of special educational needs – half of these are in mainstream schools.
- A further 18% of school children have special educational needs, but without a statement.

✓ Summary

The interaction between health and education is very important for children. Paediatricians, school nurses, audiologists, speech and language therapists and other health professionals work closely with schools and parents to minimize the impact of medical problems. Down syndrome, fragile X and squint often feature in exams.

 FOR YOUR LOG

- Observe a consultation about learning difficulties.
- Visit a school for children with particular special educational needs. or a specialist inclusion unit within a mainstream school.
- Sit in with an audiologist.

 OSCE TIP

- Examine eyes for squint, vision and eye movements (see OSCE station 10.1).
- General paediatric assessment of learning difficulties.
- Video of child with difficulties.
- Cerebral palsy: need for multidisciplinary approach.

See EMQ 10.1 at the end of the book.

OSCE station 10.1: Examination for squint

Clinical approach:

- Check child understands you and is happy to cooperate
- Note any obviously abnormal neurology

Inspection
- Do eyes look healthy?
- Symmetry
- Normal facies

Acuity
- Simple test that child can see with each eye (with glasses on if worn)
- Does the child wear glasses?

External ocular movements
- Child will follow light, toy or your face
- Test in H pattern

Ophthalmoscopy
- Red reflex
- Are discs and retinae normal? — this can be very difficult, but attempt it

Light reflection
- Hold light near your visual axis (on the end or your nose!)
- When child is fixing on light, is reflection in the middle of both pupils?

Cover test
- Cover fixing eye
- Squinting eye moves and fixes
- Uncover the eye that was covered
- **Either** return to previous eye fixing **or** previously squinting eye fixes and other eye squints

Billy is 4 years old. Please examine him and tell me if he has a squint

 He wears glasses

Acuity with glasses — identifies little pictures in book — normal

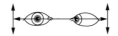

external ocular movements normal

R   L

asymmetric light reflection/right eye fixes

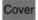

left eye now fixes (right eye must be squinting)

cover off: left eye returns to squinting + right eye fixes

Billy has a manifest, left, unilateral, convergent squint.

Never forget:

- Say hello and introduce yourself
- General health
- Quickly assess growth, nutrition and development
- Mention the obvious (e.g. drip, leg in plaster)

Look around for:

- Glasses
- Eye patch
- Eye drops

Special points

- Pseudo-squints are easily distinguished — the light reflection is symmetrical
- Almost all squints are not due to ocular disease, e.g. retinoblastoma
- Latent squints are too difficult for medical students to find in an examination

11

Emotional and behavioural problems

Chapter map

Children are unable to express their thoughts and feelings as easily as adults. Emotional disturbances are often expressed either through change in behaviour or through physical symptoms such as aches and pains. The child is part of a family, and problems elsewhere in the family may manifest as emotional and behavioural problems in the child. True psychiatric illness is rare in children. After reviewing attachment and parenting, which are foundational to children's mental health, this chapter discusses types and causes of problems. This provides the basis for management, generally and in regard to specific disorders.

Why emotional and behavioural problems are important

- They affect 5–10% of children in rural areas, 10–20% of children in urban areas.
- Up to one-third of children presenting to their GP or paediatric services have a psychological component to their presentation.

11.1 Attachment

Attachment describes the special relationship that a young child has with his main carers (usually the parents). Young children need to develop at least one secure attachment. A child may have several 'attachment figures', but for young children the most

---

intense attachment is usually to the mother. Within this attachment relationship are a typical sequence of behaviours that occur again and again:

- The child has a need, and expresses it (care-eliciting). For example, a baby cries when he is hungry, or a young child runs to her parent when she is frightened.
- The parent recognizes the need, and responds (care-giving). The baby is fed, the young child comforted.
- The child settles, his need met, and his internal balance restored.

Over the early years of life, this repeated sequence builds into the child a model of their world that affects future relationships. With 'good enough' parenting, a secure attachment forms, and the model includes fundamental concepts such as 'I am loveable', 'People will be there for me' and 'People can be trusted'. If care-giving is inconsistent, or even abusive, then the attachment is insecure or ambivalent, and the child's internal model is distorted. Such children find it difficult to form intimate, trusting relationships later on.

Stranger anxiety builds from about 6 months, is maximal at around a year, and then slowly recedes as children reach school age (this is why young children need to be examined close to their parents). A child who has not formed secure attachments may be either suspicious and hostile or overly familiar with strangers.

11.1.1 Good enough parenting

No parent is perfect, and most struggle at times with the challenges of bringing up children. Children need a certain level of care to grow and develop both physically and emotionally, and to meet their attachment needs. *Bonding* describes the special relationship that the parents (especially the mother) have with their young child. This bond allows them to love, give to, understand,

---

 RESOURCE Parenting 'handbooks'

- *Toddler Taming* by Christopher Green is full of sensible advice for the first 4 years (e.g. see the chapter on sleep).
- *How to Talk So Kids Will Listen and Listen So Kids Will Talk* by Faber and Mazlish – does what it says!
- *The Incredible Years* by Webster-Stratton is the basis for a popular parenting course (see **www.incredibleyears.com**)

---

forgive and cherish their child through good and bad times. Mothers do not necessarily love their baby at first; it may take several weeks. Ideally, parents should be alone with their new baby in quiet, happy and untroubled surroundings, but separation, for example by neonatal illness, does not prevent normal attachment.

11.2 Types of emotional and behavioural problems

Since the causes and management of these problems have much in common, the next part of this chapter will focus on a general approach. Specific problems will then be discussed in more detail.

Emotional and behavioural problems in children		
Infants and pre-school children	Older children	
Behavioural	*Behavioural*	*Stress-related*
Tantrums	Defiant	Headaches
Sleep problems	Impulsive	Abdominal
Feeding difficulties	Attention deficit	pains
Crying babies	Lying	Vomiting
Breath-holding	Stealing	Wetting
attacks	Truancy	Soiling
	Tics	

Good parenting

Positive approach
- Praise > criticism
- Rewards > punishment

Discipline
- Set limits
- Constancy
- Non-victimization
- Non-oppressive

No violence in the home

Opportunities for self-development
- Encourage learning and exploration
- Encourage independence

Stability
- Security within a family home.

11.3 Causes of emotional and behavioural problems

There are many factors which lead to these problems (Figure 11.1). Children's symptoms vary greatly and there is often no clear relationship between particular behavioural problems and specific causes. Most often it is to do with the child's interactions or relationships with important people around them. Many problems are exaggerations of normal behaviour, unintentionally

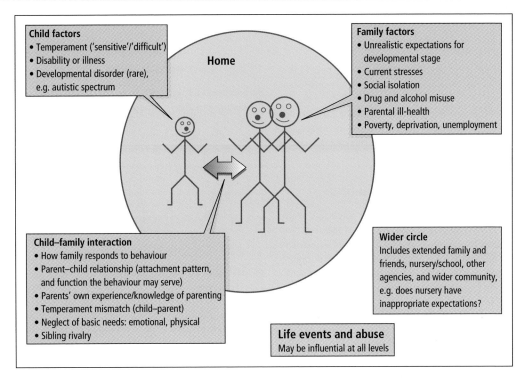

Child factors
- Temperament ('sensitive'/'difficult')
- Disability or illness
- Developmental disorder (rare), e.g. autistic spectrum

Home

Family factors
- Unrealistic expectations for developmental stage
- Current stresses
- Social isolation
- Drug and alcohol misuse
- Parental ill-health
- Poverty, deprivation, unemployment

Child–family interaction
- How family responds to behaviour
- Parent–child relationship (attachment pattern, and function the behaviour may serve)
- Parents' own experience/knowledge of parenting
- Temperament mismatch (child–parent)
- Neglect of basic needs: emotional, physical
- Sibling rivalry

Wider circle
Includes extended family and friends, nursery/school, other agencies, and wider community, e.g. does nursery have inappropriate expectations?

Life events and abuse
May be influential at all levels

Figure 11.1 Possible sources of child behaviour problems.

maintained through the way they are being handled, especially if there are inconsistencies between parents.

11.3.1 Child factors

The form that an emotional disturbance takes will depend in part upon the cause and in part upon the child's personality and the family patterns of response to stress. Some children are of a buoyant temperament and can ride almost any crisis; others are sensitive plants and bow before every emotional breeze. The way parents respond to the problem may inadvertently exacerbate or perpetuate these problems. Stress may present as headache, tempers or abdominal pain in different children. The toddler who feels challenged by the arrival of a new baby may resort to infantile behaviour.

11.3.2 Family factors

11.3.2.1 Acute separation and change

The death of a parent or of a much-loved grandparent, emergency admission to hospital, or moving house are examples of acute separations. These are most upsetting to young children around 2–4 years old who are conscious of the separation but unable to understand the reason.

11.3.2.2 Parental discord and separation

All children are conscious of the relationship between their parents and will be aware of any deterioration. Parents who attempt to get their children to take sides during conflict make this an even more difficult experience.

 RESOURCE Children and parental divorce or separation

Health professionals are sometimes asked for advice about helping children through divorce or separation. Here are some useful starting points:
- **www.divorceaid.co.uk** – this site provides advice, support and information on all aspects of divorce and has useful resources for young children, teenagers as well as for parents.
- **www.rcpsych.ac.uk** has a useful factsheet (search for 'divorce' on their site) as part of their excellent 'Mental Health and Growing Up' series.
- **www.raisingchildren.net.au** is an Australian site – search there for 'Me and my changing family', an online book, which offers tips on building healthy relationships after separation. A few items are specific to Australia.

11.3.3 Child–family interaction

11.3.3.1 Inconsistent handling

If a child is permitted something by one parent that is denied by the other, or punished on one occasion and ignored on another, this is likely to lead to behavioural problems. The intelligent child is quick to play off one adult against another, or to achieve her own ends by alarming or distressing the adults around her.

11.3.3.2 Lack of parental time

All children need regular positive attention, especially from their parents. When this is lacking, then the negative attention given for bad behaviour can become enough of a reward to reinforce the behaviour. This can lead to a vicious cycle of more negative attention (e.g. telling off, punishing) leading to worsening behaviour.

11.3.3.3 Sibling rivalry

Most toddlers, and especially first-borns, delight in the new baby, but may resent the time that their mother devotes to it. Aggression is likely to be directed against the mother rather than against the baby. When the new baby is old enough to be mobile and to interfere with the elder sibling's activities, jealousy will become more obvious. At school age, constant comparisons between siblings with different capabilities and interests can devastate the less clever or the clumsy.

11.3.3.4 Great expectations

Parents naturally want their child to do well, but may form an unrealistic idea of her capabilities or set their hearts on a career which she could never achieve. Although many a child 'could do better if she tried', not everyone is destined for an honours degree. If parents constantly nag when she is doing her best, psychological difficulties may follow. Somatization is common (e.g. abdominal pains).

11.3.4 Wider circle

Do not forget to explore the child's life outside the immediate family. Remember school, nursery and the extended family. All of these may have an impact and offer you insight into problems that are occurring. Although most schools try to minimize bullying, it is still a common and important cause of behavioural problems. Contact with the school or nursery (with the parents' permission) is often helpful.

11.3.5 Life events and abuse

Sometimes a child is witness to, or involved in, an acutely distressing situation – a road accident, a sudden death or sexual abuse. This may lead to a variety of symptoms such as disturbed behaviour (e.g. night terrors), or to acute physical symptoms (e.g. overbreathing). An event like this may have severe long-term effects.

11.4 Management

11.4.1 General approach to management of behavioural problems

Most behavioural problems in young children respond to a calm and consistent approach that emphasizes the positive. Identify and build on the strengths of the child and family. Encourage parents to work together, and to use distraction and/or change of activity when the problem behaviour is first noticed. Simple explanation helps parents realize that these problems are extremely common and part of normal experience. They do not need to feel there is something fundamentally 'wrong' or 'bad' about themselves or their child.

11.4.1.1 Strategies

- Positive reinforcement:
  - Reward desired behaviours with warmth, praise and small tokens (e.g. stars on a star chart)
  - Ignore undesired behaviours
- Time out:
  - Child removed from the situation for 3 min
  - Breaks a negative cycle
  - Calms things
- Promote positive parent–child times:
  - Good times when contentious issues are set aside
  - Affirmation of the child through gesture (e.g. cuddles)
  - Activities enjoyed together (e.g. trips, crafts)
- Set and apply clear limits, where consequences of behaviours are:
  - Clearly understood
  - Applied consistently, quickly and without argument
  - Appropriate in magnitude.

Star charts

Especially useful in early school-age children
Based on operant conditioning – reinforcing
the desired behaviour and ignoring (and thus
'extinguishing') the unwanted behaviour
The giving of stars should be:
- Achieveable – otherwise lack of stars will demoralize
- Consistent – all carers do the same
- Immediate – the younger the child, the more quickly the star should be given
- Clear – child and parents are clear what the star is for
- Contingent – only give the star for the identified behaviour.

11.4.2 General approach to management of stress-related (psychosomatic) symptoms

A large part of clinical practice involves children (and adults) with pains and other symptoms for which no satisfactory cause can be found. Deciding whether the symptoms are secondary to stress can be difficult. History, examination and growth monitoring will usually exclude serious disease. It is rarely helpful to label a pain as psychogenic, which may be interpreted as imagined or fabricated.

Adopt a comprehensive approach and accept that all symptoms result from interaction of body and mind, and that expression of physical disorder or good health is modified not just by physical factors, but also by intellectual, emotional and social factors.

11.4.2.1 Stress-related symptoms and tests

Avoid tests if possible. If tests are necessary, it is better to say:
'I think your symptoms are stress-related but I want to do some tests to make sure'
rather than:
'I will do some tests to exclude physical problems. If they are negative, it must be stress-related'
(you will end up running out of tests!).

After listening to the history, there are two useful questions, 'What sort of a boy is he?' Children with stress symptoms are more often described as nervous, worriers, perfectionists or solitary than as placid, happy-go-lucky or gregarious. 'Who does he take after?' may elicit a rueful smile and the admission

that one or both parents are cast in the same die. This helps understanding. Examination reveals no abnormal signs.

Stress symptoms do not just disappear. It is helpful to reassure that there is no organic disease. Explain the nature of the symptoms and encourage the family not to pay undue attention to them. Make it clear that you understand that the pains are real and not imaginary. Every effort should be made to identify and address stresses. Health visitors and teachers can be helpful. A careful history and examination coupled with firm reassurance is important and may be all that is needed.

Diaries – ABC approach

- A simple diary kept by parents between appointments often clarifies the problem
- Recording informed by the 'ABC approach' may lead to a solution in its own right, as parents gain a greater understanding
- For several episodes ask parents to note: **A**ntecedents (trigger/s); nature of the **B**ehaviour; the immediate **C**onsequences for the child (as well as what conclusions he/she makes about them)

11.5 Specific disorders

Some of the following disorders are covered in more detail elsewhere in this book. Follow the cross-references for more details.

11.5.1 Stress-related symptoms

11.5.1.1 Recurrent abdominal pain

Abdominal pain is a common childhood symptom, and the commonest causes are constipation and stress-related symptoms (of which some may be due to irritable bowel syndrome, non-ulcer dyspepsia and abdominal migraine) (Section 21.1.2).

11.5.1.2 Stress headaches

Stress headaches are usually frontal. In some cases, headache is the family stress symptom. (Section 17.9).

11.5.1.3 Tics

These repetitive involuntary movements are usually worse with stress. A low key reassuring approach is best (Section 17.9).

11.5.1.4 Vomiting

Vomiting is intimately connected with the emotions ('I'm sick of it all') but is less common than pain as a stress symptom. It occurs at a younger age than recurrent pains (Section 21.1.1).

11.5.1.5 Wetting problems

Both day- and night-time wetting may occur due to organic factors such as detrusor instability or urinary tract infection, but may be triggered or worsened by stress (Section 22.6).

11.5.2 Behavioural and sleep-related

11.5.2.1 Disturbance of bowel habit

Potty training may be started any time in the first 2 years, and a few parents choose to defer it for longer. If started very young, it is the parents who are training themselves to put a pot under the baby when he is going to pass faeces or urine, most commonly after a feed. This helps to establish a conditioned reflex, reinforced by praise when something arrives in the pot but not by punishing the reverse. Toddlers should not be left sitting on their pots for long periods, nor should potty training be obsessional or coercive ('You can't until…'). Faulty bowel training predisposes towards constipation, which may become life-long.

Bowel disturbances

- Chronic constipation, which may be complicated by faecal soiling (Section 21.1.5)
- Faecal incontinence resulting from neurological disorders
- Encopresis: deliberate defaecation in inappropriate places. Usually indicates emotional distress
- Toddler diarrhoea (Section 21.1.4).

11.5.2.2 Sleep difficulties

Sleepless children demoralize parents. Young children are demanding by day, but parents survive if they can enjoy peaceful nights. Sleeplessness may begin for a good reason, but persist as a bad habit. Children differ in their personalities from birth: some seem to be born 'difficult', while others are 'so easy'.

Young infants sleep most of the time, and crying usually indicates hunger, thirst, cold or pain.

Anxiety or depression in the family may make things worse. The most difficult sleep problems are usually seen in toddlers. Some do not settle down when put to bed: others sleep for a few hours and are then full of activity when the rest of the household is sound asleep. By the time advice is sought these habits have usually persisted for a long time and parents have tried both protracted and complicated bedtime routines, and the almost irreversible step of admitting the child to the parental bed. It is noticeable that whilst the parents often look worn out, the offending child has boundless energy.

Sleep disorders may date from an illness or upset in which a few broken nights were to be expected, but has been protracted by over-solicitous attention. Another common cause is putting the child to bed too early or at no fixed time.

Management of sleep problems

- Returning to sleep from the normal transient awakenings that occur through the night is a learned behaviour. If a child associates the process of going to sleep with a factor that is not there later in the night (e.g. bottle, dummy, sleeping next to parent) they are more likely to have disturbed sleep ('sleep-association disorder').
- Avoid or reduce daytime naps.
- Establish a calm bedtime routine.
- When the child wakes and cries leave him to cry for a pre-planned time, e.g. 2–5 min, then settle with as little physical contact as possible (neither kisses nor recriminations) and leave again. Continue to check on the crying child after repeating the same time delay.
- Avoid sedative medication. Behavioural techniques are far more likely to achieve a long-term solution.

11.5.2.3 Nightmares

Bad dreams are common at all ages. Parents, having experienced them themselves, are not usually very worried by them. They know that nightmares occur in normal people and that they do not mean major emotional upset. Measures such as leaving the bedroom door open, or a light on, may comfort the child who is frightened of going to bed. Nightmares occur during rapid eye movement (REM) sleep and are the culmination of a frightening dream adventure, the details of which the child can remember immediately afterwards.

11.5.2.4 Night terrors

Night terrors are not common, but are most alarming. They occur mainly in the first hour or two of sleep in children between 2 and 8 years. The child shrieks, sits up and stares wide-eyed and terrified as if being attacked by something only he can see. He may stumble out of bed and seem oblivious to the parents' soothing words. However, within a few minutes he will be sound asleep again and will remember nothing in the morning. Night terrors occur during non-REM sleep, and occur abruptly (not as the result of a dream sequence). They are accompanied by an alarming rise of the pulse and violent respirations which may at times make the parents or doctor suspect an epileptic fit. The parents can be reassured that night terrors do not indicate serious psychological abnormality, and that the child will outgrow them. Gently calming the child back to sleep is all that is needed. If they occur at a regular time of night, the child can be woken just before this.

11.5.2.5 Sleep walking

This may occur independently or as an extension of night terrors, though the sleep-walker tends to be slightly older (e.g. 6–12 years). The child gets out of bed and may walk around the house or even into the street. Although difficult to awaken, he can be guided back to bed. Regardless of that, he will usually find his own way back to bed and to sleep. Neither sleep walking nor night terrors should be considered as evidence of major emotional disturbance. Both conditions tend to be familial and to disappear before adolescence.

11.5.2.6 Crying babies

All normal babies cry. Excessive crying, especially at night, exhausts parents and is a known risk factor for physical abuse. Pain (e.g. ear ache) may be responsible for short-term crying. Persistent crying more often reflects household tensions. Mothers who seek advice about excessive crying may be afraid that they or their husbands will lose their tempers and damage the baby. The problem may sound trivial to a busy doctor but must *always* be taken seriously. The health visitor can often help.

11.5.2.7 Breath-holding attacks

Sometimes mistaken for seizures, but always triggered by some event or upset (Section 17.3, p. 161).

11.5.2.8 Tantrums

Tantrums are normal to toddlerhood. Give reassurance, telling parents how common tantrums are, and show empathy. Some tantrums are promoted by boredom, frustration, inconsistent handling and repeated unnecessary thwarting of activities which can be preventable. Explanation of normal development and the limits of children's abilities and understanding can prepare parents for the inevitable tantrum and needs for limit setting. Bad or negative attention is still more rewarding than no attention. Tantrums are best managed by distracting the child away from the tantrum to another activity. Avoid giving rewarding attention to the tantrum. Everybody who looks after the child must handle the tantrums in the same way.

11.5.2.9 Feeding difficulties in the young child (Table 11.1)

- Weigh and measure accurately.
- Base all interventions on a food diary.

11.5.3 Severe behavioural disorders

Anorexia nervosa is covered in Section 16.4.2.

Table 11.1 Common problems with feeding

Problem	Solution
Child easily distracted by TV or runs round room at meal times	Turn off TV: mealtime must be the focus and ideally family members all eat together with child in high or other safe chair and table.
Children change their mind about what they are willing to eat.	Either make only one meal for all the family, or offer child a choice of two things and, if appropriate, allow child to help in preparation.
Child very slow eater or picks at food.	If weight satisfactory, reassure parent child will not starve. Don't hurry child or force-feed. Present food for an agreed fixed period of time and then remove it.
Too much fluid, either milk almost entirely in place of food or excessive drinking of fruit juice or pop.	Give drinks and snacks after, not before, meals.

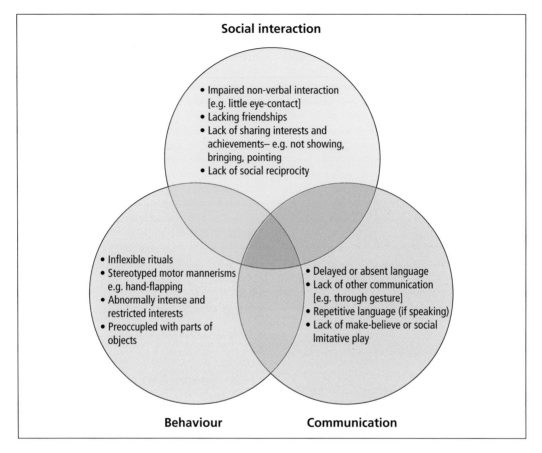

Social interaction

- Impaired non-verbal interaction [e.g. little eye-contact]
- Lacking friendships
- Lack of sharing interests and achievements– e.g. not showing, bringing, pointing
- Lack of social reciprocity

- Inflexible rituals
- Stereotyped motor mannerisms e.g. hand-flapping
- Abnormally intense and restricted interests
- Preoccupied with parts of objects

- Delayed or absent language
- Lack of other communication [e.g. through gesture]
- Repetitive language (if speaking)
- Lack of make-believe or social Imitative play

Behaviour   **Communication**

Figure 11.2 Features of autism. Note that some of these can be normal at certain ages, so assessment should take account of develomental stage. Some features in each area are needed to make a diagnosis. In Aspergers, language and cognitive development are much more normal, there are highly developed special interests, and there is more insight.

11.5.3.1 Autistic spectrum disorders

The term 'spectrum' is used because these disorders (primarily autism and Asperger syndrome) share similar characteristics and shade into each other (Figure 11.2). At their heart is an inability to read the minds of others. The normal processing of verbal and non-verbal cues and signals is impaired so that the child cannot 'think himself into someone else's shoes': he cannot imagine what someone else is thinking or feeling. Instead, the brain seems configured to process information about systems and things, to varying degrees of ability. This produces problems in communication, behaviour and social interaction (Figure 11.2). The relative level of difficulty and ability in each area determines the child's position on the spectrum, and there are formal scoring tools to help with this. A long list of other paediatric disorders have been associated with the autistic spectrum, so it is important to complete a detailed evaluation.

 PRACTICE POINT

Consider the autistic spectrum in a child who is not speaking – especially if they are silent and do not communicate non-verbally (e.g. eye-contact and pointing).

About 0.5% of children are thought to be on the autistic spectrum, although only about one-tenth of these have autism. Autistic children are often difficult to handle and always difficult to teach because of their inability to communicate. Sometimes the onset of symptoms is very early; a mother may say, 'As a baby he would never let me cuddle him'. Usually they present in the 2nd or 3rd year of life with language or behaviour problems. Classical autism is a life-long condition and can be very disabling. Early detection and skilled educational and behavioural intervention by a multidisciplinary team is recommended.

Some autistic behaviour is not uncommon amongst children with other learning disorders. There is no evidence linking autism to MMR immunization (Section 14.2).

> **TREATMENT Management**
>
> - Foster developmental progress
> - Promote learning
> - Reduce stereotyped behaviours
> - Eliminate maladaptive behaviour
> - Alleviate family distress – family support and education

Asperger syndrome is part of the autistic spectrum. Children have less severe autistic behaviour, and normal intelligence, and may merely appear odd or eccentric. They often have difficulties at school. The distress can be greater than with 'classic' autism because the child has greater insight.

11.5.3.2 Attention-deficit and hyperactivity disorder (ADHD)

Children vary greatly in the extent of their activity and concentration, and it is impossible to define the limit between physiological and pathological degrees of overactivity. Many normal children are 'always on the go', 'never still' and need relatively few hours of sleep. Beyond this is the ADHD syndrome in which these features interfere with learning or development. In children of school age this presents a grave educational problem.

> **ADHD syndrome**
>
> - **Inattention**
>   - Changes activity frequently
>   - Will not persist with tasks
>   - Short attention span
> - **Hyperactivity**
>   - Fidgetiness
>   - Restlessness
> - **Impulsiveness**
>   - Impetuous erratic behaviour
>   - Frequent accidents
>   - Thoughtless rule breaking.

ADHD is more common in boys, and in children with evidence of brain damage, which further complicates their education. Behaviour modification therapy can help. For some, methylphenidate may have a quietening effect, but drug therapy may be difficult to stop. In some children hyper-activity is caused or aggravated by particular foods or (more

often) colourings. A properly supervised exclusion diet is worth trying: any improvement in behaviour will be evident within a few days.

✅ Summary

Most emotional and behavioural problems are exaggerations of normal behaviour, unintentionally maintained through the way they are being handled. Assessment should include the context and the many potential sources of behaviour problems. Consider several appointments, use of diaries and charts, and wide consultation. Management involves addressing underlying problems where possible, but specific useful techniques include explanation, positive reinforcement, avoiding reward of undesired behaviours, time-out, promoting positive family times, and use of clear limits.

> **FOR YOUR LOG**
>
> - Observe use of star charts and symptom diaries in outpatient clinics.
> - Observe attachment behaviour in children on the wards and in clinics.
> - Discuss some of the common behaviour problems of young children with parents.

> **❓ OSCE TIP**
>
> - Stress-related conditions (e.g. pain, headache) (see OSCE station 11.1).
> - Enuresis: explain to parent, enuresis alarm.
> - Constipation and soiling: history, explanation.
> - Video of attention deficit disorder.

See Chapter 11 EMQs: 'Treatment of continence problems in children', 'Headache' and 'Abdominal pain' in the EMQ section at the end of the book.

References

Faber, A. and Mazlish, E. (2013) How To Talk So Kids Will Listen and Listen So Kids Will Talk. London: Piccadilly Press.

Green, C. (2006) *New Toddler Taming. A Parents' Guide to the First Four Years*. London: Vermilion.

Webster-Stratton, C. (2006) *The Incredible Years: A Guide for Parents of Children 2–8 Years Old*. Seattle, USA: The Incredible Years, Inc.

OSCE station 11.1: History-taking — pain

Clinical approach:

- Begin with open questions (e.g. could you tell me what worries you?)
- Then focus to more specific questions

Pain

- Nature
- Site
- First and last occurrence
- Duration of each episode
- Frequency
- Length of history
- Severity
  - How bad is it?
  - Can parents tell pain is present?
  - Does it stop him playing/going back to school?
- Timing
  - Day/night etc.
  - School days/holidays
- Modifying factors
  - Stress
  - Medicines
  - Food/starvation

Associated symptoms

- Vomiting
- Diarrhoea/constipation
- Enuresis/dysuria
- Headache

Gary is 11 years old. His mother is worried about his abdominal pain. He has not been at school for 4 weeks. Please take a brief history

- Mother's biggest worry: Gary is missing time at his new school

- Central ache
- Most of each day
- Not at night
- Better at weekends
- Appetite good
- Sleeping well
- No other symptoms

- Gary's mother is clearly very anxious
- Gary is not present. He spends most of his time watching TV
- No other significant history

Gary has stress-related abdominal pain. It may have been precipitated by the move to a new school. The mother is usually a member of staff who has been given a history

---

Never forget:

- Say hello and introduce yourself
- Tell the parent(s) and child what you aim to do
- General health — is the child ill?
- Ask, is there anything else you think I should know?

If asked or time permits:

- Full history
- Do not forget
  - Birth history
  - Development
  - Immunizations
  - Family/social history

Look around for:

- Family interaction
- Parental anxiety
- Evidence of care or neglect

Special points

- If exact answer not known (e.g. how long?) ask for approximate answer
- Ask if problem is getting better, getting worse, or staying the same
- What do the parents think about the cause of the pain?
- Does severity of pain match impact on the child's life (e.g. time off school?)

12

Nutrition

Chapter map

Infant and child nutrition is the foundation stone of healthy development. Worldwide, the most important problem is malnutrition. In industrialized societies, the main problems are eating unwisely or eating too much. In clinical practice, nutritional care is central to the management of all chronic diseases.

Nutrition is particularly important in the first year of life, when the infant is entirely dependent on his carers to feed him. Babies treble their birth weight in the first year of life; to treble it again takes 10 years. In fact, 65% of total postnatal brain growth takes place in the first year of life. Malnutrition may permanently disrupt physical and mental development.

PRACTICE POINT

Parents are often concerned about feeding, odd stools, small vomits. The first step is to plot the infant's weight in the red book (parent-held record). Normal growth is greatly reassuring.

Poor fetal nutrition and then rapid weight gain in the first years greatly increases risk of adult diabetes and cardiovascular disease: an example of nutritional programming.

12.1 Infant nutrition

Average requirements in infancy

Water	150 mL/kg/day
Calories	110 kcal/kg/day

12.1.1 Milk

Milk is a rich source of energy, proteins and minerals. It is the sole source of nutrition for the first months, and provides an essential part of energy, protein and calcium intake in pre-school children. Cow's milk has a high mineral content and osmolality. Infant formula feeds are modified to be more like breast milk.

Unmodified cow's milk should not be given in the first year: breast or formula feeding is recommended

---

to 12 months, alongside weaning foods from 6 months. As a rule, children under 5 years should drink whole milk, and not fat-reduced.

12.1.2 Breastfeeding

PRACTICE POINT

All of us in health care should take every opportunity to promote breastfeeding.

Promotion of breastfeeding

- Antenatal advice
- Put baby to breast soon after delivery
- Demand feeding
- Comfortable position for mother and baby
- Ensure good 'attachment'
- No food or drink but breast milk (unless medically indicated)
- Avoid dummies and teats
- Professional and family support and encouragement
- Promote popular awareness and support.

Women should receive information, advice and encouragement (Figure 12.1). Nobody wants to see unwilling mothers browbeaten into breastfeeding, but there is a happy medium between that and the indifference shown by many doctors and nurses.

Breast milk is nutritionally ideal for the term infant (Figure 12.2). Milk proteins are easily soluble (whey) or tend to curdle or precipitate (casein). Breast milk is whey dominant (70%). It is free, readily available and convenient. Breastfeeding, even for a few months, gives an infant an excellent start to life. Protection from infection is important for survival in developing countries.

RESOURCE

- **www.nhs.uk** – search '*pregnancy and baby*', click any link, then choose '*Your newborn*' from the main menu for resources on breast and bottle feeding, with useful links. Alternatively search '*breastfeeding*' for other resources including a 'video wall' with a good animation.
- **http://newborns.stanford.edu/breastfeeding** – a useful set of resources on breastfeeding from Stanford School of Medicine USA.

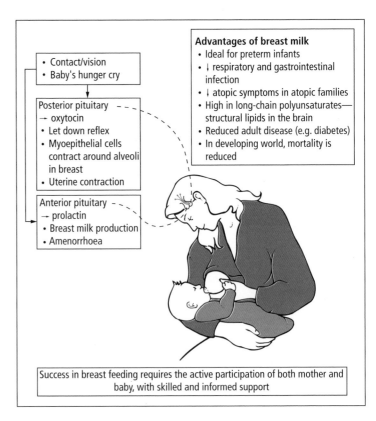

Advantages of breast milk
- Ideal for preterm infants
- ↓ respiratory and gastrointestinal infection
- ↓ atopic symptoms in atopic families
- High in long-chain polyunsaturates— structural lipids in the brain
- Reduced adult disease (e.g. diabetes)
- In developing world, mortality is reduced

- Contact/vision
- Baby's hunger cry

Posterior pituitary ---
→ oxytocin
- Let down reflex
- Myoepithelial cells contract around alveoli in breast
- Uterine contraction

Anterior pituitary ---
→ prolactin
- Breast milk production
- Amenorrhoea

Success in breast feeding requires the active participation of both mother and baby, with skilled and informed support

Figure 12.1 Breastfeeding.

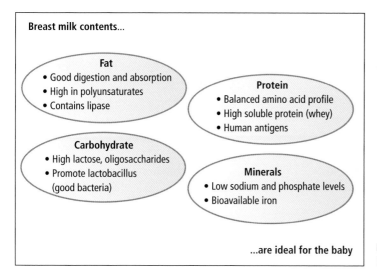

Breast milk contents...

Fat
- Good digestion and absorption
- High in polyunsaturates
- Contains lipase

Protein
- Balanced amino acid profile
- High soluble protein (whey)
- Human antigens

Carbohydrate
- High lactose, oligosaccharides
- Promote lactobacillus (good bacteria)

Minerals
- Low sodium and phosphate levels
- Bioavailable iron

...are ideal for the baby

Figure 12.2 The composition of breast milk.

Anti-infection properties of breast milk

- Sterile feed
- Maternal antibody (IgA)
- Lactoferrin
- Lysozyme
- Promotes colonization with lactobacilli and bifidobacter.

Breast-fed babies are usually fed on demand but may be fed by the clock. To establish lactation, most recommend frequent *demand feeding*: after a feed the infant is allowed to rest, and the next feed is given when the infant wakes and appears hungry. Crying does not necessarily mean hunger: sleep does not necessarily mean satiation. Breastfeeding is a highly satisfying experience for the mother and infant. Seldom is there true failure of lactation. In the UK, rates have been rising but there is room for improvement: 80% of all mothers begin to breast-feed, 55% continue some breastfeeding at 6 weeks, and 34% at 6 months. Variation in rates is large: almost 90% of social class I mothers choose breast-feeding. In the UK, breastfeeding usually stops at 4–9 months; in the developing world, 2 years is the rule. There is, however, no evidence to suggest that bottle-fed European babies are either nutritionally or emotionally deprived.

Many drugs are excreted in breast milk, but maternal medication is rarely a contraindication to breastfeeding. The *British National Formulary* offers advice on most drugs. Breastfeeding is contraindicated with high-dose steroids, cytotoxic and immunosuppressive agents. Breast milk contains very little vitamin K (Section 7.3). Viral transmission means that breastfeeding is contraindicated in known maternal HIV infection in developed countries (but not in the developing world, where the benefits still outweigh the small risk). 'Breast milk jaundice' is not a reason to stop (Section 8.4.2.1, p. 77).

 RESOURCE

- Child and Maternal Health Intelligence Network: **http://atlas.chimat.org.uk** – choose 'Breastfeeding profiles' for rates of breastfeeding by UK area
- UNICEF: **www.unicef.org.uk/babyfriendly** gives information on the UNICEF/WHO 'Baby Friendly Hospital' initiative, which promotes breastfeeding worldwide.

12.1.3 Bottle feeding

Formula feeds are available in two forms: whey dominant (60% whey) like breast milk and casein dominant (30% whey). The former is more akin to breast milk and should be first choice. Each of the four UK milk manufacturers makes two milks so that a mother can change milks without changing company. There are no major advantages to different manufacturers' milks, and parents should be dissuaded from constantly changing milk. Follow-on formula should not be used before 6 months. Their use after that age is popular but not necessary. Attention to detail in making up the feed is essential. Extra scoops, heaped scoops, packed scoops or additional cereal should be avoided. They add calories which encourage obesity, and extra solutes which cause thirst, irritability and hypernatraemia. It is conventional to warm feeds to approximately body temperature, but this is not always needed.

Bottle feeding requirements

Meticulous care in hygiene
Sterilizing bottles
Correct feed reconstitution for a 4-oz bottle (110 mL)
- Take 4 oz of cooled boiled tap water
- Fill scoop without compressing powder
- Scrape scoop level with clean knife
- Add four scoops of powder
- Dissolve, allow to cool to about 37 °C
- May be refrigerated
- Only rewarm once.

 PRACTICE POINT

Soya-based formulae do not prevent food allergy or atopic disease. Soya formulae should not be used under 6 months.

Feeds should be given either 4 hourly or on demand. The newborn baby will require feeding round the clock, but within a few weeks will drop the night feed. As long as a night feed is demanded, it should be given. Leaving him to cry is pointless and unkind.

12.1.4 Mixed feeding

The term *weaning* is variously used to mean taking the baby off the breast or introducing solid foods (Figure 12.3). A full-term baby receiving milk will not develop any nutritional deficiency within 6 months of birth. The WHO and UK advice is that solids should be given at 6 months, although in practice a majority of European infants receive solids from 4 months onwards. Solids before 3 months are ill-advised. Early weaning is linked to later obesity.

- Use pureed fruit, vegetable and rice as first foods.
- Ensure an adequate introduction of food containing protein and iron.
- Introduce one new food at a time in small quantities.
- Increase solids in diet as chewing begins around 6 months.
- The average 1-year-old will be having three main meals a day, with a small drink or snack mid-morning, mid-afternoon and at bedtime. Milk intake 20–30 oz/day (600–900 mL).

 PRACTICE POINT

Many parents (and doctors) still use ounces:
1 fluid ounce = 28 mL
1 pint = 560 mL.

12.1.5 Iron and vitamin supplements

In the UK vitamins A, C and D are provided free to children aged 6 months to 5 years in low-income and at-risk groups via the 'Healthy Start' programme. Supplements may be made available to the wider population (already happening in some countries), because targeted provision is logistically difficult, and there is increasing concern about widespread subclinical vitamin D deficiency. Clinical vitamin deficiency states are rare. Some parents may choose to give a children's multivitamin supplement, and this is safe.

Folic acid is provided by leaf vegetables and fruits. Vitamin D may be derived from cholesterol

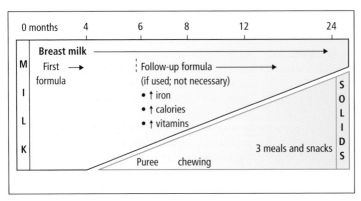

Figure 12.3 Weaning.

through the action of sunlight. It is contained in oily (non-white) fish, liver and margarines. An increasing proportion of vitamin intake comes from 'fortified' foods: formula milk, bread, breakfast cereals and fruit-flavoured drinks. In prematurity, chronic illness or poor diet, vitamin supplements are important.

Energy requirements (kcal/kg/day)	
Maintenance	80
Growth	5
Physical activity	25
Total	110

 Iron-deficiency anaemia occurs in around 15–25% of toddlers in areas of socioeconomic deprivation. It can be prevented with use of iron-enriched formula.

12.2 Nutrition of toddlers and school children

Changing social patterns in industrialized countries have had profound influences, not necessarily beneficial, on the nutrition of children. A tradition of home cooking, and indeed home growing of vegetables, has given place to supermarket shopping, fast and convenience foods, and takeaway meals. This pattern is now established across the socioeconomic groups and persists even in the areas or times of deprivation.

Recent concerns about food additives (artificial flavourings, colourings, sweeteners, preservative), food provenance, and food allergies have turned some families towards 'natural' food and a return to home cooking.

The chief nutritional requirements of children are protein for building new tissue as they grow, and sufficient fat and carbohydrate to meet their substantial energy needs. Protein requirements (milk, egg, fish, meat, cereals and pulses) are about 1–1.5 g/kg/day. Energy requirements are high compared with most adults, who need less than a third of a child's requirements/kg.

The dietary basis of obesity, dental caries and much constipation in childhood is well accepted. Refined sugar should be eaten in moderation, and sticky sweets preferably not at all (or at least not continuously!). An excess of fried foods (e.g. hamburgers and french fries) encourages obesity, and public opinion has now forced recognition of this in fast-food outlets. Fibre helps prevent constipation. Most fizzy drinks ('pop') have little or no nutritional value and help to rot teeth. Milk is highly nutritious (400 kcal/pint) but an excessive intake can contribute to obesity.

12.3 Feeding problems

 PRACTICE POINT

Beware of modifying a young child's diet without dietetic help!

12.3.1 Early problems

Difficulties with feeding are common and may cause great anxiety. Feeding problems may present with vomiting, disturbed bowel habit, unsatisfactory weight gain or crying. Most difficulties arise from one or more of three factors:

1 *Quantity* of food. Both underfeeding and overfeeding may lead to vomiting and crying. In the first, weight gain is consistently poor. An overfed baby gains weight excessively to begin with, but may later lose. Overfeeding is more common in bottle-fed babies, partly because they are often fed as much as they can take, partly because food has a sedative effect, and partly because of the mistaken belief that the biggest babies are the best.

PRACTICE POINT

Luke is 8 days old and is at home. He is breastfeeding. He is unwell, quiet and lethargic. On examination he has lost 14% of his birthweight, but does not look clinically dehydrated. Investigations show a high serum sodium (154 mmol/L) and he is quite jaundiced.

Luke has hypernatraemic dehydration which is often difficult to detect because the clinical signs of dehydration may not be present. The problem is lactation failure and the clue is his weight loss. After slow rehydration and breastfeeding support, lactation was established and he thrived well.

2 *Kind* of food. Early mixed feeding may lead to vomiting, diarrhoea and crying. A return to a milk diet will allow recovery, followed by cautious reintroduction of solids. Changing from one milk to another rarely achieves anything.

3 Feeding *technique*. The mother who wishes to breastfeed should be given help, support and practical advice. This comes from experienced professionals or groups such as the National Childbirth Trust (NCT: www.nctpregnancyandbabycare.com). Difficulties with bottle feeding can only be recognized by watching the baby feeding. The baby may not be held comfortably; the bottle may be held at the wrong angle; the hole in the teat may be too small or too big; the milk may have been wrongly prepared. Instruction and advice provide the remedy.

> **PRACTICE POINT Always check growth**
>
> You can quickly estimate expected weight: birthweight is regained after 10 days (normal loss is 5–7% of birthweight, max 10%). Then babies gain 200 g/week (an ounce a day).

12.3.2 Infantile colic

Infantile colic, or evening colic, is a common problem arising in early life. It is usually better by 4 months. An otherwise placid baby devotes one part of the day, most commonly between the 6 p.m. and 10 p.m. feeds, to incessant crying. He may stop when picked up, but certainly cries again if put down. Attention to feeds, warmth, wet nappies, etc. does not help. The cause is unknown. First reassure and monitor growth. Anti-bubbling agents (Infacol) may be helpful. In severe colic, some infants respond to a diet free of cow's milk with a formula feed containing hydrolysed proteins.

12.3.3 Sucking and feeding

Most babies take a feed in 20–30 min. Some drain a bottle in 5–10 min and may then have filled their stomachs. Infants may find comfort in non-nutritive sucking on a thumb or a dummy, but the latter should be avoided in the first few weeks while breastfeeding is being established.

From 6 months, an increasing diversity of foods and textures should be tried, and the child allowed to learn the joy of eating – even if this is not the tidiest of processes. Major conflict is best avoided. There is a delicate distinction between encouraging the conservative child to try something new, and coercing the reluctant child to eat 'what is good for him'. Parents are best advised to back off from

conflict and to developing good mealtime rituals. It is helpful to note that no normal child with access to food will starve; that children of some ages are dominated by the need for food, but at other ages it may be a low priority; that wise parents do not start battles with their children that they are bound to lose; and that a parent will often achieve most by doing least.

12.4 Defective nutrition

12.4.1 Obesity

> **UK Government policy**
>
> A sustained downward trend in the level of excess weight in children by 2020, as part of a broader strategy to tackle obesity in the population as a whole.

Obesity in childhood is a common and important problem – important to the child, the family and public health. The tendency to excessive weight gain may appear in infancy, toddlerhood or during school years. Obese children often come from overweight families and are likely to become obese as adults. The proportion of the population overweight or obese rises with age: 1/4 of 4–5 year olds, 1/3rd of 10–11 year olds, and 60% of adults in England. The essential problem is energy intake exceeding energy needs. Deficiency of leptin, which normally signals calorie sufficiency, may be important but, in the vast majority of obese children, no cause is found. Obese children are nearly always tall for their age.

> **PRACTICE POINT**
>
> Obesity combined with short stature suggests an underlying pathology, such as endocrine disease, and merits investigations.

> **Obesity in childhood and adult life**
>
> • Psychological: poor self-esteem
> • Poor exercise tolerance
> • Obstructive sleep apnoea
> • Slipped upper femoral epiphysis
> • Non-insulin-dependent diabetes
> • Hypertension
> • Abnormal blood lipids.

Obesity may limit exercise tolerance. The dominant symptoms in childhood are psychological. The fat child may be teased and ostracized, losing self-esteem. In boys the disappearance of the penis into a pad of suprapubic fat may lead to a mistaken diagnosis of hypogonadism.

A body mass index (Section 3.2.4, p. 30) (kg/m²) over the 97th centile is diagnostic. In the obese child, weight reduction is advisable but impossible to procure without the enthusiastic collaboration of the child and their family.

12.4.2 Malnutrition

> 🔑 Marasmus is due to energy (calorie) and protein starvation.
>
> Kwashiorkor is the result of protein malnutrition.

12.4.2.1 Marasmus

Nutritional deficiency ranges from starvation to lack of specific nutrients: in Europe, starvation is seen in children who have been grossly neglected, but in parts of the world afflicted by poverty, famine or war, *infantile marasmus* is all too common. Breastfeeding continues for about 2 years, but when supply of breast milk is inadequate, starvation ensues. The infant with marasmus is prey to intercurrent infection, and mortality is high. There is also evidence that starvation in the first year of life, even if subsequently corrected, may cause permanent mental handicap.

12.4.2.2 Kwashiorkor

This is seen in the same parts of the world as marasmus but in older children, usually 2–4 years old. At this age, the next baby often displaces the older sibling from the breast. Milk is replaced by a low protein, starch- (rice or maize) based diet. The child is listless, the face, limbs and abdomen swell, the hair is sparse, dry and depigmented, and there are areas of hyperpigmentation ('black enamel paint') especially on the legs. Diarrhoea is sometimes a feature.

12.4.2.3 Vitamin deficiencies

Worldwide, vitamin deficiencies remain an appalling problem for children. Vitamin A deficiency is the single most important cause of childhood blindness worldwide. Initial loss of dark adaptation is followed by corneal disease (xerophthalmia), which may lead to irreversible corneal perforation. An estimated 250 000 young children each year suffer from xerophthalmia and nearly 10 million suffer from lesser degrees of deficiency. Supplementation is cheap, protective and reduces infection.

Some European families adopt bizarre diets for their own reasons, and growing children fed on such diets may be malnourished. In contrast, children on a vegetarian diet are usually healthy (and most unlikely to be obese). Specific nutritional deficiencies such as scurvy (vitamin C deficiency with bleeding into gums and subperiosteum) are very rare in otherwise healthy children.

12.4.2.4 Rickets

Nutritional rickets results from dietary deficiency of vitamin D coupled with inadequate exposure to sunlight (Figure 12.4). It presents at times of active growth – in the pre-school years of life and at puberty. It is more common in Asian children in the UK because the traditional diet is poor in calcium and they receive little sunlight on their skin.

Deficiency of calcium, phosphorus or vitamin D interferes with bone maturation, leading to a build-up of osteoid tissue. Thickening of the metaphyses where active growth is most rapid is seen at the wrists, ankles and costochondral junctions ('rickety rosary') (Figure 12.5). Toddlers develop bow legs: older children become knock-kneed. There is hypotonia. In children with malabsorption, rickets declares itself when growth is rapid because it is a disease of growing bones. Serum calcium is normal or reduced, and the alkaline phosphatase is raised. Some present with hypocalcaemic fits. Adequate vitamin D intake prevents rickets.

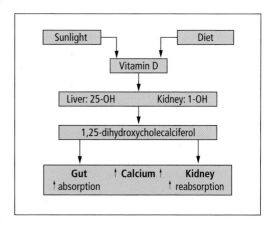

Figure 12.4 Vitamin D metabolism.

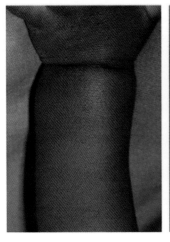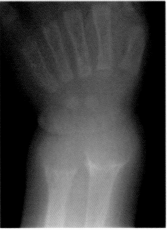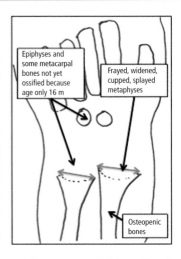

Epiphyses and some metacarpal bones not yet ossified because age only 16 m

Frayed, widened, cupped, splayed metaphyses

Osteopenic bones

Figure 12.5 Rickets. The widened metaphyses at the distal ends of the radius and ulna can cause visible swelling of the wrist, as seen in this child.

All baby milk foods and most cereals have vitamin D added. Treatment of rickets requires dietary education and supplementary vitamin D.

Renal rickets has two main origins:

- *Glomerular* disease in chronic renal failure leads to failure of hydroxylation of vitamin D in the kidney to the active form (1,25-dihydroxycholecalciferol).
- *Tubular* renal rickets. Failure of normal tubular reabsorption of phosphate occurs (e.g. vitamin D-resistant rickets).

12.5 Nutrition in chronic disease

In many chronic diseases of childhood, nutritional care is an essential part of management (Table 12.1). Careful monitoring of growth is mandatory. The paediatrician should be a source of support, information and advice for the family. A multidisciplinary approach is needed.

Table 12.1 Nutritional aspects of some childhood conditions

Condition	Problems	Management
Severe cerebral palsy	Poor oromotor skills Gastro-oesophageal reflux Constipation Family stress Family support	Protein/energy supplements Avoid obesity Treat reflux/constipation Nasogastric/gastrostomy feeding
Cystic fibrosis	Protein fat malabsorption Recurrent infection High energy demands Loss of appetite Fat-soluble vitamins Aggressive management of infection	High energy intake (150% of average needs for age) Do not use a low-fat diet Pancreatic enzymes
Chronic renal failure	Anorexia/ill-health Renal osteodystrophy Poor vitamin D hydroxylation Poor phosphate excretion Low calcium Hyperparathyroidism	Energy supplements Nasogastric/gastrostomy feeding Controlled protein intake Phosphate restriction Vitamin D and Ca
Childhood malignancy	Anorexia Recurrent ill-health Vomiting	Protein/energy supplements Intensive nutritional support Anti-emetics

Summary

Feeding and nutritional concerns account for a good deal of paediatric practice. You need to know what is normal in order to be able to give appropriate advice. The problems of defective nutrition are a window into our unequal world. Obesity is a problem of plenty in resource-rich countries, while malnutrition is a major cause of childhood morbidity and mortality in poorer countries. Rickets is on the rise, and you should recognize the typical features and X-ray findings.

 OSCE TIP

- Feeding problems, normal infant nutrition, weaning
- Red book and use of growth charts, e.g. failure to thrive
- Make up an infant's formula feed
- Childhood obesity: plot BMI, talk to child, talk to parent (see OSCE station 12.1).

See EMQ 12.1, EMQ 12.2 and EMQ 12.3 at the end of the book.

 FOR YOUR LOG

- Ask to help make up a feed, and feed some babies. Few educational activities are as delightful!
- Talk to a breast-feeding counsellor and if appropriate observe her give advice.
- Plot children's measurements (including working out and plotting BMI) on growth charts and interpret.

OSCE station 12.1: Obesity

Task: Charlie, age 8 years, has been referred because he is overweight (BMI 24 kg/m^2). His height is 75–90th centile, and his weight is over the 98th centile. His growth charts (BMI, height and weight) are provided.

His parents are convinced that there is a 'glandular' problem. Take a history and make an initial assessment to discuss with the examiner.

Don't forget:

Is Charlie obese?	Interpret chart
Is Charlie's growth satisfactory?	Interpret height and weight together
Family history?	Do other members of the family have a similar problem?
Is diet satisfactory?	Take a brief history, a dietitician will be needed to do this properly
Are there symptoms of ill-health?	Look for short stature, as well as secondary problems (e.g. poor exercise tolerance, obstructive sleep apnoea)
How does obesity affect Charlie?	Look for social, psychological consequences. Does he have friends, a socially supportive network? Are there problems at school?
What does Charlie think about it?	This is essential. Charlie needs to understand and be keen to be thinner

Charlie is obese with BMI >98th centile; he has simple obesity. His weight is above the 98th centile and his height is normal on the 75–90th centile. An endocrine problem is most unlikely. Explain a limited-calorie diet, encourage exercise and give ample moral support. Do not forbid any foods, but the second slice of buttered toast must be avoided. Charlie could join a group activity. Drugs are best avoided. Try to help alleviate any emotional stresses at home or school. If he loses weight, keep following him up for support.

13

Abnormal growth and sex development

Chapter map

Concerns about growth feature commonly in paediatric outpatient clinics, and sometimes result in admission. You need to be comfortable in assessing normal growth so that you can identify the abnormal. Common problems include failure to thrive in young children, and short stature in teenagers. Problems of sex development are less common, but distressing. An understanding of the range of causes informs investigation and management.

13.1   Abnormal growth

13.1.1   Failure to thrive

13.1.1.1   What is failure to thrive?

This applies to a young child who is not growing well, usually for weight gain (Figure 13.1). In practice, this means:

- Weight crossing down through two centile lines
- Weight on or below the 2nd centile line and falling away.

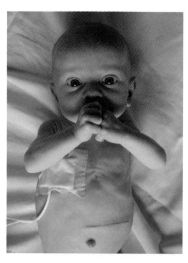

Figure 13.1 Failure to thrive. Loss of subcutaneous fat is seen in this boy who is failing to thrive.

Paediatrics Lecture Notes, Ninth edition. Simon J. Newell and Jonathan C. Darling. © 2014 John Wiley & Sons, Ltd. Published 2014 by John Wiley & Sons, Ltd.

Causes of failure to thrive

Inadequate food intake
- Feeding problems or neglect
- Poor appetite
- Mechanical problems, e.g. cleft palate, cerebral palsy

Vomiting
- Gastro-oesophageal reflux, pyloric stenosis
- Feeding problems
- Food intolerance

Defects of digestion or absorption
- Cystic fibrosis
- Food intolerance (including coeliac disease)
- Chronic infective diarrhoea

Failure of utilization
- Chronic infections
- Heart failure, renal failure
- Metabolic disorder

Genetically determined
- Constitutionally small
- Genetic syndrome, e.g. Turner's in girls

Emotional deprivation.

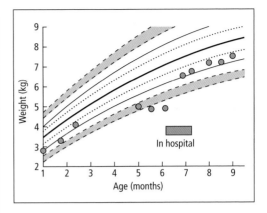

Figure 13.2 Sadie was admitted at 6 months of age with failure to thrive. In hospital she gained weight well with normal feeding and was discharged with intensive community-based support.

 PRACTICE POINT Common reasons for a failure to thrive referral

- Weights measured or plotted incorrectly: do not forget to allow for gestation in the preterm (<37 weeks).
- Over the first few months of life, uterine influences 'wear off' and the child finds his own centile for weight. This may result in tracking upwards or downwards on the centile chart, and the latter may appear as failure to thrive.
- Child drinking excessive amounts of fluid – especially milk or juice. Remedy – reduce fluid intake, especially before meals.
- Poor intake and socioeconomic deprivation.

13.1.1.2 Approach to failure to thrive

Careful history and examination are essential. Sometimes the main reason for failure to thrive is obvious – inadequate food intake or chronic vomiting or diarrhoea. Often there is no clear reason apparent at the first consultation: parents appear caring and competent, adequate food is given, and there are no clues to a particular disorder. Solving the problem is difficult, and unfocused investigation

is not helpful. The parent-held child health record (the red book) gives invaluable information about growth. It is helpful to work with a dietician who will quantify intake and help with management. The health visitor can provide a reliable account of the home and whether both food and emotional nourishment are available there. A home visit can be most revealing. Sometimes the child is admitted to hospital to be fed standard amounts of food and observed to see if weight gain occurs, and to note symptoms (Figure 13.2). Investigations may be performed, looking for common problems first (see box). The single greatest challenge is to distinguish those with organic pathology from the many children with *non-organic failure to thrive* – an important group whose problems are social, emotional or economic in origin.

 PRACTICE POINT Investigations to consider in failure to thrive

Depending on severity and clinical pointers, the following may be helpful:

- Urinalysis (dipstick and microscopy and culture) – for infection
- Full blood count
- Renal and liver function
- Acute phase response (ESR, CRP or plasma viscosity)
- Thyroid function
- Coeliac disease antibodies
- Chromosomes (in girls) – for Turner's.

Causes of short stature

Physiological causes
- Constitutional
- Delayed puberty

Pathological causes
- Defects of nutrition, digestion or absorption
- Social and emotional deprivation
- Most malformation syndromes
- Chronic disease (e.g. renal insufficiency, malignancy)
- Genetic syndromes (e.g. Turner syndrome in girls)
- Endocrine (e.g. deficiency of thyroid or growth hormone)
- Iatrogenic (e.g. long-term steroid therapy)
- Disorders of bone growth (e.g. skeletal dysplasias).

13.1.2 Short stature

There are many causes of short stature (see box), but the majority of children presenting with short stature are normal, short children. Some of them were born small for gestational age and many have short relatives, including one or both parents.

In healthy short children, growth velocity is normal, as shown by serial measurements plotted on a

---

 PRACTICE POINT How to calculate the mid-parental height (MPH) and target centile range (TCR)

Example: Abigail has short stature, height is on the 0.4th centile at age 11. Parents' heights: mother 154 cm, father 170 cm.

Prompts to assist you with the calcuations feature on most growth charts. Essentially you are averaging the parents' heights, but adjusting for difference between the sexes.

- Reduce father's height by mean difference between male and female heights of 14 cm. Father (adjusted) = 156 cm.
- MPH = mean of mother and father (adjusted) = 155 cm.
- TCR = MPH ± 8.5 cm.
- Plot TCR + MPH on growth chart at 18 years.
- The TCR extends to below the 0.4th centile, and her height is growing along the 0.4th centile, indicating a normal growth velocity within the target centile range.
- She is likely to be *constitutionally small*.

For boys do the same but adjust the mother's height by adding 14 cm, and calculate a slightly wider TCR by using ± 10 cm.

---

centile chart. Growth velocity (Section 3.2.3) can be measured more accurately over 6–12 months and plotted on a growth velocity chart. The most common reason for a child being short is having short parents. The child's height centile should be compared with their 'target centile range' which is calculated from their parents' heights (see box).

Delayed puberty (often familial) with delayed bone age is common; the later pubertal growth spurt allows these children to catch up. These children have a delayed 'bone age', i.e. their skeleton is less mature (Section 3.2.5). Children whose height is below their TCR, who are obese or who have a reduced height velocity require careful assessment. Congenital hypothyroidism is detected by neonatal screening (Section 27.3.1), but acquired hypothyroidism in older children commonly presents with short stature. Growth hormone (GH) deficiency may be isolated or part of a wider pituitary insufficiency, and it may be complete or partial. Random GH levels are of little use. Diagnosis of GH deficiency requires complex tests, and secretion can only be tested by measurement after stimulation of secretion. However, it is unlikely if height velocity is normal. Bone age is delayed in both pituitary and thyroid deficiency.

Catch-up growth is seen in young children in whom the cause of retarded growth has been removed or corrected (Figure 13.3). In infants and young children,

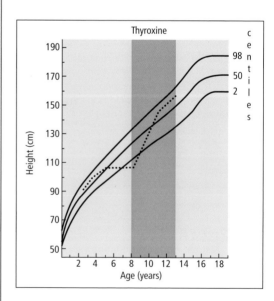

Figure 13.3 Catch-up growth. This boy developed hypothyroidism which was diagnosed at the age of 8. He showed excellent catch-up growth with replacement therapy.

catch-up growth can be complete: thus a 4-year-old whose growth has been suppressed by high doses of prednisolone will regain normal height once the steroid therapy is decreased or stopped. However, as puberty nears catch-up, growth may be incomplete so that temporary factors may result in permanent reduction of stature.

> **PRACTICE POINT Investigations in short stature**
>
> - Bone age (X-ray of the left wrist) (see Section 3.2.5 under Section 3.2.4)
> - Thyroid function tests
> - Cortisol studies
> - GH stimulation test (e.g. glucagon/clonidine).

13.1.3 Tall stature

Children who are entering puberty early or who are overweight tend to be relatively tall (90–97th centile). Children with heights well above the 97th centile usually come from tall families. If height is going to exceed socially acceptable limits, exceptionally hormone therapy is used to finish the growth process prematurely.

> **Two important but rare causes of tall stature**
>
> **Klinefelter syndrome**
> (see below, this chapter)
>
> **Marfan syndrome**
> - An autosomal dominant disorder of connective tissue.
> - Features: tall and slim, arachnodactyly (long, slender fingers), typical facial appearance, prolapsing mitral valve, propensity to dislocated lenses and dissecting aneurysm of the aorta.
> - When this is suspected, children should be referred for cardiology review.

13.2 Abnormal sex development

13.2.1 Intersex

The external genitalia at birth are not clearly male or female: some are masculinized genetic females; others are incompletely masculinized genetic males. The diagnostic problem is urgent, partly because the most common underlying disorder is dangerous congenital adrenal hyperplasia (Section 27.4.1) and partly because prolonged uncertainty about the true sex is intolerable for the parents. No-one should assign sex at birth if they are not sure; much harm may be done if the wrong sex is assigned: later reversal may be traumatic. The 'right' sex is determined by anatomy (functional possibilities), genetics and multidisciplinary discussion with the family. Intersex is rare. True *hermaphrodites* (with ovarian and testicular tissue) may have indeterminate genitalia. Investigation of intersex begins with karyotyping, ultrasonography and steroid chemistry.

13.2.2 Testicular feminization (androgen insensitivity) syndrome

The embryonic 'default' for genitalia is female unless a testosterone signal is received to switch them to male pattern during embryogenesis. Thus, abnormalities at the androgen receptor result in genetic males with testicles, but external genitalia of a female pattern. Inguinal hernias are typical and sometimes testes are palpable in the labia majora. At puberty, normal female secondary sexual characteristics develop with amenorrhoea. Orchidectomy is advised later because of a risk of malignant change. The androgen receptor is on the X chromosome and there is a recurrence risk for siblings.

13.2.3 Turner syndrome

Turner syndrome occurs in 1 in 2500 girls (Figure 13.4). The characteristic karyotype is 45XO (one X chromosome is lacking), but deletions or mosaicism involving the X chromosome may also be found. At birth the only noticeable abnormality may be lymphoedema of the legs. More characteristic features may be apparent later. Coarctation of the aorta should be excluded. Secondary sexual characteristics rarely appear: the uterus and vagina may be small and the gonads rudimentary streaks in the edge of the broad ligament. Breast development and menstrual periods may be induced by hormone therapy. Affected individuals remain infertile and short (few exceed 1.5 m or 5 feet), but in some girls GH may improve stature. Intelligence is normal in most.

13.2.4 Klinefelter syndrome

Characteristic karyotype is 47XXY, but mosaicism may be found. Although this condition occurs in 1 in 500 males, most are not detected until late childhood or adult life. The small testicles, long limbs

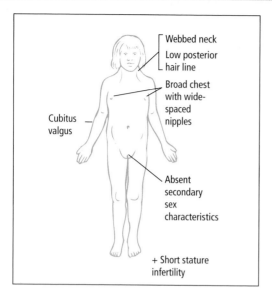

Webbed neck

Low posterior hair line

Broad chest with wide-spaced nipples

Cubitus valgus

Absent secondary sex characteristics

+ Short stature infertility

Figure 13.4 Turner syndrome.

and female habitus are rarely noticed early in life. Spermatogenesis is always impaired and infertility is usual.

13.2.5   Late and early puberty

Girls reach puberty on average a year before boys (see Figure 13.5).

The age of puberty is influenced by genetic and environmental factors (Section 3.4).

Children (especially boys) and their parents frequently seek advice about 'late puberty'. The absence of any signs of puberty at the age of 14 in girls and 16 in boys does not necessarily require investigation especially if there is a family tendency to late puberty. The measurement of height

is useful because physiological delay is more probable in short boys. In short girls with delayed puberty, it is important to exclude Turner syndrome. The vast majority of children with 'late' puberty are normal: they need reassurance, moral support and patience. Exceptionally, induction of puberty is indicated if there is pituitary or gonadal insufficiency.

13.2.5.1   Precocious puberty

🔑 *Precocious puberty* is the development of secondary sexual characteristics before 8 years in a girl or 9 years in a boy. True precocious puberty is more common in girls, while in boys it is more likely to be due to underlying pathology (e.g. brain tumour).

True (central) precocious puberty results from premature secretion of gonadotrophins and follows the normal pattern of development. In gonadotrophin-independent precocious puberty (e.g. congenital adrenal hyperplasia, adrenal tumours, gonadal tumours) the sequence of pubertal changes may be abnormal. Isolated precocious development of breasts (*thelarche*) is less rare and commonly resolves, followed later by normal puberty. Intracranial tumours, hydrocephalus, meningitis and encephalitis may lead to precocious puberty.

🔑 *Gynaecomastia* in adolescent boys is almost always physiological and self-limiting. This does not prevent it being a considerable social embarrassment.

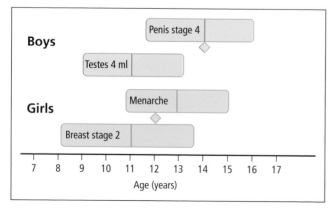

Boys

Penis stage 4

Testes 4 ml

Girls

Menarche

Breast stage 2

7   8   9   10   11   12   13   14   15   16   17

Age (years)

Figure 13.5 Age of puberty in boys and girls. Each bar represents the 2nd (left hand end) to 98th centiles, with the median shown by the vertical line in the middle of the bar. The diamonds indicate maximal growth velocity. Note that puberty starts earlier in girls, and there is an earlier growth spurt. The first sign of puberty in boys is enlargement of the testes to 4 mls, while in girls it is usually breast stage 2.

Summary

Failure to thrive may be due to nutrients (lack, loss), nature (genes), nuture (emotional/neglect) or any chronic disease. Careful history is essential. You should know about growth velocity and midparental height to assess children with short stature. Although many are constitutional, there are important pathologies to look out for, such as Turner syndrome and hypothyroidism. Marfan and Klinefelter syndrome are rare but important causes of tall stature. Precocious puberty is the commonest disorder of sex development, and usually needs investigation. It is more often due to underlying pathology in boys than girls.

 OSCE TIP

- Growth, nutrition and physical development (see OSCE Station 13.1).
- Child with short stature – history or discussion with parent.
- Failure to thrive history.
- Growth chart with normal growth and worried parent.
- History of a child presenting with early or late puberty.

See EMQ 13.1 and EMQ 13.2 at the end of the book.

 FOR YOUR LOG

- History of child with failure to thrive
- Practice using and interpreting growth charts showing abnormal growth patterns
- Learn how to stage puberty
- Approach to child with short stature.

OSCE station 13.1: Failure to thrive

Task: Take a history from a parent whose 14-month-old girl Rebecca has been referred to out-patients with failure to thrive.

Don't forget the following:

- Who is concerned? Sometimes the concern is mainly the health professional's rather than the parents'.
- Duration? Originally grew well, but poor weight gain for last 4 months.
- Note birth weight, ask to see parent-held record for previous growth plots.
- Careful dietary history: drinks large amounts of milk, fussy eater, poor appetite for solid food.
- Vomiting or loose stools/diarrhoea? No.
- Recurrent or chronic illness? No, generally very well except three or four coughs/colds in last 6 months.
- Other family members small? Yes, mother and father both small, don't know exact heights. Three-year-old brother has always been on bottom line of centile charts for weight and height.

Optional extra task or separate linked station
You are shown Rebecca's centile chart (height steady on 9th centile, weight falling from 9th to below 0.4th centile over last 4 months) and are told that examination is otherwise normal. You are asked to discuss the likely cause for Rebecca's failure to thrive, and what to do next.

In this case, the cause is likely to be a combination of constitutional (small parents and sibling) and excessive milk intake. Say you would like to measure parents' heights and plot the mid-parental height and target centile range. Suggested initial management: arrange dietary assessment and advice, contact health visitor for more information and her help with management, advise reduction in milk feeds especially in the 2–3 h before meals.

14

Immunization and infections

Chapter map

Immunity is first lost (waning maternal antibodies) and then gradually regained, through exposure to infection and immunization. Immunization is a key public health measure of great importance to child health worldwide. Anaphylaxis is considered here because it is a rare risk when giving vaccines. Infections are a common reason for children to present to hospital or primary care. Most are non-specific viral, but you should be able to recognize the key infective syndromes which are outlined in this chapter.

14.1 Immunity

Immunological mechanisms in childhood are essentially the same as in adults but are not fully developed at birth. Cellular immunity is effective from birth. For the first 2 or 3 years of life, the total white cell count is relatively high, and lymphocytes predominate over polymorphs in the circulating blood. Pus can be formed at any age.

Humoral (antibody-mediated) immunity is slower to develop. Maternal IgG is transferred across the placenta from early fetal life. This gives the full-term infant passive immunity to many infections, including measles, rubella and mumps. This gradually wanes from a few months to a year of age. In contrast, the larger molecules of IgM do not cross the placenta and the neonate is therefore fully susceptible to some bacterial infections including pertussis.

> IgM stays in the Mother, IgG crosses to the fetus.

The fetus is capable of mounting its own IgM in response to intrauterine infection, e.g. rubella, but synthesis of other immunoglobulins gets off to a rather sluggish start after birth. Total immunoglobulin levels in all infants are at their lowest at about 3–4 months of age, which is another susceptible period. A reasonable level of humoral immunity is established by the age of 6–9 months (Figure 14.1).

Paediatrics Lecture Notes, Ninth edition. Simon J. Newell and Jonathan C. Darling. © 2014 John Wiley & Sons, Ltd. Published 2014 by John Wiley & Sons, Ltd.

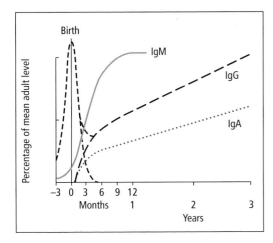

Figure 14.1 Immunoglobulin levels in early life.

 Increased susceptibility to infection

- Preterm infants
- Socioeconomic deprivation
- Chronic/debilitating illness, e.g. cystic fibrosis, chronic renal failure
- Immunodeficiency, primary or secondary, e.g. treatment of malignancy
- Congenital abnormality, e.g. urinary tract anomalies.

14.2 Immunization

As infectious diseases account for a large part of the mortality and morbidity of early childhood, it is essential to make the maximum use of all available preventative measures.

 PRACTICE POINT

Never miss a chance to check on, and encourage, immunization. It is every child's right to be protected against infectious diseases.

Immunization protects the individual but also prevents disease in the community. *Herd immunity* occurs with widespread immunization in the community. If a large proportion of the population is immune, the disease cannot find a host or spread. This reduces the chances of transmission of infection between children, protects any small proportion who have not had effective immunization and may even

allow disease eradication (e.g. smallpox). No child should be denied immunization without serious thought as to the consequences, both for the individual child and for the community. Almost 2 million children die each year worldwide as a result of disease which can be prevented by vaccination.

Immunization scares can have a serious impact on immunization uptake. They are often based on little evidence, but amplified by unbalanced media reporting. The resulting fall in immunization levels leads to a rise in the number of cases, with increased morbidity and deaths. Pertussis was linked with encephalopathy in the 1970s, and MMR with autism in the 1990s (Figure 14.2). Extensive research found no basis for the original concerns.

 OSCE TIP

When counselling about immunization scares, consider the following summary line:
'If there is any risk, it is very small, and far outweighed by the benefits.'

Design of immunization schedule

Two key questions:
1. What diseases to immunize against?
The following favour immunization:

Disease
- Frequency – common
- Severity – severe, dangerous

Vaccine
- Effectiveness – high
- Risks – low
2. What age to immunize?
- What age are children susceptible to the disease?
- What age do they best respond to the vaccine?

Often immunization schedules have to compromise: for example, the greatest danger of pertussis disease is in the first 6 months of life, but the immunological response is relatively poor before 3 months of age. The programme runs between 2 and 4 months of age (Table 14.1).

In the last 10 years, immunizations against Meningococcus C, *Haemophilus influenzae* and *Pneumococcus* have greatly reduced the numbers of children admitted with these life-threatening infections. Human papilloma virus (HPV) vaccination has recently been added to the UK schedule for girls to prevent cervical cancer. Current innovations include immunization against RSV bronchiolitis and rotavirus (Table 14.2), and a multicomponent Meningococcal B vaccine is in development.

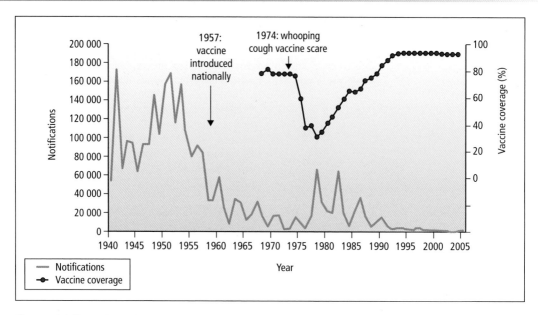

Figure 14.2 Pertussis notifications and uptake of vaccine in England and Wales 1940–2005. Note the increase in notifications after the drop in vaccine uptake. This was associated with an increase in deaths from pertussis (12 children died in the 1978 peak). (Source www.hpa.org.uk.)

Table 14.1 UK immunization schedule

Age	Immunizations
Birth	↘BCG –high-risk groups (e.g. immigrant families), all infants in high-risk areas ↘Hepatitis B for infants born to infected mothers (usually given immunoglobulin too)
2 months	↘DTP/Hib/Polio + ↘pneumococcus + ◊rotavirus
3 months	↘DTP/Hib/Polio + ↘MenC + ◊rotavirus
4 months	↘DTP/Hib/Polio + ↘pneumococcus
12 months	↘Hib/Men C
13 months	↘MMR + ↘pneumococcus
2 years and upwards	◊Influenza*
3 years 4 months	↘DT/Polio + ↘MMR (pre-school booster)
10–14 years	↘BCG for at-risk children (if tuberculin test negative) ↘MenC (around 14 yrs)
12–13 years (girls only) – three injections over 12 months	↘↘↘HPV
13–18 years	↘MenC (around 14 yrs) ↘DT/Polio (school-leaving)

↘ indicates one injection; ◊ indicates an oral or nasal vaccine; * influenza vaccine is to be offered annually (autumn dose) to all children age 2 years from 2013, then gradually extending to include all children age 2–16 years.

Details and contraindications are in 'The Green Book' — *Immunization against Infectious Disease* (HMSO). This can be accessed online at www.gov.uk/government/organisations/public-health-england/series/immunisation-against-infectious-disease-the-green-book or simply search for 'the green book' in your browser.

Table 14.2 The vaccines

Vaccine	Protection	Nature	Live	Route
BCG (*bacille Calmette–Guérin*)	Tuberculosis	Attenuated mycobacterium	Yes	Intradermal
DTP	Diphtheria, tetanus, pertussis	Toxoid and bacterial antigen	No	Intramuscular or deep subcutaneous
Hib	*Haemophilus influenzae* B	Conjugated capsular antigen	No	Intramuscular or deep subcutaneous
HPV	Human Papilloma Virus	Conjugated antigen	No	Intramuscular or deep subcutaneous
Influenza	Seasonal influenza	Live attenuated	Yes	Intranasal spray
Men C	Meningococcus group C	Conjugated antigen	No	Intramuscular or deep subcutaneous
MMR	Measles, mumps, rubella	Attenuated viruses	Yes	Intramuscular or deep subcutaneous
Pneumococcus	*Strep. pneumoniae*	Conjugated capsular antigen	No	Intramuscular or deep subcutaneous
Polio	Poliomyelitis	Killed virus	No	Injection (has replaced oral live attentuated vaccine)
Rotavirus	Rotavirus gastroenteritis	Attenuated virus	Yes	Oral (new from 2013)

 RESOURCE

* The Department of Health website at **www.dh.gov.uk** is a useful source of information source on immunization (search for 'immunisation' on the site), and includes links to the UK 'Green Book', a key reference source.

In the USA, the Centers for Disease Control and Prevention provides equivalent information at **www.cdc.gov/vaccines**, with a link to the 'Pink Book' (the USA immunization key reference).

 Contraindication myths

The following are *not* contraindications to immunization:

* Minor infections without fever or systemic upset
* A history of seizures (fits)
* A history of eczema or allergies
* Egg allergy is not a contraindication to MMR.

14.2.1 Contraindications

* Acute illness
* Major reaction to a previous dose of vaccine
* For live vaccines only:
  * Depressed immunity (disease or drugs)
* Risk to other family member (live vaccine viruses may be transmitted within a household)
  * Pregnancy
  * Immunosuppression
* *Extreme* hypersensitivity to certain antibiotics (should have been clearly documented in patient records):
  * oral polio (penicillin, streptomycin, neomycin or polymyxin)
  * measles (neomycin or kanamycin).

14.2.2 Reactions to immunization

14.2.2.1 Mild

* Common after all immunizations
* Restlessness, fever and crying
* Lasts a few hours
* Sore injection site, small area of erythema (2–3 cm)
* Mild fever, rash and malaise common 1 week after MMR
* Treat with paracetamol as necessary.

14.2.2.2 Severe

* Unusual
* Large area of swelling/inflammation involving most of the injected limb
* High fever

- Prolonged high-pitched crying
- Do not immunize again but obtain specialist advice.

PRACTICE POINT

Although anaphylaxis is a rare complication, immunizations should only be given if appropriate facilities for its treatment are available.

The killed pertussis vaccine previously administered in the UK used to be the most common cause of minor and more severe reactions. It has now been replaced by an acellular vaccine which is less likely to cause reactions.

BCG is injected *intradermally* over the insertion of the deltoid muscle. After 3–6 weeks there is local erythema, induration and sometimes ulceration. The axillary glands may be large and painful. The local signs disappear in 2–6 months. In school children, BCG is given routinely only if the prior tuberculin skin test was negative.

14.3 Anaphylaxis

This is a rare reaction to immunizations, drugs and also to foods and insect stings. Early intramusuclar adrenaline is essential for a severe reaction. Oxygen is always given, along with hydrocortisone, antihistamines and saline in some cases. The offending allergen should be removed if possible. Children should be referred to an allergy clinic for further evaluation. Epipens (adrenaline autoinjector pens) may be provided for use in the event of a future reaction (Figure 14.3). Training for parents and other carers is important.

14.4 Infections

Assessment and management of infection is a key skill in acute paediatrics. The presentations of infections are protean, and there are a wide range of specific and supportive therapies. Infection is by far the most common cause of acute illness.

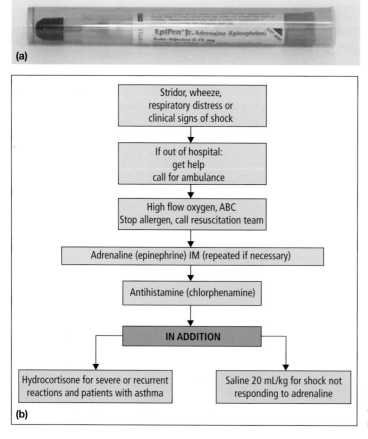

Figure 14.3 **(a)** Epipen containing adrenaline and **(b)** anaphylaxis protocol.

14.4.1 Recurrent infections

Most illness in childhood is infective. In the early years of life, children meet and establish immunity to a wide variety of infecting organisms. Recurrent infections in early childhood are troublesome for children and worrying for parents, but in the vast majority of cases the child is essentially healthy, and reassurance is all that is needed. A few children need investigation for an underlying cause such as immunodeficiency. Most recurrent infections are of the upper respiratory tract.

Recurrent infections: when to consider further investigation

Failure to thrive
Unusual infections
- More severe
- More frequent
- More protracted
- Two or more episodes of pneumonia or meningitis
- Unusual organisms
- Unusual sites of infection.

Unusual features in the history
- Family history of immunodeficiency
- Risk factors for HIV
- Persistent diarrhoea.

Unusual features on examination
- Large or hard cervical or inguinal nodes, any axillary nodes
- Hepatosplenomegaly
- Persisting rashes.

14.4.2 Diagnosis of infections

Always begin with history, examination and then investigations. Symptom patterns and indicative signs are found in some infections. Often the presentation is non-specific. In children with unexplained fever and in some in whom a firm 'disease diagnosis' has been made (e.g. meningitis), it is important to try to establish the responsible organism.

Infection is found by:
Clinical history and findings
Identification of the organism
- Microscopy
- Culture
- PCR (polymerase chain reaction)
- Rise in specific antibody titre.
Other supportive laboratory results (e.g. CRP, white cell count).

Swabs should be taken thoroughly (especially throat swabs) and transported to the laboratory swiftly. Material for virological culture must be put straight into transport medium. Immunofluorescent techniques allow rapid, positive viral identification, e.g. rotavirus in stool, RSV in nasal secretions. Skin scrapings are needed to identify skin fungi. Demonstration of a significant rise in antibody titre, whether bacterial (e.g. anti-streptolysin O titre, ASOT) or viral, requires at least two specimens, one taken early in the illness, another 10 days to 3 weeks later. A single convalescent sample showing a high antibody titre must be interpreted more cautiously.

 Take all necessary bacteriological specimens before giving antibiotics, unless this will delay treatment that is urgently needed.

Proof of some infections (e.g. HIV, hepatitis B, meningococcus and pertussis) may be possible by PCR tests which detect the relevant DNA/RNA material, and provide a rapid result.

14.4.3 Infections in childhood

14.4.3.1 Important childhood infectious diseases

Table 14.3 shows key characteristics for important childhood infectious diseases. In general, infectivity is maximal in the prodromal stage (i.e. between the onset of first symptoms and appearance of the rash) and ends within a week of definitive signs appearing. Note that all can have unpleasant complications (although rubella's impact is on the fetus).

Measles and international child health

Measles is a devastating illness in malnourished children (especially if vitamin A deficient). It is the leading vaccine-preventable childhood killer. Measles vaccination resulted in a 78% drop in measles deaths between 2000 and 2008 worldwide. However, in 2008, there were still 164 000 measles deaths globally, mostly children under the age of five.

Whooping cough and immunization

Efficacy of the vaccine is above 80%, but if immunized children do get the disease, it is much milder. Whoop and lymphocytosis may be absent, so the diagnosis is easily missed. Since the illness is much worse in infants, high rates of coverage are needed to protect those too young to be immunized.

Table 14.3 Important childhood infectious diseases

	Main features	Rash	Important complications	Laboratory findings	Treatment
Measles	• Incubation period 7–12 days (average 10) • Misery and fever • All the Cs: catarrh, coryza, cough, conjunctivitis • Koplik's spots (like grains of salt glistening on the buccal mucosa)	• Blotchy, red, maculopapular • Starts behind ears about day 4 • Spreads to face and trunk	• Pneumonia • Otitis media • Encephalitis (rare but serious).	• Rise in antibody titre • Immunofluorescence of nasopharyngeal aspirate	• Symptomatic only (fluids and paracetamol) • No antibiotics unless complications
Rubella	• Incubation period 10–21 days (average 18) • Upper respiratory catarrh • Cervical and suboccipital adenopathy • Usually mild illness	• Erythematous rash, mainly on trunk • Small, pink macules • May be confluent and resemble scarlet fever	• Virtually none in childhood • Children do not get arthralgia (common in adolescent and adult females) • Encephalitis very rare • Included in immunization to prevent fetal rubella syndrome (Chapter 8).	• Virus culture from stool or nose • Rise in antibody titre	• Symptomatic only (fluids and paracetamol)

Chickenpox (varicella) (see Figure 14.4)	• Incubation period 10–21 days (average 14)
	• Fever
	• Itchy rash
		• Predominantly on trunk, also perineum and scalp (Figure 21.9)
		• Lesions evolve: papules, vesicles, pustules, then scabs
		  • fever at pustular stage
		  • consider infected papular urticaria (Chapter 24) as differential diagnosis, but these lesions are peripheral
			• Complications rare
			• Conjunctival lesions
			• Encephalitis
			  • presents as ataxia a week or so after the rash appears
			  • prognosis good.
			• Maternal infection around the time of delivery can be life threatening to the baby
				• Electron microscopy of vesicular fluid demonstrates virus
				• Virus culture
				• Monoclonal antibody
					•Symptomatic only (fluids, paracetamol, soothing lotion such as calamine)
					• Aciclovir for severe infection/complications
					• Human varicella zoster immune globulin at birth to infants at risk from maternal infection

Mumps	• Incubation period 14–28 days (average 18)
	• Parotitis with swelling that is nearly always bilateral
	• Swelling of the orifice of the parotid ducts
	• Involvement of other salivary glands (less common)
	• Do not confuse with cervical adenitis
		• Rarely – a morbilliform (measles-like) rash	• Meningitis
			  • can occur without parotitis
			  • rarely may cause unilateral nerve deafness
			• Pancreatitis — rare before puberty
			• Orchitis after puberty.
				• Virus from saliva
				• Rise in antibody titre
				• Lymphocytosis
					Symptomatic only:
					• Fluids
					• Paracetamol
					• Warm/cold packs to inflamed parotid region

Whooping cough	• Incubation period 7–14 days (average 10)
	• Paroxysmal cough with vomiting; upper respiratory catarrh
	• Inspiratory 'whoop' of air intake after paroxysm (but not usually in babies)
	• Conjunctival haemorrhages (due to capillary rupture)
	• Serious disease in the very young infant
	• In infants, apnoeas may be presenting feature (cough develops 1–2 days later)
		No rash	• Pneumonia
			• Lobar collapse
			• Convulsions due to hypoxia from long paroxysms
			• Haemorrhage (nose, eyes, brain)
				• Bordatella pertussis from nasal swab
				• Immunofluorescence
				• Lymphocytosis +++
				• PCR test
					• Erythromycin
					  • Helps prevent infection of others
					  • Does not alter the course of the disease
					• Young infants may require admission, and even intensive care

Scarlet fever	• Incubation period 1–7 days (average 3) • Tonsillitis (pharyngitis) • Tongue sore and coated • Circumoral pallor	• Diffuse, erythematous, initially axillae and groins, then mainly on trunk • Facial flushing with circumoral pallor	• Otitis media • Rheumatic fever • Acute nephritis	• Throat swab grows group A haemolytic streptococcus • Rise in ASO titre	Penicillin (10 days)

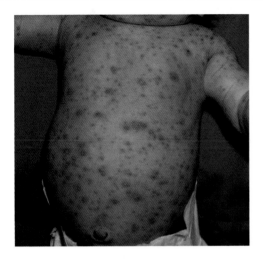

Figure 14.4 Chickenpox rash.

> **PRACTICE POINT** **Exclusion from nursery/school**
>
> Parents are advised to allow their child, once well, to return to school:
> - 5 days after appearance of rash for chickenpox, measles and rubella
> - 5 days after starting antibiotics for whooping cough.

14.4.3.2 Viral infections

Roseola infantum (exanthem subitum)

Roseola infantum, caused by herpes virus 6 and 7, is a mild disease of infants and young children, and rarely severe enough to need admission. Catarrhal symptoms and fever for 3 or 4 days are followed by the abrupt appearance of light red, discrete macules on the trunk. As the rash appears, the fever rapidly settles and the child is greatly improved. A few days later, the illness is over.

Erythema infectiosum (fifth disease/ slapped cheek disease)

This mildly contagious disease is caused by a human parvovirus. It commences on the face with bright red cheeks ('slapped face'). Maculopapular red spots appear on the limbs with a symmetrical distribution beginning on the extensor surfaces and spreading to the flexor surfaces and then to the buttocks and trunk. The rash subsides over the course of a week but may recur in response to a variety of skin irritants. Parvovirus may cause marrow aplasia in the fetus or in the child with chronic haemolytic anaemia (e.g. sickle cell disease).

Infectious mononucleosis (glandular fever)

Glandular fever results from infection with Epstein–Barr virus (herpes virus 4), but a similar clinical picture may result from infection by cytomegalovirus or *Toxoplasma gondii*. The presentation is very variable. Onset may be gradual, with malaise, anorexia and low-grade fever for 1–2 weeks, or it may begin abruptly with high fever and headache.

> **Glandular fever – specific signs**
> - Pharyngitis, often exudative and oedematous
> - Lymphadenopathy – multiple, firm, non-tender glands especially in the neck
> - Hepatosplenomegaly and hepatitis
> - Rash, macular or urticarial
> - Meningeal involvement, with headache, stiff neck, and raised cells and protein in the CSF.

> **PRACTICE POINT**
>
> Do not give ampicillin or amoxycillin when glandular fever is suspected since this will cause a florid rash.

In classic glandular fever, the blood shows an increased number of mononuclear cells (lymphocytes and monocytes) with atypical lymphocytes ('glandular fever cells'). There may be thrombocytopenia. The Paul–Bunnell (heterophil antibody) test is positive after the first week or two of illness. In practice, a simplified version of this test (Monospot) is generally used. Specific EBV serology is more reliable.

Hepatitis A (infectious hepatitis)

Worldwide, this is the most common cause of childhood jaundice. It is seen most frequently where hygiene is poor. It is milder in children than in adults.

> **TREATMENT** **Hepatitis A**
>
> **Prodrome (week 1)**
> - Anorexia, malaise
> - Nausea/abdominal pain
>
> **Jaundice (weeks 2–3)**
> - Tender hepatomegaly
> - Pale stools, dark urine
> - Urine urobilinogen ↑ and bile ↑
>
> **Serum**
> - Bilirubin ↑
> - Liver enzymes (AST, ALT) ↑.

Differential diagnosis in the pre-icteric and non-icteric cases is from other causes of abdominal pain and vomiting. Once jaundice has developed, diagnosis is not difficult. Urobilinogen may be detected in the pre-icteric stage and may be the sole diagnostic clue in the mildest cases without clinical jaundice. Serum bilirubin is raised, with roughly equal parts conjugated and unconjugated. Complications are rare. Jaundice usually fades in 1–2 weeks but exceptionally persists for months.

Transmission is usually by the faecal–oral route, therefore cross-infection should be prevented by good hygiene. Infectivity is greatest before jaundice appears and it is quite common to have more than one case in a household. In the average case, the child will be in bed for a few days and kept off school for 2–3 weeks.

Herpes

Herpes simplex virus (HSV) type I infections are very common, and usually asymptomatic. Spread is by infected saliva: primary infection involves the mouth, skin or eye.

HSV type II is a genital infection in adults. Transmission in the birth canal can cause serious neonatal infection. In children, it implies sexual abuse.

Herpetic stomatitis results from a primary infection with HSV I, and is most common in toddlers. There are vesicles, ulcers and scabs on the lips and tongue, the gums are inflamed and the child drools. There is cervical adenitis. Because of pain, the child may not eat or drink, and admission to hospital may be necessary to maintain fluid intake. The condition is self-limiting, the discomfort easing after a few days; the lesions have healed within 2 weeks.

Reactivation of herpes simplex infection commonly presents as a *cold sore* on the lip, tending to recur at times of infection, exposure to sunshine or other stress. Topical aciclovir is effective if given early. Someone with gingivostomatitis or a cold sore may easily auto-inoculate themselves, or another person, causing a herpetic whitlow of the finger, eye infection (keratoconjunctivitis) or vulvovaginitis. People with cold sores should not kiss children.

Herpes encephalitis may occur during primary infection, or reactivation of the virus, and in the absence of other features of herpes infection. It is a severe encephalopathy with a high morbidity and mortality despite treatment with aciclovir.

Enteroviruses

Coxsackie and echo viruses are common causes of brief febrile illnesses associated with respiratory and gastrointestinal symptoms. Faecal–oral transmission is usual, and outbreaks are most common in the autumn. Some are associated with ulcers confined to the posterior pharynx – *herpangina*. In addition to mouth ulcers, some coxsackie A group viruses are associated with vesicles on the hands, feet and buttocks – *hand, foot and mouth disease*. Complications from enteroviral infection are rare in healthy children.

HIV

> AIDS causes about 0.5 million child deaths per year worldwide, and in 2005 there were 2.3 million children living with HIV or AIDS. Africa has 12 million AIDS orphans.

In children, HIV type I is usual, and vertical transmission from mother to child is the usual route of infection (35% risk of transmission without treatment). Infection from blood products still occurs in developing countries. Infected babies appear normal at birth, but without prophylaxis nearly 25% develop AIDS or die in the first year. The rest show a much slower disease progression, with some showing no evidence of indicator diseases (e.g. pneumocystis carinii pneumonia) until the teenage years.

> **Conditions that suggest AIDS**
> - Opportunist infection
> - Recurrent bacterial infections
> - Failure to thrive
> - Encephalopathy
> - Malignancy.

The HIV antibody test is unreliable in infancy because of maternal antibody transmission. Children over 18 months who have HIV antibody are infected. PCR tests for viral RNA are increasingly used for diagnosis. Prophylactic treatment is begun as soon as HIV infection is suspected, and some units give prophylaxis to all children born to HIV-positive mothers from birth.

> **HIV: reduction of vertical transmission to <10%**
> - Maternal antiretroviral therapy in pregnancy
> - Caesarean section
> - Avoid breast feeding (in developed countries)
> - Antiretroviral treatment for infant in first weeks.

14.4.3.3 Bacterial infections

Meningococcal disease

The Gram-negative diplococcus (*Neisseria meningitidis*) (meningococcus) is divided into several sero-groups: groups B and C are most prevalent in the UK. Meningococcal disease is an important cause of morbidity in the UK (nearly 2000 cases per year) and has a case fatality rate of just over 10%. Transmission is via close contact with nasopharyngeal droplets. Infections are more common in winter. The peak incidence is at 6–8 months of age, with a smaller second peak in teenagers (of whom 25% are nasopharyngeal carriers). The incubation period is 2–10 days. The presentation varies according to the dominance of either septicaemia or meningitis.

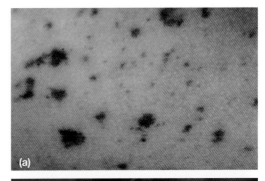

> **Meningococcal infection**
>
> - 25% septicaemia
> - 60% septicaemia and meningitis
> - 15% meningitis alone.

Septicaemia

> **PRACTICE POINT**
>
> A young child may be well in the morning and dead in the evening as a result of meningococcal septicaemia.

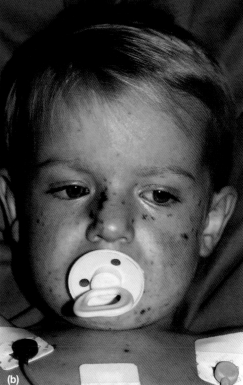

Mild non-specific symptoms are followed within days, or within hours (in severe cases), by severe illness and fever and the rapid appearance of a widespread red, macular rash which soon becomes purpuric (not blanching on pressure) (Figure 14.5). The rash may be sparse or profuse. Typically, it appears before your eyes. It varies from tiny petechial spots to large purpuric lesions which coalesce to form large ecchymoses. Septic shock follows in 30% of cases and requires prompt diagnosis and treatment. Severely ill children require treatment in a paediatric intensive care unit; others can be treated safely with antibiotics and antipyretics on the children's ward.

> **PRACTICE POINT**
>
> A feverish ill child who has a purpuric rash should immediately be given benzylpenicillin IV or IM and then transferred urgently to hospital.

Figure 14.5 Meningococcal rash. Make sure you can recognize this rash. Recognition saves lives.

Meningococcus may be grown from pharyngeal swab, blood culture, aspirate of skin lesions or CSF. PCR tests provide confirmation of diagnosis.

There is an increased risk of disease in the child's close contacts at home or in the nursery, though such secondary cases are rare. Close contacts are given a 2-day course of rifampicin (as is the affected child before leaving hospital) to lessen the risk of such secondary infection. They should be warned that rifampicin makes their urine pink.

Meningococcus is the most common cause of bacterial meningitis in Europe (features are described in Section 17.5.1). Children are now immunized against group C meningococcus, but not against group B.

Tuberculosis

Tuberculosis is common wherever poverty, malnutrition and overcrowding are prevalent, and rare where standards of hygiene and nutrition are good. In the developing countries of the world, tuberculosis appears in forms that were common in Europe 50 years ago. TB is rampaging through the African population along with HIV. The chief sources of infection are adults with sputum-positive pulmonary tuberculosis (*Mycobacterium tuberculosis*) and milk from infected cattle (*Mycobacterium bovis*). Erythema nodosum may be caused by tuberculosis (Section 24.2.8).

In Europe, childhood tuberculosis is becoming more common again. Primary complexes in the lung are seen more often in immigrant children from Asia than in others.

> The WHO estimates an annual incidence of over 8 million cases of TB in the world, of whom 95% live in developing countries. The WHO Global Tuberculosis Control Programme now reaches half of the world population. Early detection of infection and treatment is key.

Prevention depends first upon general improvement in socioeconomic conditions, and secondly upon specific measures including the prompt recognition and treatment of infectious adults, BCG immunization, tuberculin testing of cattle and pasteurization of milk.

> Three million of the world's population die from TB each year.

The initial infection is in the lungs if conveyed by droplets, or in the bowel if conveyed by milk. The first site of infection is known as the *primary focus*. The *primary complex* comprises the primary focus and the enlarged lymph nodes draining it. Spread of infection beyond the local nodes may result in tubercle bacilli reaching the blood stream, causing either tuberculous septicaemia (*miliary TB*) or infection of distant organs (meninges, kidneys, bones and joints). Tuberculous cervical lymph nodes are thought to be infected via the tonsils.

The child with a primary complex has minimal symptoms. Haemoptysis and systemic symptoms are exceptional. Children with TB, traced through their contact with infected adults, are often symptom-free. Diagnosis is based on the X-ray appearances and a positive tuberculin test. Sputum is not usually present, but tubercle bacilli may be recovered from gastric washings.

Tuberculous meningitis

This disease is dangerous and may lead to death or permanent disability. The onset is insidious and diagnosis difficult, with weight loss, vague malaise, anorexia and perhaps slight fever. Evidence of meningeal involvement may be shown by headache, drowsiness, irritability and neck stiffness. Later, there may be convulsions, focal neurological signs and impairment of consciousness.

> **PRACTICE POINT**
>
> A child with a lymphocytic meningitis, and low CSF glucose, should be treated for TB until proved otherwise.

Cervical adenopathy

Tuberculous neck glands are rare in the UK. Unilateral, firm lymph nodes are characteristic. In TB, the tuberculin test is positive.

> **PRACTICE POINT Diagnosis of TB**
>
> **Tuberculin test**
> - Intradermal tuberculin is injected in the forearm.
> - A skin reaction occurs if child has been exposed to TB.
> - Size of reaction checked 2–3 days later.
> - Children who have been immunized should have some reaction.
> - Strong reaction indicates active TB.
>
> **Chest X-ray** may show lesions of pulmonary TB
> **PCR**, e.g. on CSF sample
> **Bacterial culture** – slow (several weeks)
> **Gastric washings** may yield the organism.
> **TB blood tests** based on the immune response to the bacteria (inteferon-gamma release) are increasingly useful.

Management

Regardless of the site, the management of tuberculosis can be divided into three parts.

Notification of the case: immunization of contacts and identification of possible sources.

Anti-tuberculous drugs: rifampicin, pyrazinamide and isoniazid form the basis of treatment. Treatment should be continued for at least 6 months.

General management: children should not be admitted to hospital or kept off school without good reason. A pulmonary primary complex is rarely infectious, and isolation is unnecessary. If nutrition is unsatisfactory, it should be improved.

14.4.3.4 Other infections/ infection-like syndromes

Malaria

> **Malaria and international child health**
>
> Malaria kills a child somewhere in the world every 30 s. Malaria accounts for one in five of all childhood deaths in Africa. It is a major cause of childhood anaemia, which leads to poor growth and development. Maternal disease leads to low birthweight infants. 'Roll Back Malaria' is a global campaign to reduce the world's malaria burden by 75% by 2015. It focuses on proven strategies: insecticide-treated nets, prompt treatment of malarial disease and treatment of pregnant women.

Malaria is endemic in many parts of the world and may be seen in immigrants from malarious areas or in persons who have visited such places within the preceding 4 months. It usually presents with fever, which does not necessarily show the classic periodic pattern. The spleen may be enlarged. Diagnosis depends on identification of parasites in blood smears, and may be easier *between* peaks of fever. It may be necessary to examine several smears.

> **PRACTICE POINT**
>
> Think of malaria in the ill febrile child with a positive travel history.

Plasmodium can develop resistance to drugs. The appropriate treatment varies according to the local sensitivity of the responsible organism. Prophylactic drugs must be taken throughout residence in a malarial area and for at least 4 weeks afterwards (Figure 14.6).

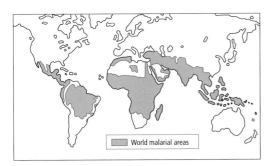

Figure 14.6 Distribution of malarial endemic areas.

Kawasaki disease

This is a rare but important disease. It presents as a systemic febrile vasculitis affecting children under the age of 5. No causative organism has been identified. It is the most common cause of acquired heart disease in childhood in developed countries (where rheumatic fever is rare). Coronary arteritis leads to the formation of aneurysms in up to 30% of children, which can be fatal.

> **Diagnostic criteria for Kawasaki disease**
>
> At least five of the following six:
>
> - Fever >5 days
> - Inflamed mouth, cracked lips, red pharynx
> - Bilateral conjunctivitis, non-purulent
> - Polymorphous rash
> - Hand/foot reddening, oedema and later desquamation (Figure 14.7)
> - Cervical lymphadenopathy >15 mm.

If diagnosis is made early, intravenous immunoglobulin, given within 10 days of illness onset, decreases the incidence and severity of coronary aneurysms. Aspirin is also given.

14.4.4 Notification of infectious diseases

Doctors are required, for public health and epidemiological reasons, to notify certain infectious diseases to the local authority or Health Protection Unit. Common ones are shown in Table 14.4.

> **RESOURCE**
>
> - You can see more information and the full UK list by searching the Health Protection Agency's website at **www.hpa.org.uk** for 'notifiable diseases'.
> - The American equivalent is at **www.cdc.gov**.

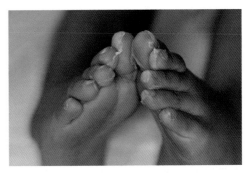

Figure 14.7 Peeling of the toes in Kawasaki disease.

Table 14.4   **Common notifiable diseases**
Encephalitis
Meningitis
Infectious hepatitis
Food poisoning
Haemolytic uraemic syndrome (HUS)
Infectious bloody diarrhoea
Invasive group A streptococcal disease and scarlet fever
Measles
Meningococcal septicaemia
Mumps
Tuberculosis
Whooping cough

syndromes of infection in children. Make sure that you recognize meningococcal disease and take appropriate action – one day you may save a child's life!

 FOR YOUR LOG

- Listen to discussion of immunizations with parents.
- Clerk a child with suspected infection.
- Recognise the rash of meningococcal disease.

 OSCE TIP

- Counsel parent about immunizations (e.g. parental concern, previous reaction, immunization scare).
- Parent not giving consent for immunizations.
- Photo or video of chicken pox, whooping cough, primary herpes.
- Photo or video of meningococcal disease.

✅ Summary

Know the immunization schedule and be prepared to discuss it with parents, including immunization myths and scares. This can prevent some of the most serious infections in childhood. Learn the common

See EMQ 14.1 at the end of the book.

OSCE station 14.1: Fever and a fit in an infant

Two linked stations: (a) History-taking; and (b) Management.

History-taking station

Take a history from the parent of this 7-month-old boy John who has presented to A&E at 4 p.m. with a seizure and fever. He now appears reasonably well with no rash, but is irritable.

Seizure

What exactly happened?
Obtain a clear description of the fit, its timing and duration.
Timing in relation to fever?
What was he like afterwards?
Has he had a seizure before?
Any head trauma?

Take a careful, clear history so that you are sure what has happened. Decide if it was a fit, and whether there was a fever. Think: is this meningitis, febrile convulsion or something else?

This illness

When did he become unwell?
Has temperature been measured – how high?
Duration of fever?
Irritability and feeding
Other symptoms (especially respiratory, gastrointestinal, urinary, rashes)

John had an episode at 3.15 p.m. at home where his eyes rolled back, all four limbs jerked rhythmically, and his body was stiff for about 2 min. This occurred just after his temperature had been measured at 38 °C. He recovered spontaneously and was then sleepy. He is now irritable. He has never had anything similar before. He has not suffered any trauma.

Past medical history

Birth or neonatal problems
Immunizations
Development

He has been unwell for 24 h with a fever measured with a digital thermometer in the axillae up to 39.0 °C. He has been irritable and off his feeds, taking half his usual amounts. He has no other symptom and is fully immunized. Other history is unremarkable.

FH&SH

Any family history of seizures or neurological problems?

Management station

Present and summarize your history. You will then be told any key points in the history that you have not elicited, and the examination findings. The examiner will then ask you about diagnosis, further investigation and management.

Present and summarize your history
(Get in the habit of summarizing your histories concisely when you write notes or present patients.)

This station depends on you having a reasonable differential diagnosis, and being able to bring all the information together to decide about management. You are told that examination is normal apart from the irritability and a fever of 39°C.

Diagnosis?

John's history is convincing for a seizure associated with a fever. Causes include:
- *Meningitis – likely and treatable, look for it first*
  - ◊ *Lack of focus*
  - ◊ *High fever*
  - ◊ *Seizure*
  - ◊ *Irritability*
- *Febrile convulsion*
  - ◊ *Bacterial sepsis*
  - ◊ *Viral infection*
- *Other less likely:*
  - ◊ *Metabolic cause of fit (always check for hypoglycaemia)*
  - ◊ *Head trauma with subdural*
  - ◊ *Epilepsy – first seizure*
  - ◊ *Other CNS lesion*

Investigations?

Septic screen (i.e. looking for a focus of sepsis)– blood culture, urine microscopy and culture; chest X-ray; lumbar puncture for microscopy, culture, protein and glucose; swabs as indicated

Blood tests – for seizure: glucose, U&E, calcium, magnesium
– for infection: FBC, ?CRP

Management?

Broad-spectrum antibiotics, e.g. cefotaxime needs to be given promptly (don't wait for the results to come back). Paracetamol can be used to control the fever. Consider IV fluids if John is not feeding well.

In fact John actually had a meningococcal meningitis. What findings would you expect in the CSF (Chapter 17)? What medication should be given to family members (Chapter 14)? He makes a good recovery. What test would you arrange on discharge (Chapter 17)?

The CSF showed a polymorph leucocytosis, high protein, low glucose and Gram-negative diplococci. Household members and kissing contacts were given rifampicin or ciprofloxacin as prophylaxis with public health involvement.
He needs a hearing test.

OSCE station 14.2: Allergic reaction

Task: You are working in General Practice. Mrs Phillips rushes in with Luke who is 3 years old. She is sure he has eaten peanut to which he is allergic.

Luke is a manikin held by the examiner. Ask the examiner anything you wish to know about Luke. Assess Luke and decide on his immediate treatment.

Don't forget:

Luke's history: key points

Rapid assessment	Airway, Breathing, Circulation	
? respiratory distress	*How fast is he breathing? How hard is he working to breathe – recession increased effort?*	**Luke is breathing fast at 70 bpm.** **He is working hard with some intercostal recession.**
	Is he maintaining his airway?	**His airway is maintained.**
? respiratory failure	*Is he alert and conscious, or blue?*	**He responds to his parents, but is not talking**
? added noises	*Is there stridor or wheeze?*	**Luke has audible stridor.**

Other features of anaphylaxis

? angio-oedema	*Is his face or tongue swollen?*	**Luke's parents are sure his face is swollen.**
? urticarial skin rash	*Does he have a widespread red rash?*	**He has a rash that is red and blanches but is otherwise pale.**
Progression	*When did it start, what has happened?*	**The reaction started about 40 min ago. The funny noise started about 15 min ago.**
	Is he getting better or worse?	**Luke is getting worse.**

Luke has anaphylaxis. You must act quickly. He has respiratory distress and is getting worse. If he is agitated, this means he is likely to be hypoxic. Ask someone to dial 999. Luke needs IM adrenaline treatment, usually in a preloaded syringe.

15

Accidents and non-accidents

Chapter map

Accidents are common and important. Non-accidents are rarer, and are part of the spectrum of child abuse. This chapter will describe the main types of both. Although sudden infant death syndrome does not fit either category, there are areas of overlap.

15.1 Accidents

Accidents are a common cause of death in children over the age of 1 year (Chapter 1). In the UK, around 300 children die each year; 70% are boys. Every year over 2 million children are taken to a hospital after having an accident.

Accidents vary by age group:

- Road traffic accidents involve mainly children of school age.
- Accidents in the home involve mainly children under the age of five.

 By the age of 11, one in four children has experienced a serious accident.

The risk of accident is influenced by social circumstances. The child in a large family in poor housing, on the street much of the day and ostensibly supervised by another child only marginally older, is at great hazard; and the mother trying to care for young children

> **RESOURCE**
>
> Children of parents who have never worked, or who have been unemployed for a long time, are 13 times more likely to die from unintentional injury than children of parents in higher managerial and professional occupations.
>
> See 'Better safe than sorry' (2007) which is available online from The Audit Commission at **www.audit-commission.gov.uk**.

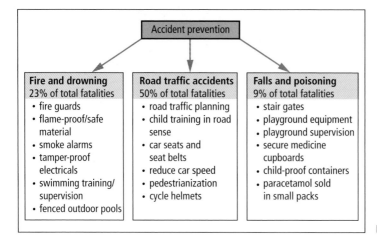

Figure 15.1 Accident prevention.

at the top of a tower block, without the privilege of an enclosed garden or play space, has a difficult task.

Pedestrian accidents are most common in the 5–9 age group when parents are falsely confident about their child's skills: it is wiser to underestimate, rather than overestimate a child's abilities. In general, children cannot cross a busy road safely, even at a traffic light, on their own until the age of 8 or 9 years, and cannot ride a bicycle safely on a main road until 13.

There is great need for better education of children and parents about safety, and for legislation to minimize the opportunities for accidents (Figure 15.1).

> The UK government has targeted accident prevention as a key policy area over the past 20 years, and there has been a steady reduction in number of accidents in children. However, accidents remain one of the leading causes of morbidity and mortality in childhood.

15.1.1 Head injury

 KEY POINTS

- Apparently trivial injuries can lead to intracranial bleeding that only becomes clinically apparent after an interval of time.
- Intracranial bleeding may occur without a skull fracture.
- CT head scan is the first-line investigation after significant head injury.

15.1.1.1 Management

- Airways, Breathing and Circulation
- Observe
  - Pulse
  - Respiratory rate
  - Blood pressure
  - Level of consciousness
- Pupillary size and reactions
- CT head scan if risk factors for serious intracranial injury (Figure 15.2)
- Consider spinal imaging (X-rays +/− CT depending on suspicion and severity of injury)
- Admit and observe (usually overnight) if:
  - Severe injury
  - Any neurological symptom or sign including depressed conscious level
  - Persisting symptoms:
    - Headache
    - Vomiting
    - Altered behaviour
- Consider non-accidental injury if injuries and history don't match, or other suggestive features (see Section 15.2).

 RESOURCE

National guidelines for management of head injury (CG 56) are available at **www.nice.org.uk** (**www.nice.org.uk/CG56**). These or similar are used by most A&E departments.

15.1.2 Burns and scalds

15.1.2.1 Scalds

- Caused by hot fluids
- Predominantly loss of epidermis
- Blistering
- Peeling.

The skin of young children sometimes suffers full thickness loss from comparatively minor scalds. There is a strong argument for limiting the maximum temperature of hot water in the home to 54 °C (129 °F). Most scalds occur in the kitchen.

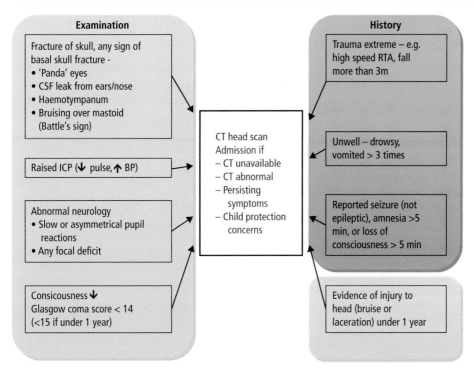

Examination

Fracture of skull, any sign of basal skull fracture -
• 'Panda' eyes
• CSF leak from ears/nose
• Haemotympanum
• Bruising over mastoid (Battle's sign)

Raised ICP (↓ pulse, ↑ BP)

Abnormal neurology
• Slow or asymmetrical pupil reactions
• Any focal deficit

Consicousness ↓
Glasgow coma score < 14 (<15 if under 1 year)

CT head scan
Admission if
– CT unavailable
– CT abnormal
– Persisting symptoms
– Child protection concerns

History

Trauma extreme – e.g. high speed RTA, fall more than 3m

Unwell – drowsy, vomited > 3 times

Reported seizure (not epileptic), amnesia >5 min, or loss of consciousness > 5 min

Evidence of injury to head (bruise or laceration) under 1 year

Figure 15.2 Management of head injury. Use the Acronym 'FRACTURE' to remember when to do a CT Scan in a child with head injury.

15.1.2.2 Burns

• Caused by
  • Direct contact with very hot objects
  • Clothes catching fire
• Often full thickness skin loss
• Shock – fluid is lost through the damaged skin surface (Figure 15.3).

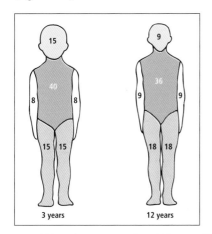

Figure 15.3 Skin surface areas at 3 and 12 years. The figures indicate the percentage of total body surface represented by each part.

If more than 10% of the body surface is involved, intravenous fluid therapy will be required. Burns involving 50% or more of the body surface carry a grave prognosis, although children have survived more extensive burns than this.

 PRACTICE POINT

Burns and scalds are more serious than they seem, and hospital admission is advisable for all but the most trivial. Severe injury needs specialized multidisciplinary care in a Burns unit.

15.1.2.3 Prevention

• Use cordless kettles or those with short coiled flexes (reduces risk of child reaching up and pulling the kettle over).
• Place pans on back of hob, handles turned inwards.
• Take care of children in the kitchen or use door gate to keep children away when cooking.
• Run cold water into bath before hot water.
• Use fireguards, radiator guards.
• Use smoke alarms.

15.1.3 Poisoning

15.1.3.1 Accidental poisoning (see Table 15.1)

- Common
- Toddlers aged 2–4 years
  - agile enough to find and swallow things
  - do not appreciate the dangers
- Less than 15% of children develop symptoms
- Death is very rare.

In the UK, things plucked from the hedgerows and ditches hardly ever cause serious illness. Occasionally younger children are given poisons by their parents (Table 15.2).

15.1.3.2 Deliberate poisoning

Older children may ingest drugs to self-harm, or recreationally (see Section 16.4.1), while rarely children may be deliberately poisoned by parents or carers (Table 15.1).

15.1.3.3 Management

> **TREATMENT**
> - Identify poison.
> - Check with poisons information center.
> - Estimate maximum amount/toxicity.
> - Minimize absorption (? emesis, lavage, charcoal).
> - Promote excretion (fluids/purgatives).
> - Combat symptoms.

If a large amount of a potentially dangerous poison has been ingested in the previous 6 h, the stomach should be emptied. Emesis usually follows the administration of 20 mL of ipecacuanha syrup in orange juice, repeated if necessary. Gastric lavage may be needed if emesis does not occur, or if the child is unconscious.

Table 15.1 Substances children swallow accidentally

Tablets and medicines*	Household and horticultural fluids	Berries and seeds
Sleeping tablets	Bleach	Laburnum
Tranquillizers	Turpentine	Deadly nightshade
Antidepressants	Paraffin	Toadstools
Iron	Cleaning fluids	
Analgesics	Weedkillers	

Table 15.2 Characteristic patterns in different types of poisoning

	Accidental	Self-harm	Deliberate (by parent)
Occurrence	Very common	Common	Uncommon
Age (years)	2–4	>10	0–5
Substance	Anything	Analgesic	Prescribed drug
Quantity	Small	Variable	Large
Recurrence risk	Small	Medium	Large

Do not induce emesis if:

- The child is not fully conscious
- Caustics (bleaches, acids)
  - (↑ risk of perforation)
- Hydrocarbons (turpentine)
  - (↑ risk of pneumonitis).

Other measures:

Discourage absorption
- Dilute the poison
  - Milk - usually available
- Absorbent agent
  - Activated charcoal absorbs the poison
- Specific antidote (e.g. desferrioxamine chelates iron, thus reducing absorption).

Encourage excretion
- Purgatives
- Forced diuresis in selected cases (rare).

Admit poisoned children to hospital for observation for at least a few hours.

> **RESOURCE**
> - Toxbase (**www.toxbase.org**) – an online resource for the NHS – should be consulted for any poisoning.
> - The National Poisons Information Service (**www.npis.org**) is available for more detailed expert help and advice. (Contact details are in the *British National Formulary* and the *BNF for Children*.)

15.2 Child abuse and neglect

Abuse: deliberately inflicted injury.
Neglect: inadequate or negligent parenting, failing to protect the child.

Many children suffer a combination of abuse and neglect. The definitions suggest that abuse is an active

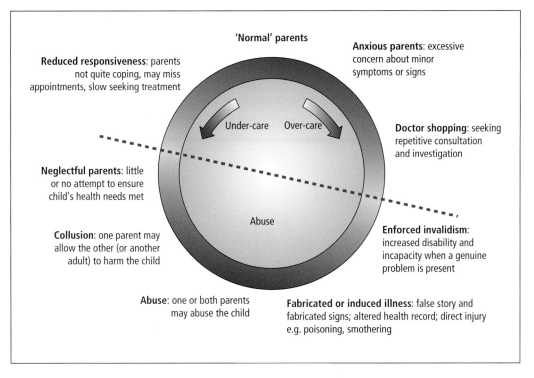

Figure 15.4 The spectrum of parental behaviour towards illness.

process and neglect a passive one, but for most forms of abuse the parents, who are the usual perpetrators, contribute to the abuse by both active and passive roles (Figure 15.4). Thus the spouse who fails to intervene when their partner sexually abuses the child is a passive partner to the abuse and colluding with it. A parent who passively fails to provide food or love may also indulge in active physical assault.

> **Types of abuse**
>
> - Physical abuse
> - Neglect
> - Sexual abuse
> - Emotional abuse
> - Factitious and induced illness (Munchausen syndrome by proxy).

A child is considered to be abused if he or she is treated by an adult in a way that is unacceptable in a given culture at a given time. It is important to recognize that children are treated differently not only in different countries but in different subcultures of one city and that there will be various opinions about what constitutes abuse. With the passage of time, standards change: corporal punishment is much less acceptable than it was. These factors contribute to the

difficulties of determining changes in the prevalence of abuse.

15.2.1 Physical abuse (non-accidental injury)

This is usually short-term and violent, though it may be repetitive. Infants and toddlers are most at risk. Soft tissue injuries to the skin, ears and eyes are common, as well as injuries to the joints and bones (Figure 15.5).

15.2.1.1 Common patterns of injury

- Bruising
  - Especially face and trunk
  - Multiple
  - Different ages

Note: a normal active toddler will often have five or six bruises of different ages, usually on the shins.

- Fractures
  - Especially ribs, humerus and femur
  - Different stages of healing denote repetitive injury
  - Infants do not often sustain accidental fractures
  - Often no clear history

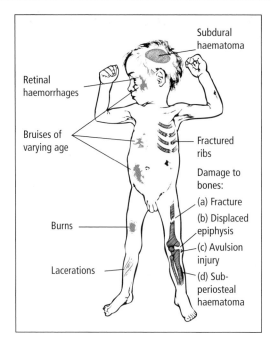

Figure 15.5 Characteristic injuries caused by physical abuse.

- Head injuries
  - Due to direct injury or shaking (shaken baby syndrome)
  - Skull fracture
  - Subdural haematoma
  - Fractures especially if depressed or complicated (as opposed to simple linear)
  - Retinal haemorrhages
  - Severe, intracranial haemorrhage leads to death or permanent brain damage
- Burns
  - Cigarettes
  - Holding a child close to a fire
- Scalds
  - Immersion in very hot water
  - Usually involve hand, foot or buttock.

15.2.2 Neglect

> **Neglect**
> - Failure to provide the love, care, food or physical circumstances that will allow the child to grow and develop normally
> - Exposing a child to any kind of danger.

Neglect and injury are closely associated, and both are indications of parental inadequacy. The child may show evidence of poor standards of hygiene or nutrition; height and weight, when plotted on a growth record, may be well below the expected centile (*non-organic failure to thrive:* Section 13.1.1). Neglect is often combined with emotional abuse.

 Features suggesting non-accidental injury
- Delay in seeking medical advice.
- Explanation incompatible with injury (a baby's skull does not fracture if he rolls off the sofa onto a carpeted floor).
- Story varies.
- Child brought by someone other than the person in whose presence the injury occurred.
- Unusual parent or child behaviour.
- Parents more interested in their own feelings, and in returning home, than in concern for the child (sometimes the parents will leave the child in hospital before the senior doctor has arrived).
- Abnormal parent–child interaction, with the child looking frightened or withdrawn.

15.2.3 Sexual abuse

Child sexual abuse includes any use of children for the sexual gratification of adults. It ranges from inappropriate fondling and masturbation to intercourse and buggery. Children may be forced to appear in pornographic photographs or videos, or participate in sex rings or ritual abuse. *Organized abuse* is the term used to describe abuse involving either a number of children, or a number of abusers.

15.2.3.1 Presentations of sexual abuse

- Disclosure by child or carer
- Local
  - Trauma
  - Infection
  - Perineal soreness
  - Discharge or bleeding
- Behaviour change
  - Anorexia
  - Encopresis
  - Self-harm
  - Sexual behaviour inappropriate for the child's age or environment.

Children of all ages, and either sex, are abused, though the most common is for a girl to be abused by a male who is either a relative or a member of the household.

15.2.4 Emotional abuse (psychological abuse)

> The child receives the repeated message that he is worthless, unloved or unwanted, or only of use in meeting the parents' needs.

Emotional abuse ranges from the failure of parents to provide consistent love, to overt hostility including spurning, terrorizing, isolating, corrupting and exploiting, or merely denying the child the right to emotional responsiveness. For an infant, this may result in failure to thrive with recurrent minor infections and frequent attendances at hospitals and health centres, general developmental delay and a lack of social responsiveness. The older child is likely to be short, developmentally immature and with delayed language skills. Her behaviour is likely to be overactive, impulsive and aggressive. All abuse entails some emotional ill-treatment, but currently it is uncommon for emotional abuse alone to be the sole reason for child protection measures through legal action, even though its consequences can be more severe than occasional episodes of physical abuse.

15.2.5 Factitious and induced illness (Munchausen syndrome by proxy)

This term encompasses a range of behaviour in which false illness in the child is invented or induced for the benefit of the abuser. It commonly includes both physical and emotional abuse. The harmful behaviour lies at the far end of the spectrum of inappropriate ways in which parents may behave in relation to childhood illness.

The consequences for the child can be disastrous:
- Unpleasant and harmful investigations and treatments
- Induction of genuine disease
- Effects of poisoning or suffocation
- Longer-term effects on child
- Child assumes illness role, believes himself to be disabled
- Misses school
- Somatoform or factitious behaviour (e.g. Munchausen syndrome) as an adult.

15.2.6 Prevalence of child abuse and neglect

- Four per cent of children up to the age of 12 are notified to social service departments because of suspected abuse.
- At least 1 child per 1000 under the age of 4 suffers severe physical abuse, e.g. fractures, brain haemorrhage or mutilation (Figure 15.6).
- This week at least four children in the UK will die as a result of abuse or neglect.

There is some evidence that there may have been an increase in child abuse in recent years, but the apparent increase may be more the result of greater unwillingness by society to tolerate child abuse, increased public awareness and professional recognition.

15.2.7 Perpetrators

- Most child abuse occurs in the home.
- The parents are the usual abusers.
- Physical abuse, emotional abuse and neglect are often inflicted by both parents.
- Sexual abuse is more common by fathers than mothers.
- Poisoning, smothering and factitious and induced illness are most commonly perpetrated by the mother.

Abuse occurs in all sections of society, but probably occurs more commonly in poor families. Abused deprived children are more likely to become abusing, neglecting parents – *the cycle of deprivation*.

The motives for abuse are complex. We can all understand how a weary parent in an overcrowded home, where the children are on top of one another, and the father is on shift work attempting to sleep, hits out impatiently at a fractious overdemanding child. However, much abuse is repetitive and, seemingly, premeditated. Often it is an expression of the parent's inner violence and their wish to exert power over their child. It is common for normal parents to have mixed feelings about their children and to have moments when they hate their child. Most parents can control their feelings, but a minority injure their child during those feelings of hatred. Most are not suffering mental illness.

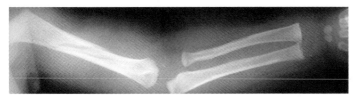

Figure 15.6 Spiral fracture of the humerus in a young child. These are often caused non-accidentally due to wrenching and twisting forces across the limb, and there may be little or no history of any significant injury.

15.2.8 Management of child abuse and neglect

Unless you think of the possibility of abuse, you won't diagnose it. When you suspect abuse, you need to know what action to take, and where to refer for more detailed assessment. Know about local policies and referral routes (usually general or community paediatric departments, and/or social services).

> In suspected abuse, consider the following:
> - Record history carefully (and who provided it) – always!
> - Sketch of injuries
> - Photographs
> - Skeletal survey (X-rays of skull, chest and limbs)
> - Check whether known to Social Services.

Multidisciplinary involvement is key to all steps in management. The following may be asked to provide information, or be involved in discussion:

- Child
- GP
- Parents
- Health visitor
- Family
- Hospital staff
- Neighbours
- Social services
- School/nursery
- Police.

If abuse is likely, the doctor (or other concerned person) will contact the Social Services Department who usually convene a case conference (Figure 15.7). The aim is to form a clear picture of the child and family relationships. Then, making the child's interests paramount, recommendations are made for the child's future safety, including decisions about future legal proceedings.

If the child is in imminent danger, an *Emergency Protection Order* may be sought from a magistrate. This allows the child to be detained in a hospital or foster home whilst enquiries are made. In view of the high incidence of abuse in siblings, it is mandatory to check the other children in the child's home. Subsequent court action may be needed to take a child into the care of the local authority if the risk of further abuse at home is too great (Section 1.5).

More commonly the child is made subject to a *Child Protection Plan* and skilled help arranged for the family so that the child can be supervised at home

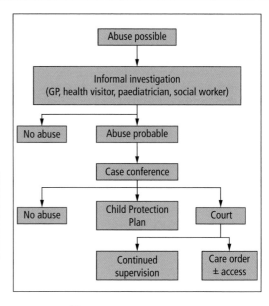

Figure 15.7 The usual course of investigation of alleged child abuse.

and the family helped to modify their behaviour. This help and supervision is normally provided by local authority social workers or the *National Society for the Prevention of Cruelty to Children (NSPCC)*. Further abuse occurs in up to 20% of cases; the recurrence rate is a sensitive index of the effectiveness of management.

The police are represented at case conferences and may be asked to investigate more serious or difficult cases. Only a minority of cases end with a criminal prosecution.

15.3 Sudden infant death syndrome (SIDS, cot death)

 KEY POINTS

- Sudden death of an infant
- Unexpected by history
- Thorough postmortem examination fails to demonstrate an adequate cause
- 0.4 per 1000 live births (Figure 15.8)
- Causes one-fifth of infant deaths in the UK
- Peak age 4 weeks to 4 months
- Most occur at home
- Most occur at night.

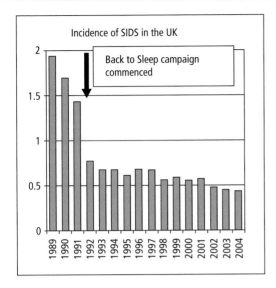

Figure 15.8 Incidence of SIDS in the UK 1989 to 2004. Rates are per 1000 live births from birth to 1 year.

Risk factors

Urban rather than rural areas
Social and economic deprivation
Younger mothers
Parental smoking
• During pregnancy (mother)
• After pregnancy

Co-sleeping (parent and baby)
• On a sofa
• In a bed if parent drunk, tired or a smoker

Excess heat
• Room temperature
• Too much bedding

Prone sleeping.

SIDS is a categorization rather than an explanation. It is a label of exclusion. Many hypotheses have been proposed to explain SIDS. It is likely that there are several different causes. Hyperthermia or overheating is an important factor, and is the reason for some of the preventative measures. The 'Back to Sleep' campaign (commenced in the UK in 1991), where parents are told to put infants on their back to sleep, and not prone, has brought about a dramatic reduction in SIDS deaths. Accidental 'overlaying' (*smothering*) by a parent is uncommon.

A small proportion of infants labelled as SIDS have been murdered. Suspicious features in the history or examination (such as injuries or bleeding around the mouth or nose) may raise concerns.

 Parents are advised: Do not sleep with your infant:
• Under the influence of
  • Alcohol
  • Drugs
  • Medications
• If you smoke
• On a sofa.

Sudden unexpected death causes a profound family crisis and the bereaved parents need expert counselling and help. Commonly such parents are invited to enrol in the CONI (Care of Next Infant) programme when they have a subsequent baby. Many are lent an apnoea alarm; though this may be reassuring, evidence is lacking that the alarms prevent cot death.

 RESOURCE

SANDS (Stillbirth and Neonatal Death Society) **www.uk-sands.org** supports affected parents.

Prevention of SIDS

Back to sleep
• Avoid sleeping prone

Not too hot, light bedclothes
• 16–20 °C overnight head exposed, no hat

Feet to foot
• Baby's feet touching foot of cot

Smoke-free zone
• Avoid smoking in pregnancy and in the home

Prompt medical advice
• If unwell, feverish, or less responsive.

See EMQ 15.1 at the end of the book.

 Summary

Accidents are part of childhood, and most are trivial. Management of more serious accidents is an important part of paediatric practice. Any doctor working with children needs training in child protection, so that they can take appropriate action when child abuse is suspected.

FOR YOUR LOG

- Discuss accident prevention advice with health visitor.
- Observe advice being given following head injury.
- Listen to discussion about a case where there are child protection issues.

 OSCE TIP

- Counsel about accident prevention in a young child or toddler.
- Identify signs of physical abuse on photographs or X-rays.

OSCE station 15.1: Accidental poisoning

Task: Sarah, almost 3 years of age, arrives with her father who is distraught. Her mother has left some paracetamol elixir open in Sarah's sister's bedroom, and Sarah has been found with the bottle and spoon. There is medication on her clothes and the carpet. Sarah looks very well and has no significant past medical history.

Take a history. Discuss what you need to do next with Sarah's father.

Don't forget:

Clarify the history	When did it happen? What is the poison?
Ascertain amount of drug	Have the parents brought the bottle?
	How much was in it, is it new?
Any evidence that poison was ingested?	Any evident effects or side effects on child?
If caustic, is the mouth sore?	
Get expert advice	Discuss with your registrar or consultant
	Contact the national poisons advice service
Plan management	This will depend upon the poison taken, timing, amount and expert advice
Explain and reassure if possible	Parents will be worrried, and feel guilty

Sarah has probably not taken much paracetamol. The bottle was not new and there remains about the same amount in it. She is well but this does not help in acute assessment. It is now nearly 3 h since the incident. You decide to measure the blood paracetamol level at 4 h. You reassure the father that dangerous effects are rare, but admission now and an urgent test is needed to be safe. Paracetamol can be dangerous. You discuss that this is a common event. The level is then found to be low and no further treatment is needed.

The Poisons Information Service can tell you what poisons are contained in most substances as long as you can identify what the child has ingested (e.g. a certain cleaning agent). They will give expert advice on management.

16

Adolescent health

Chapter map

Adolescents are different from children or adults, and have different needs. In the consultation, the best overall approach is to show equal respect and attention to the young teenagers and their parents. As they get older, we talk principally with the young patient, and involve them in decision-making (including consent issues). This chapter will consider issues of consultation and consent, and the particular challenges of adolescence.

> 🔑 No decisions about me without me. Equity and Excellence: Liberating the NHS, 2010

> 🔑 One in every five people in the world is an adolescent, and 85% of them live in developing countries (WHO).

Adolescence is the period of transition from childhood to adulthood. It begins with the first signs of puberty, and ends when the young person is 'mature' – physically (end of growth and sexual development) and emotionally. Societal recognition of when maturity is reached varies across cultures, and some do not recognize adolescence at all.

Dimensions of maturity

- Biological maturity – completion of physical growth and sexual development
- Psychological maturity – development of an identity separate from parents and family
- Social maturity – an ability to contribute to, and interact with, society (e.g. through relationships, in the workplace).

The phase of adolescence roughly corresponds to age 10-19 (WHO definition).

16.1   Approach to consultation

Efforts to make paediatric areas child friendly may result in an environment that is unsuitable for the adolescent patient. At the very least, pack away the toddler toys before your 16 year old patient walks in! Dedicated adolescent areas are best, but not always available. Give opportunity for the young person to talk and ask questions, listening carefully to what they say and respecting their views. The monosyllabic adolescent may be much happier to talk if you offer to see him without his parent. Arranging to see him on his own first next time may send a powerful message that you see his role as key. But this will not always be appropriate or possible – the overriding principles

Paediatrics Lecture Notes, Ninth edition. Simon J. Newell and Jonathan C. Darling. © 2014 John Wiley & Sons, Ltd. Published 2014 by John Wiley & Sons, Ltd.

are sensitivity, respect and flexibility. These also apply to physical examination and any procedures. Check whether the young person would like their parent present, and consider the need for a chaperone (p. 25, 'Chaperones').

Consultations with adolescents

Time – take time (see on own?)
Respect – for privacy, assure confidentiality (providing their well-being or that of another is not jeopardized)
Understanding – avoid judgmental or glib statements
Sensitive – work extra-hard to read the situation, body language, to hear what is said and unsaid
Thoughtful – how can I put the young person at their ease?

16.2   Consent

In England and Wales a young person of 16 years or over is deemed legally competent and able to make decisions about their own medical treatment. *The Gillick Principle* allows a teenager under this age to give consent for treatment if the doctor is satisfied that they are competent to do so.

PRACTICE POINT
Competency – 4 Cs

Comprehend – to retain and understand the information
Consider – to be able to weigh up the risks and benefits
Choose – to be able to arrive at a choice
Consequences – to understand the implications of not consenting.

Treatment overrides non-treatment in dispute. If despite careful counselling and discussion, there remains disagreement between a competent young person and their parent(s), and refusal of treatment will result in serious harm then treatment should be given. This applies up to age 18. So treatment should go ahead if either party (child or parent) wants the treatment, even if the other dissents. In practice, it is difficult or impossible to force treatment on an unwilling adolescent, and agreement through sensitive negotiation and compromise is better.

PRACTICE POINT

Take careful account of all children and young persons' views, whatever their age.

16.3   Physical problems

16.3.1   Puberty and growth

Problems of growth and sex development are considered in chapter GD.

16.3.2   Periods, pregnancy and contraception

Primary amenorrhoea (never having had a period) is usually physiological due to delay in onset of puberty (Section 13.2.5). However, think of Turner syndrome (Section 13.2.3). Primary or secondary amenorrhoea may be due to pregnancy, eating disorders (especially anorexia nervosa), chronic illness, stress, and intense physical training. It may also be seen in hyperthyroidism, and rarely brain tumours. Dysmenorrhoea (painful periods) can usually be controlled with simple analgesics, but sometimes the combined oral contraceptive pill is used.

Around 30% of teenagers in the UK have sexual intercourse before their 16th birthday (Section 6.1.1). Teenage girls who become pregnant have higher rates of postnatal depression, and their babies are 60% more likely to die in infancy. Prevention is through appropriate and accessible sex education, promotion of self-esteem, delaying age at first sex, and provision of contraception. Condom use will also reduce rates of sexually transmitted infections.

16.3.3   Acne

Pubertal androgens increase skin sebum production, which tends to block pores and promote infection and inflammation.

TREATMENT Treatment of acne

- Regular use of a mild cleanser
- Water-based moisturizer
- Avoid picking/squeezing spots
- If resistant:
  - Consider topical/systemic antibiotics (erythromycin, oxytetracycline)
  - Topical or systemic retinoids may be used

16.3.4   Chronic illness

16.3.4.1   Adolescence and pre-existing chronic illness

Chronic illness brings special challenges in adolescence. Part of finding a new psychological identity may involve risk taking and rejection of parental and professional advice. The perfect diabetes control chart may go haywire (or not be kept at all). The well-controlled asthmatic starts to have frequent exacerbations. Parents (and doctors) have to tread the difficult tightrope of promoting independence and respecting autonomy, while maintaining reasonable disease control. Often some compromise is needed, but not always reached. Adherence issues are common, and are best approached without blame or pressure, with matter of fact acknowledgment of the difficulties of treatment regimes. It is better to agree a less-than-ideal treatment plan that can be kept to, than to go for something too demanding that results in the young person feeling there is no point trying at all.

16.3.4.2 Chronic fatigue syndrome (myalgic encephalitis)

This disease of unknown cause is rare before adolescence. It may follow a non-specific viral infection. Tiredness is the most prominent feature. It may sometimes have a psychological cause.

> **Symptoms in chronic fatigue syndrome**
>
> * Tiredness
> * Headaches
> * Dizziness
> * Poor sleep
> * Earache

Consider investigations for inflammatory conditions, brain tumour, infection (glandular fever) and hypothyroidism. Treatment is through cognitive behavioural therapy combined with a gradual planned increase in exercise and activity. Recovery can take months to years.

16.4 Psychological problems

Families have an invisible web (Figure 16.1) that usually helps to support the adolescent journey, but can sometimes malfunction. The cross-cords of protection, nuture and support all have to be gradually relaxed as the young person reaches maturity and independence. At the same time, they must be held in the right amount of tension to provide at different times: (a) a *platform,* to reach new goals; (b) a *shock absorber,* to absorb the repeated impacts of the young person working out their new identity; and (c) a *safety net,* to catch them safely when things are difficult. The circular cords of the web are contributed by the young person's own personality, health, and experiences; the parental or family beliefs and supports; and external factors including wider family and professionals (including health). Sometimes the 'cords' become 'sticky', for example due to chronic illness in child or parent, psychological difficulties or due to a combination of other stressors. The web can then function as a *trap,* which can limit the young person's journey to independence, or even lock them into an illness role. As the adolescent struggles, the cords become tighter. The longer this goes on, the more complex the 'knot', and the family situation might be called 'enmeshed'. Sometimes it is serving particular needs

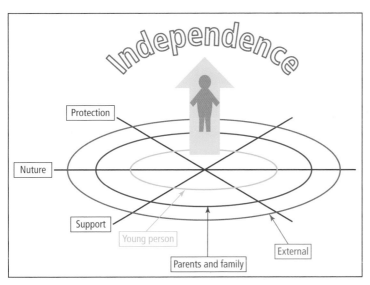

Figure 16.1 The family and the young person.

of parents or teenager (secondary gain). Experienced psychological help is needed to gradually undo the knot and find a way forward.

16.4.1 Deliberate self-harm

Adolescents (and sometimes younger children) swallow poisonous substances (usually drugs) because of emotional upset. Most often it is done as a gesture of defiance, or a wish for temporary oblivion, rather than with serious intention to commit suicide. Nevertheless, some are pathologically depressed. Review by the adolescent mental health team before discharge is advisable. See Section 15.1.3, for management.

16.4.2 Anorexia nervosa

This is uncommon in children, but important. It occurs more commonly in girls (1 in 200) than in boys (1 in 1000), and rarely before puberty. It is now seen less rarely in boys and younger children. A central feature is a disturbance of body image, so that the teenager is convinced that they are fat. In contrast to children who eat poorly because they are depressed, children with anorexia nervosa appear to have an abundance of energy strangely at variance with their microscopic food intake and steadily falling weight. They may look ill but insist that they feel well. It is a serious disease, which is fatal in 5% of sufferers.

16.5 Social problems

16.5.1.1 School refusal

Poor school attendance, particularly if over weeks or months, indicates serious physical, psychological or behavioural issues. Early action pays dividends. Consider a joint approach: involve the young person and their family, health services and education and look for a solution together.

16.5.1.2 Drugs, alcohol and smoking

Drugs of abuse are now relatively cheap and widely available. Solvent abuse (inhalation of glues and aerosols) is becoming less prevalent. Tobacco and alcohol should not be overlooked. There is growing concern and awareness of teenage alcoholism, and its combination with other agents may be lethal. Young people who binge drink in adolescence are more likely to abuse other substances, have lower educational attainment and be involved in crime.

Currently the aim is to give children honest, realistic information (Table 16.1). There is no point in pretending to the child who knows how to procure drugs that they harm all who take them. Drugs education in school is seen by some as contentious. Parents may be alerted by finding drug-taking equipment or by noticing changes in their child's behaviour. The national drugs helpline or local organizations are helpful contacts.

Table 16.1 Recreational drugs

Name	Street names	Formulation	Undesired effects
Opiates	Scag; smack; dragon; tiger	Methadone: liquid, powder, wrapped in foil/prescription opiates	Respiratory depression Coma Pin-point pupils Hypotension
Hallucinogens	Tabs; LSD; acid; trips; magic mushrooms	Small squares of absorbent paper with pattern/microdots (tiny pellets)/ mushrooms	Psychotic symptoms Accidents
Cocaine	Coke; snow; base; crack; wash; rocks	White powder Paper wrapped or twisted	Agitation Dilated pupils Tachycardia Hypertension
Amphetamines	Speed; uppers; sweets; whiz; ecstasy; Es; doves	Powder Tabs Capsules Homemade tabs	Agitation/paranoia Hallucination Hypertension Dehydration Hyperthermia Delirium/coma Convulsions/coma
Cannabis	Pot; dose; grass; ganja; weed; spliff; joint	Resin blocks; dried leaves	Anxiety attacks Panic disorder

PRACTICE POINT

FRANK is the national drugs helpline offering free, confidential information and advice 24 hours a day, seven days a week. Anyone can call FRANK on 0800 77 66 00 or text a question on 82111.
www.direct.gov.uk

In children who become ill after taking such agents, it is important to be aware that adverse effects arise from the drug, contaminants or other agents added to the mixture. Solvents may lead to asphyxia, cardiac dysrhythmias and hepato-renal failure.

16.6 Transition to adult services

Some teenagers (and parents) find the transition from paediatric to adult care challenging, especially those with chronic conditions.

Transitional care for adolescents

- Plan carefully
- Arrange gradual transfer into adult services
- Involve both paediatric and adult services
- Agree timing with the young person
- Strike the right balance for each family between:
  - Fostering independence of the child
  - Maintaining the parents' involvement.

 Summary

Adolescent health services are relatively underdeveloped in the UK. All professionals working with children and young people need to be sensitive to the particular problems of adolescence, so that health problems do not thwart the young person's successful transition to adulthood.

 FOR YOUR LOG

- Take time to talk to young people about what they think about their illness and health care.
- Take a history from a young person with a chronic illness.
- Discuss the ethics of consent.

 OSCE TIP OSCE pointers

- Consent for contraception
- History in anorexia.

Reference

Department of Health (2010) *Equity and Excellence: Liberating the NHS*. London: DoH.

OSCE station 16.1: Discussion of asthma treatment

Emily is 16 years old and is attending the paediatric asthma clinic. She usually attends with her mother, but has come on her own today. The GP has written a short note recently expressing concern about regular attendances to the surgery and the Emergency Department over the last 3 months with asthma symptoms, and asking if her treatment should be increased. You have 10 minutes to see her.

(Note that clinical examination should not be performed – assume it is normal. Her inhaler technique has just been checked by the clinic nurse and is satisfactory, but peak flow is only 70% of predicted).

Opening

- Introduction
- Establishes rapport
- Reason for parent not being present
  – is she happy to proceed?

The simulated patient will be uncommunicative at first, but will respond positively to an open and empathetic approach. She will then reveal more information. Try to read verbal and non-verbal cues, give time, and avoid judgemental comments.

Asthma

Progress
- Open questions initially

Clarifies recent exacerbations
- Severity
- Response to treatment
- Any admissions

Ask about peak flow chart

She has not brought this.

Triggers
- Ideas about what could be making things worse?
- Mention smoking

If this is explored sensitively she will reveal she has been smoking for 3 months.

Treatment
- Clarify what she is taking
- Acknowledge difficulties

Again with a sensitive approach you will discover that she hardly takes her regular brown (preventer) inhaler because it seems to make little difference, but is taking her blue (reliever) inhaler two to three times most days.

Discussion
- Pros and cons of treatment
- Explanation of key points, without dictating solutions

Emily hadn't realized that the brown inhaler is a preventer that has to be taken regularly to work. Exercise (especially PE) is a problem – could take salbutamol beforehand.

Agree plan
- Overcoming difficulties in taking regular treatment, doing peak flow diary (why this is useful)

E.g. Emily thinks of her own way to avoid forgetting to take her brown inhaler. She finds doing the peak flow chart too much, but agrees a compromise.

Closure

- Summarize
- Anything else?
- Close consultation

Overall marks for rapport, empathy, organization, communication

Part 3

Systems and specialties

This section is organized approximately anatomically, from head to chest and abdomen, then skeleton and skin and other body systems.

17

Neurology

Chapter map

Normal variation in child development and minor neurological symptoms are common and usually benign. Fits, faints and funny dos are common in children and need careful assessment. Most seizures are febrile convulsions. In meningitis and other CNS infections, early detection is important. Many conditions result in neurological or neurodevelopmental problems in children that can impair lifelong or shorten life. Important neurological conditions manifest as seizures (fits), cerebral palsy, learning disorders or behaviour problems. Cerebral palsy is a broad descriptive term with many causes and a wide range of disability. Progressive, degenerative brain disorders are rare. The spinal cord may be affected by congenital abnormality, infection or trauma.

Paediatrics Lecture Notes, Ninth edition. Simon J. Newell and Jonathan C. Darling. © 2014 John Wiley & Sons, Ltd. Published 2014 by John Wiley & Sons, Ltd.

Brain growth and development occur early in life. Neurone formation is completed within 6 months of conception. Half the increase in head circumference between birth and adult life occurs in the first 18 months. Myelination is largely complete by the age of 3 years, and the establishment of dendritic connections by 5. The brain is particularly vulnerable in the fetus and young child.

Factors affecting brain development

Genetic
- Polygenic (e.g. epilepsy, intelligence)
- Single gene defects (e.g. tuberous sclerosis)
- Chromosome abnormality (e.g. Down syndrome)

Prenatal
- Drugs (e.g. alcohol)
- Infections (e.g. rubella, HIV)

Perinatal
- Extreme prematurity
- Metabolic disturbances (e.g. hypoxia)

Postnatal
- Infections (e.g. meningitis)
- Trauma.

17.1 Seizures

A seizure is the result of an abnormal paroxysmal discharge by cerebral neurones. The terms seizure, fit and convulsion are interchangeable. The pattern and prognosis varies with age (Figure 17.1). A seizure is a symptom, it has many potential causes and it may indicate epilepsy.

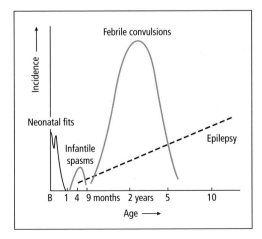

Figure 17.1 The incidence and type of seizure at different ages.

Fits are common in childhood

- 1 in 20 febrile convulsion
- 1 in 200 school age epilepsy
- 1 in 2000 severe epileptic disease.

17.1.1 Febrile convulsion

 Febrile convulsion: a seizure without other known cause occurring between 6 months and 6 years of age with fever.

Almost 5% of pre-school children have had a seizure; the most common cause by far is a febrile convulsion. A family history of febrile seizures is often present. They are precipitated by febrile illness and tend to occur at the start of the illness. Upper respiratory tract infections are the most common association. The seizures are generalized, with clonic movements usually lasting less than 5 min. There are no neurological signs after the seizure.

Temperature should be reduced to normal. Remove excess clothing or covers and in some tepid sponging is used. Paracetamol is usually given. Most commonly, shortly after the fit, the child appears well, while parents who thought their child might die may be desperately worried. One-third will have further febrile convulsions with future illnesses, but only 1–2% will develop epilepsy.

Management includes explanation of the relatively benign nature of febrile seizures. We need to make sure the family know about: recognition and management of fever (temperature control by removing clothing); future seizures (first aid, and when and how to seek emergency assistance). Antipyretics are not now recommended routinely (since they do not prevent further convulsions) but may be given to treat discomfort. Long-term prophylactic anticonvulsant therapy is occasionally used with recurrent febrile convulsions.

PRACTICE POINT

Do not forget that some children with a fit and fever have meningitis.

17.1.2 The child with fits

Non-febrile seizure in a previously healthy child should prompt consideration of epilepsy. In between attacks, most children are perfectly well. It is exceptional for the doctor to have an opportunity to witness a fit, and the diagnosis rests principally on the history. A video on the parent's phone can be very helpful.

PRACTICE POINT

There is no reliable diagnostic test for a seizure. A good history and eye-witness account is essential.

Careful examination and appropriate investigation are essential; the EEG is abnormal in 60%. Diagnosis can be difficult and it is important not to diagnose seizures without good reason. If the episodes are not typical, ask yourself 'are these really fits?' It is unusual for serious brain disease or metabolic abnormality to present solely with a fit in a child with no other neurological or developmental abnormality.

TREATMENT Management of fitting

- Call for help, this is a potentially serious situation
- Recovery position
  - Semiprone with slight neck extension so that secretions drain out of the mouth.
- If respiratory distress
  - Open the airways by gently extending the neck, lifting the jaw forward
  - Do not put anything in the mouth
  - Give O₂ if available.
- If fit continues >5 min, escalate up through these steps:
  - Buccal midazolam or IV lorazepam (repeat after 10 mins if need)
  - IV diazepam
  - IV phenytoin (or if on phenytoin maintenance, phenobarbitone)
  - Rectal paraldehyde
  - Anaesthesia with thiopental and intensive care
- Always check blood sugar

17.1.3 Epilepsy

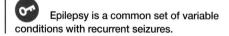

Epilepsy is a common set of variable conditions with recurrent seizures.

Epilepsy classification provides a helpful basis to approach therapy and support. Children with epilepsy should only be managed by a doctor trained to do so. The full classification is key in complex disease or where fits are hard to control. In infants and children there are 3 main axes of classification:

- *Seizure type.* This includes description of precipitating factors in reflex epilepsy.
- *Epilepsy syndromes,* patterns of disease with recognized characteristics. No single syndrome is common, but up to half of childhood epilepsy may be placed

in a syndrome (e.g. West syndrome with infantile spasms; benign centrotemporal (Rolandic) epilepsy).
- *Aetiology or cause.* This includes genetic disease and importantly seizures symptomatic of other disease.

An additional axis describes impairment and relates to the impact of the condition on the child's functioning, disability and health. The section below will focus on the main seizure types you should be able to recognize, but will not cover the other axes.

17.2 Seizure types

- **Generalized**
  - tonic clonic
  - absences
  - myoclonic
  - atonic
  - infantile spasms
- **Focal**
  - sensory
  - motor
  - with secondary generalization
  - ± impaired consciousness
- **Precipitating factor**
  - e.g. flickering lights

17.2.1 Generalized seizures

17.2.1.1 Tonic–clonic

These fits comprise a tonic phase (continuous muscle spasm) which may start with a cry and, if prolonged, lead to cyanosis: then a clonic phase (jerking) which may be associated with tongue-biting and frothing at the mouth: then relaxation, unconsciousness and a period of drowsiness and/or confusion. Children often sleep after an attack. Recurrent episodes which are regularly followed by sleep suggest epilepsy. Most occur for no apparent reason. Flashing lights trigger fits in some children, usually when they are watching a malfunctioning TV screen or sitting very close to the TV. The EEG may show bilateral, slow-wave, subcortical seizure discharges. Major fits can last from less than 1 min to over 30 min (*status epilepticus*). Uncontrolled prolonged fits can cause hypoxia, and may lead to brain damage, especially in the temporal lobes.

17.2.1.2 Absences

Typical absence seizures (*petit mal*) begin in childhood. Most affected children are otherwise healthy with normal intelligence. An attack consists of a very brief absence of awareness lasting less than 5 s and accompanied by blinking. The eyes may roll up. The child does not fall down. He may present with school difficulties because of 'daydreaming' or inattention.

Absences may be provoked by encouraging the child to hyperventilate for 2 min. The characteristic EEG shows a three per second spike and wave pattern.

Atypical absence seizures tend to be longer, and associated with other movements, sensations or altered awareness of consciousness. The prognosis is less good than typical absences.

17.2.1.3 Myoclonic

The sudden brief jerks affect one part of the body, commonly an arm or leg. They are a common feature in children who have other neurological disorders. Single jerks as we fall asleep are normal (*physiological myoclonus*).

17.2.1.4 Atonic

Atonic (astatic) seizure are known as drop attacks. Sudden decrease in muscle tone makes a child lose postural control and drop to the floor.

17.2.1.5 Infantile spasms

Infantile spasms are a rare and serious form of seizure usually at age 1–6 months. The infant doubles up, flexing at the waist and neck, and flinging the arms forward – a flexor spasm; less commonly it is an extensor spasm. Associated developmental delay is common. The EEG usually shows a characteristically disorganized picture – *hypsarrhythmia* (Figure 17.2). Anticonvulsants or corticosteroids may suppress the fits. The final outcome is related to the cause, which may be metabolic, malformation or cerebral damage. The single most common cause is tuberous sclerosis. Idiopathic infantile spasms is West syndrome.

17.2.2 Focal seizures

The seizure discharge starts in a focus in the brain. Sometimes the focus is at the site of previous cerebral damage. Focal (also known as partial) seizures may be motor (e.g. twitching of one limb), sensory (e.g. paraesthesia), autonomic (e.g. pallor) or psychic (e.g. strange thoughts or funny smells). Diagnostic problems are common and EEG and brain imaging are used.

Focal seizures may occur with or without loss of consciousness and awareness.

17.2.2.1 Temporal lobe epilepsy

Motor, sensory or emotional phenomena occur singly or in combination, together with impaired consciousness. These seizures vary widely in description, but in each child the pattern is usually the same each time. The diagnosis is confirmed by temporal lobe discharges on EEG.

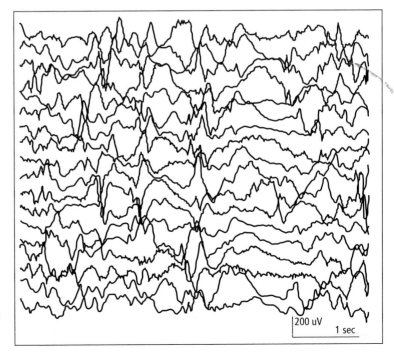

Figure 17.2 Hypsarrhythmia EEG with chaotic spike and wave.

200 uV

1 sec

17.2.2.2 Benign centrotemporal (Rolandic) epilepsy

Short focal fits, characteristically at night, affect the face or arms. School age children most commonly have a small number and the condition resolves. Frequent or numerous attacks may need treatment.

17.2.3 Neonatal seizures

Seizures are common in the first month as a result of birth injury, metabolic and infective causes or developmental abnormalities (Section 8.4.5).

17.2.4 General management of epilepsy

Epilepsy is the most common cause of childhood seizures, but it is important to search for a primary cause through careful history and examination. Seizures can be caused by space-occupying lesions, meningitis, hypoglycaemia, hypertension and many other factors.

Prophylactic anticonvulsant therapy is given to children with recurrent seizures, usually until the child has been fit-free for at least 2 years. The lowest dose of the safest drug that suppresses fits is used. The prognosis is good for children who are otherwise healthy, have a normal EEG and respond promptly to preventative therapy: less good for those with learning problems or cerebral palsy, with persistent seizure activity on EEG, and in whom a variety of drugs, alone or in combination, fail to give adequate control. Children's epilepsy should be managed by team with appropriate expertise, often offering support through a specialist nurse.

 TREATMENT Prophylactic anti-epileptic drugs (AED)

Drugs of first choice
- Valproate–generalized (tonic–clonic, absence, myoclonic)
- Carbamazepine–focal and generalized (tonic–clonic, focal)

Reserve drugs
There are many other AED. These include: Lamotrigine, Vigabatrin, Ethosuximide, Clonazepam, Topiramate, Levetiracitam. Phenobarbitone is used in newborns.

Most children with epilepsy attend normal school: it is important that teachers know how to recognize and deal with any seizure. Children should take part in most activities but may need extra supervision for swimming, and it may be wise to prevent them from doing activities such as fishing, rope or rock climbing, and canoeing. Some doctors forbid cycling in traffic if the child has had a seizure in the previous 2 years, though seizures are uncommon during concentrated activity.

 RESOURCE

The Epilepsy Society has a useful site. Go to **www.epilepsysociety.org.uk** and look at 'Children' under the A-Z of topics (**www.epilepsysociety.org.uk/AboutEpilepsy/A-Zoftopics**).

17.3 Conditions which may be mistaken for seizures

Many children have unusual periodic events as a result of other conditions (Table 17.1). A careful history from more than one observer should lead to an accurate diagnosis (Table 17.2).

17.3.1 Habit spasms (tics)

There may have been a reason for the movement initially – a twist of the neck in an uncomfortable collar, a forceful blink because of eyelid irritation – but the movement persists when the reason has gone. Reassurance that it is likely to improve with time, and a low-key supportive approach is usually all that is necessary.

Tics
- Repetitive
- Involuntary
- Stereotypic (the same each time)
- Often head and neck
- Not rhythmical
- Worse with stress
- Most frequent in boys aged 8–11 years.

Table 17.1 Other episodic events.

Age	Event
Age 1–4	Reflex anoxic seizures (brief cardiac asystole from vagal inhibition — pain)
	Breath-holding attacks
	Gastro-oesophageal reflux, writhing or back arching
Age 4–8	Benign paroxysmal vertigo
	Night terrors
Age 9–16	Faints
	Migraine
	Habit spasms (tics)
	Behavioural disorders — psychosomatic

Table 17.2 Features differentiating a seizure from a faint (syncope)

	Seizure	Faint
Age	Any	8–15 years
Timing	Day or night	Day
Situation	Commonly during inactivity	Standing (school assembly)
Prodrome	Brief (twitching, hallucinations, automatisms)	Long (dizziness, sweats, nausea)
Duration	Variable	Under 5 min
Tonic–clonic movement	Common	Rare
Colour change	May be cyanosis	Pallor
Injury (e.g. tongue-biting)	Common	Rare
Incontinent of urine	Common	Rare
After event	Drowsiness, confusion or headache Rarely partial paralysis	Quick full recovery Never paralysis

17.3.2 Breath-holding attacks

Breath-holding attacks are common but harmless; they occur in 1–2% of children up to 3 years, and are precipitated by frustration or pain. After one lusty yell the child holds his breath, goes red in the face, and may later become cyanosed and briefly lose consciousness. He then starts breathing again and is soon back to normal. Sometimes cerebral hypoxia is sufficient to cause brief generalized twitching, and the possibility of epilepsy may then be raised. A careful history will usually resolve any doubts. The attacks are benign and self-limiting, The parents require explanation and reassurance, and should ignore the attacks as far as possible. Distraction at the right moment may help.

17.4 Neurodermatoses (neurocutaneous syndromes)

Neurodermatoses are rare but important conditions that affect the skin and CNS. Diagnosis can be difficult and presentation is variable. Many of these are genetically determined and associated with learning difficulties. It is important to examine the skin of the child with fits, neurological or developmental problems. It is helpful to ask if 'birthmarks' run in the family.

The two most common conditions are both autosomal dominant. In neurofibromatosis (Figure 17.3) the café-au-lait skin lesions are typical. Children with tuberous sclerosis have seizures, developmental delay and skin lesions: depigmented *ash leaf*-shaped macules on the trunk and, later on, papules over the nose and face (*angiofibroma*); periventricular tubers (the white spots at the edges of the ventricles) are seen on CT (Figure 17.4).

The other condition to be aware of is *Sturge–Weber syndrome*, where there is a port wine stain (Section 24.1.1.2).

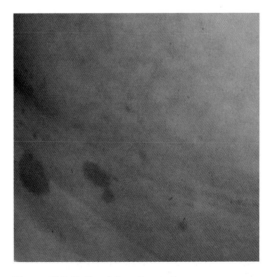

Figure 17.3 Café au lait spots seen in neurofibromatosis.

(a)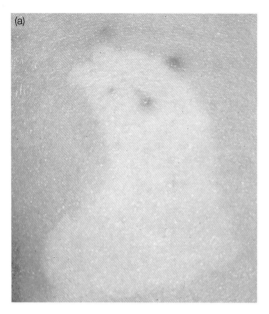

(b)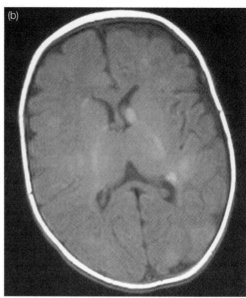

Figure 17.4 (a) Depigmented skin macule and (b) CT of tuberous sclerosis.

17.5 Infections and infection-related

17.5.1 Meningitis

A majority of meningitis occurs in the first 5 years of life (Table 17.3). The younger the child, the more difficult the diagnosis, and the greater the risk of residual brain damage. In infants, a delay of only hours in diagnosis can make the difference between complete and incomplete recovery. If meningitis is possible, you must perform a lumbar puncture, unless there is raised intracranial pressure (see below).

Always consider the *possibility* of meningitis in any sick child (see also Section 14.4.3.3).

In children, *meningism* (the classic signs of meningeal irritation) may not be present. Neck stiffness – a reluctance to flex the neck –may be demonstrated by encouraging the child to look at his feet or kiss his knee. Kernig's sign (with the child lying down, flex the hip and then extend the knee: spasm or pain in the hamstrings occurs with meningism)

is often present, but its absence does not exclude meningitis. Head retraction is a sign of advanced meningitis.

Meningism alone is not diagnostic of meningitis. It may be caused by otitis media, tonsillitis, cervical adenitis, arthritis of the cervical spine or pneumonia.

Table 17.3 Causes of meningitis		
1/3 Bacterial		**2/3 Viral**
Child	**Newborn**	**All ages**
Neisseria meningitidis (Gram -ve diplococcus)	Group B streptococcus	Enterovirus
Streptococcus pneumoniae (Gram +ve diplococcus)	Listeria	Adenovirus
Haemophilus influenzae (Gram -ve coccobacillus)	*Escherichia coli*	Epstein–Barr
Mycobacterium tuberculosis	Other coliforms	

Symptoms of meningitis are non-specific:

All ages
Fever
Vomiting
Drowsiness
Seizures

Infant
Fretfulness
High-pitched cry
Bulging fontanelle

Child
Headache
Photophobia
Neck stiffness.

17.5.1.1 Investigation

Prompt lumbar puncture is imperative. If there is raised intracranial pressure (see box), lumbar puncture is not performed because of risk of coning. A CT scan may be needed. Usually it is possible to differentiate between a viral meningitis and a bacterial meningitis from the CSF examination (Table 17.4). Recent antibiotics may make this difficult. CSF culture is key, while PCR amplification allows rapid testing for bacteria and viruses. If in doubt, it is usual to treat as if there is a bacterial pathogen. Faeces, CSF and throat swabs can be cultured for viruses, and in all cases blood culture should be performed.

The rare, but serious tuberculous meningitis (Section 14.4.3.3, p. 133) may present as a lymphocytic meningitis.

 PRACTICE POINT Signs of raised intracranial pressure

These can mean raised intracranial pressure:
• Papilloedema
• Altered level of consciousness
• ↑ blood pressure and ↓ pulse
• Full fontanelle
• Focal neurological signs, neck retraction.

17.5.1.2 Treatment

 PRACTICE POINT

The main causes of childhood meningitis are preventable by immunizations (see Section 14.2).

Children with bacterial meningitis are treated initially with intravenous antibiotics, using cefotaxime until cultures are available. This is combined with supportive and symptomatic therapy – antipyretics, analgesics or intravenous fluids. Improvement should occur within 36 h, and early treatment is usually associated with complete recovery. After meningococcal infection, antibiotics are given to contacts to prevent carriage (Section 14.4.3.3, p. 133). Viral meningitis is treated symptomatically.

17.5.1.3 Outcome

Bacterial meningitis is a serious condition: 5–10% of children die and 10% of survivors incur permanent brain damage resulting in deafness, cerebral palsy, hydrocephalus or epilepsy. Recurrent meningitis is rare and should provoke a close search for a dermal sinus: a small defect connecting the skin and the meninges.

Viral meningitis has a much better prognosis; complete recovery is usual. Paralyses resulting from *poliomyelitis*, or deafness from *mumps meningitis* is hardly ever seen in the immunized population.

17.5.2 Encephalitis

Encephalitis (inflammation of the brain) causes cerebral symptoms (e.g. fits and drowsiness) and neurological signs. Meningism is variable. The CSF usually has raised protein and/or lymphocytes. Most cases are viral and mild, but occasionally it is severe and brain damage results from demyelination. The more severe form in childhood is acute disseminated encephalomyelitis (*post-infectious encephalitis*)

Table 17.4 Characteristics of CSF in infants and children

	Normal	Viral meningitis	Bacterial meningitis
Appearance	Clear	Clear or hazy	Cloudy or purulent
Cells (×10⁶/L)	0–4	20–1000	500–5000
Type	Lymphocytes	Lymphocytes	Neutrophils
Protein (g/L)	0.2–0.4	↑	↑↑
Glucose (mmol/L)	3–6	Normal	↓

usually occurring about a week after infection, e.g. chicken pox. Encephalitis very rarely follows immunization (pertussis, measles); the risk is many times smaller than with the corresponding infection.

Herpes simplex encephalitis produces a wide variety of neurological symptoms and is one of the most serious encephalitides. PCR, CT scan or MRI of the CSF together with serology may be diagnostic. In suspected encephalitis, give aciclovir while awaiting results. Intensive care is often needed. Around half the children acquire brain damage or die.

Chronic encephalitis may occur with HIV or following measles (*subacute sclerosing panencephalitis, SSPE*).

17.5.3 Acute post-infectious polyneuropathy (Guillain–Barré)

This is an uncommon condition, which follows acute infections. Ascending paralysis starts in the legs and moves up the body over 2–4 weeks. The symmetrical peripheral neuritis leads to motor loss, sensory loss and absent tendon reflexes. If bulbar or respiratory muscles are involved, intensive care and ventilatory support are needed. Nearly all children recover fully, though this may take months. The CSF is either normal or shows a high protein but normal cell count, and nerve conduction is abnormal.

17.5.4 Bell's palsy

The most common cranial nerve lesion is unilateral, post-infectious facial nerve (Bell's) palsy (Figure 17.5). It is a lower motor neurone lesion with sparing of the forehead muscles. The eye needs to be protected as it does not close, and most cases will resolve spontaneously over a few weeks. Early treatment with steroids may be beneficial.

17.6 Hydrocephalus

In hydrocephalus, excess CSF results in accelerated head enlargement (Figure 17.6). It arises from obstruction of the normal CSF circulation either as a result of congenital abnormality (e.g. aqueduct stenosis) or from postnatal causes (e.g. meningitis, intracranial haemorrhage or tumour). Congenital neurological abnormalities are often associated with hydrocephalus (e.g. spina bifida). As the CSF accumulates under pressure the head enlarges rapidly, the skull sutures separate, the anterior fontanelle is full and the scalp veins appear prominent. The eyes turn downward (*setting sun sign*). The large head is the most common

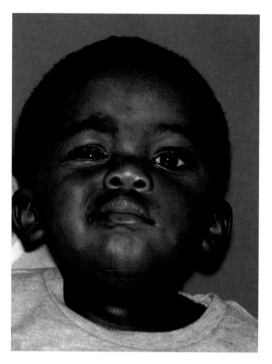

Figure 17.5 This boy has a left-sided facial palsy.

presentation, although the most common cause of a big head is having parents with big heads. The rate of skull expansion is very important (Figure 17.6). In the older child whose skull sutures are united, obstruction to CSF pathways causes headache, vomiting and other symptoms of raised intracranial pressure.

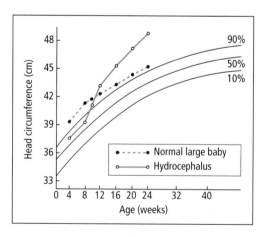

Figure 17.6 The head circumference of a normal large baby increases at a rate parallel to the centile lines; in the child with hydrocephalus, head circumference increases at an abnormal rate.

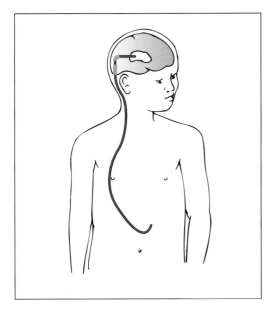

Figure 17.7 If hydrocephalus is progressive, CSF can be drained from the lateral ventricle to the peritoneal cavity. The ventriculo-peritoneal shunt is tunnelled under the skin, and can be felt behind the ear.

Prompt surgical treatment is often needed. The obstruction is relieved by inserting a ventriculo-peritoneal shunt. Depending on the cause of the obstruction and the success of treatment, normal brain development and function is possible. Low grade infection and other technical problems are important complications of shunt insertion (Figure 17.7).

17.7 Neural tube defects (spinal dysraphism)

17.7.1 Spina bifida

Spina bifida is less common due to:

- Improved nutrition
- Increased folic acid intake
- Prenatal diagnosis.

Spina bifida is due to failure of closure of the posterior neuropore, which normally occurs around the 27th day of embryonic life.

The most common and most severe form is a *meningomyelocele* (myelocele) in which elements of the spinal cord and nerve roots are involved. It may occur at any spinal level, but the usual site is the lumbar region.

The baby is born with a raw swelling over the spine in which the malformed spinal cord is exposed.

It is often associated with hydrocephalus, particularly as a result of the *Arnold–Chiari malformation* where the cerebellar tonsils protrude into the foramen magnum, blocking flow of CSF from the 4th ventricle.

 Meningomyelocele

- Legs – paralysis with sensory loss below the level of the lesion. Hip dislocation and leg deformities (club foot).
- Head – hydrocephalus with learning problems.
- Bladder – neuropathic bladder with incontinence, recurrent urinary tract infections, renal damage.
- Anus – faecal incontinence.

The emotional and social problems for the child and family are considerable, varying from the frequent hospital admissions and attendances to the problems of providing suitable education for a paraplegic, incontinent child. Children with this condition need the care of a large multidisciplinary team. Fetal detection usually leads to termination of pregnancy.

17.7.2 Meningocele

This is rare and less serious. The swelling over the lower back is covered by skin and contains no neural tissue. Cosmetic surgery is not urgent.

17.7.3 Encephalocele

Encephaloceles are protrusions of brain through the skull, covered by skin, usually in the occipital region. They are often associated with severe brain abnormality.

17.7.4 Spina bifida occulta

Minor defects of the posterior arches of the lower lumbar vertebrae are common and do not matter at all. Sacral dimples in the natal cleft are normal. Intraspinal pathology is rare but slightly more likely if there are external 'markers' in the lumbar region (hairy tuft, naevus, lipoma). The main concern is tethering of the spinal cord, which may result in traction on the cord as the child grows.

17.8 Cerebral palsy

 A disorder of posture and movement resulting from a non-progressive lesion of the developing brain.

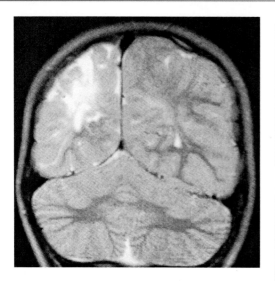

Figure 17.8 This brain MRI shows a neonatal stroke which led to a hemiplegic cerebral palsy.

Incidence is 2 in 1000. The basic pathology may be a developmental abnormality, pre- or postnatal brain infection, physical or chemical injury to the brain, or a vascular accident (Figure 17.8). The brain lesion is fixed and non-progressive, but the clinical picture changes with CNS maturation. A hypotonic neonate may become hypertonic during the first year of life.

Presentation varies according to severity. In the severe cases, poor sucking or altered muscle tone is present soon after birth. More often cerebral palsy is suspected during the first 2 years. Follow-up surveillance of high risk newborns (e.g. extreme preterm delivery, birth asphyxia) aims to allow earlier detection and intervention.

Causes of cerebral palsy

Prenatal
    70% primary brain malformation; congenital viral infection (Section 8.4.4)
Perinatal
    15% birth asphyxia; trauma; stroke
Postnatal
    15% intraventricular haemorrhage and periventricular leukomalacia (preterm); meningitis; trauma; metabolic.

 PRACTICE POINT

CP presents with:

- Delayed motor development
- Gait problems
- Feeding difficulties
- Hand preference in infancy
- Abnormal movements.

These presentations also have many other potential causes.

17.8.1   Classification (Figure 17.9)

Terminology in cerebral palsy

Diplegia. Predominant involvement of the legs, though the arms may also be affected.
Quadriplegia. Involvement of all four limbs.
Hemiplegia. Involvement of one arm and one leg on the same side (Figure 17.10).

Cerebral palsy covers a very broad spectrum of disability, ranging from problems playing football to complete dependency. Classification across axes (including

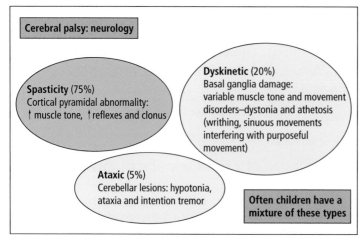

Figure 17.9 Neurology of cerebral palsy.

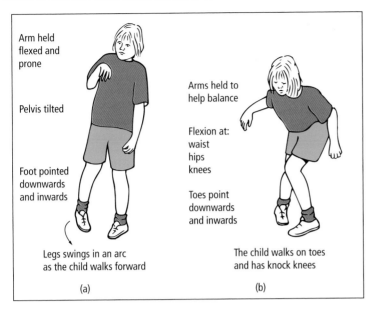

Arm held
flexed and
prone

Pelvis tilted

Foot pointed
downwards
and inwards

Legs swings in an arc
as the child walks forward

(a)

Arms held to
help balance

Flexion at:
waist
hips
knees

Toes point
downwards
and inwards

The child walks on toes
and has knock knees

(b)

Figure 17.10 Abnormal gaits in children with (a) hemiplegia and (b) diplegia.

pattern, severity, disability, associated problems, and cause) assist care and support of the individual child.

17.8.2 Management

Early comprehensive assessment and where necessary investigation is essential because:

- Other disability is common: learning difficulties, epilepsy, defects of vision and hearing, behavioural problems.
- Disordered posture and movement can lead to permanent deformities.
- Cerebral palsy can present major problems at home and at school.

Assessment, family support and therapy are organized by the multidisciplinary team in the *Child Development Centre*. Early physiotherapy (and sometimes botulinum toxin injections) aims to establish a normal pattern of movement and to prevent deformity. Orthopaedic surgery may correct deformity to improve function. Speech therapy is needed for feeding and speech. The team also includes occupational therapist (aids, wheelchairs), educational psychologist, health visitor/social worker. Usually the community paediatrician takes a leading role.

17.8.3 Prognosis

This depends mainly on the pattern and severity of CP, associated handicaps, and in particular on the intelligence of the child. With normal intelligence, the problems of even severe motor handicaps may be overcome.

The quality of the management itself affects the prognosis. A severely affected child may require education in a special school where expert physiotherapy, occupational therapy, teaching and other facilities are available.

Children less severely affected, often those with hemiplegia, manage at normal school. The least severely affected of all do not always reach the specialist. Their clumsiness or educational problems may not be recognized as mild cerebral palsy.

17.9 Headaches

 If headache wakes the child at night, is present on waking or worse in the early morning, this may mean raised intracranial pressure. Brain imaging may be needed.

Headaches are a common outpatient symptom but are unusual in younger children.

> **PRACTICE POINT Causes of headaches**
>
> - Stress/tension
> - Migraine
> - Eye strain
> - Dental problems
> - Sinusitis
> - Space occupying lesion

17.9.1 Stress headaches

- Common
- Daytime
- Not present on waking
- Timing relates to stress (school, etc.)
- Frontal
- No associated symptoms.

17.9.2 Migraine

Migraine is classically unilateral, the headaches are throbbing in nature and associated with nausea or vomiting and photophobia; a visual aura is much less common in children than in adults with migraine. Migraine sometimes results from sensitivity to food (chocolate, cheese) or food additives. It is unusual to diagnose migraine in the absence of a family history.

17.10 Space-occupying lesions

Symptoms vary greatly in pattern, severity and timing. Headache, misery and irritability are common early symptoms and are followed by unsteadiness, vomiting and visual disturbances. Fits may occur.

> **Space-occupying lesions**
>
> - **Neoplasm**
> - **Subdural haematoma**
>   - Accidents
>   Non-accidental injury, shaking (Section 15.2.1)
> - **Cerebral abscess**
>   - Meningitis
>   - Infected emboli (Section 20.5.4.1)
>   - Chronic otitis media.

> **PRACTICE POINT**
>
> If a space-occupying lesion is suspected, CT or MR brain imaging must be carried out promptly (Section 26.3).

Focal seizures or signs should always make you think of a space-occupying lesion. Management demands a multidisciplinary approach including: paediatrics, neurology, radiology, neurosurgery.

17.10.1 Abnormal head shape Craniosynostosis (craniostenosis)

Premature fusion of one or more of the skull sutures results in an unusual-shaped head and may compress the brain or cranial nerves. The prognosis depends upon which sutures are affected. Premature fusion of all sutures results in a bulging forehead, proptosis and brain compression, and requires surgery. Syntostosis of a single suture may require surgery for cosmetic reasons. The cause is unknown. Sometimes there is a hereditary factor with associated skeletal abnormalities.

17.10.1.1 Plagiocephaly and skull flattening

Natural skull asymmetry is common in early infancy, but the sutures and fontanelles are normal. In the more obvious plagiocephaly, one side of the forehead and occiput are displaced forward (Figure 17.11). The asymmetry becomes less with growth and does not cause problems. There may be associated chest asymmetry.

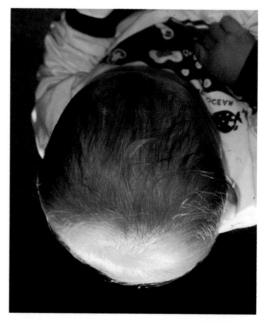

Figure 17.11 Plagiocephaly. The left forehead is more prominent than the right, while the left occiput is flattened.

Flattened occiput is common in infants nursed on their backs and resolves with time. Head shaping helmets preserve shape but have no medical benefit.

17.11 Progressive neuromuscular disorders

Among the most distressing disorders of childhood are those that strike a previously healthy child and progress inexorably towards incapacity and death over months or, more often, years. They may affect principally the brain, the spinal cord or the muscles; many are genetically determined and few are open to effective treatment. Onset is usually in the first 2 years; in general, the earlier the onset, the more rapid the progress.

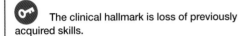 The clinical hallmark is loss of previously acquired skills.

Progressive brain degeneration conditions are often due to autosomal recessive genes (Section 5.2.1). They can be grouped into those that affect the grey matter (e.g. the *lipidoses* such as *Tay–Sachs disease*) and those that affect the white matter (*leucodystrophies*).

17.11.1 Spinal muscular atrophies

- Autosomal recessive
- Proximal muscle weakness
- Tongue fasciculation
- Normal facial movement
- Variable age of onset and progression.

The infantile form (*Werdnig–Hoffmann disease*) is evident from birth and progresses to death within a year or so; forms with later onset progress more slowly. Those with a condition with onset in late childhood enjoy a reasonably active adult life.

17.11.2 Myopathies (muscular dystrophies)

The muscular dystrophies vary in their age of onset, rate of progress and mode of inheritance.

17.11.2.1 Duchenne muscular dystrophy

This is the most common type of muscular dystrophy. It only affects boys because it is due to an X-linked recessive gene. The genetic abnormality is a deletion in the gene for dystrophin, a protein essential for muscle function. The condition presents at 1–6 years with difficulty walking, an abnormal waddling gait or difficulty climbing stairs. Affected boys develop enlargement of the calves due to fatty infiltration (*pseudohypertrophy*) with absent knee jerks. There is often marked lumbar lordosis.

The ability to walk is lost at about the age of 10 years, and death occurs in early adulthood due to pneumonia or myocardial involvement. A proportion have intellectual impairment. A grossly elevated serum creatine phosphokinase level is present, and genetic testing is diagnostic.

> In Duchenne dystrophy, boys asked to stand up from sitting on the floor turn over onto all fours, and then 'climb up their legs'. This is *Gower's sign* (Figure 3.11).

There is no cure for the dystrophies and therapy is supportive: physiotherapy, prevent deformity, maintain mobility. Obesity is to be avoided. Clinical and genetic diagnosis allows genetic counselling and antenatal diagnosis in future pregnancies. Research focuses on gene therapy or modulation.

In a milder form of pseudohypertrophic muscular dystrophy (*Becker*), symptoms develop later and disability is mild.

17.11.3 Other progressive disorders

17.11.3.1 Rett syndrome

- Severe mental and physical handicap in girls
- Normal early development
- Slow psychomotor development by 1 year
- Loss of manipulative skills and speech
- Repetitive hand movements, e.g. hand wringing.

Many progressive neuromuscular diseases of adult life have their onset in childhood. Examples are *myotonic dystrophy* (which may be lethal in the newborn) and *Friedreich's ataxia*.

17.12 The floppy infant

Degrees of infantile hypotonia are common and usually resolve with maturation. Infants present with poor head control, floppiness or feeding problems. In severe hypotonia there is paucity of movement and respiratory problems.

> When picked up under the arms the baby tends to slip from one's grasp. In ventral suspension, the baby flops like a rag doll.

Floppy infants fall into two main groups.

17.12.1   Benign hypotonia

Temporary floppiness characterized by gradual improvement over months. There may be a helpful family history.

17.12.2   Paralytic with weakness

Severe weakness accompanies hypotonia in conditions due to spinal or muscular disease. These infants make few movements and may be unable to raise their arm upwards against gravity. It can be caused by a number of rare neuromuscular or spinal cord disorders (e.g. spinal muscular atrophy, see above).

17.12.3   Non-paralytic without weakness

Hypotonia with mild weakness. Possible causes include:

- Severe/neurodevelopmental delay
- Cerebral palsy - children with spasticity are initially floppy
- Certain syndromes - Down, Prader–Willi (obesity, hypotonia, hypogonadism)
- Systemic disorders - malnutrition, rickets, hypothyroidism.

 ## Summary

Neurological problems in a developing fetus, infant or child may have lifelong consequences. You should know about fits, cerebral palsy and meningitis, and understand a little about the wide spectrum of neurological disorders. All are very worrying for the child and her family: while many resolve, a few are progressive and even lethal. For more severe conditions, the key is early detection, accurate diagnosis, and access for the child and family to the multidisciplinary team.

 FOR YOUR LOG

- Febrile fits are a common cause for admission to see when you are on call.
- Talk to a child or family who have had fits or have epilepsy.
- Visit the Child Development Centre or community based neurodisability team.
- Attend a multidisciplinary meeting.
- Ask to visit a child with cerebral palsy at home during your GP attachment.

? OSCE TIP

- 'Tommy was admitted with a febrile fit last night. He now appears well. Please talk to his mother about febrile fits.'
- Function, tone, power and reflexes in the lower limbs (see OSCE station 16.1).
- Manikin: management of the fitting child.
- Video: recognize epileptic seizures and non-epileptic events.
- Results of a lumbar puncture.
- Cerebral palsy: assess gait, type of cerebral palsy, limb distribution.
- Examine gait, coordination, cognitive function.

See EMQ 17.1, EMQ 17.2, EMQ 17.3, and EMQ 17.4 at the end of the book.

OSCE station 17.1: Neurological examination of the legs

Clinical approach:

- Observe for other neurological or neurodevelopmental problems
- Is the child generally alert and aware?
- Is she behaving as you would expect?

Gait
- Ask mother/child if happy to walk
- Best to observe in underwear, no shoes
- Observe for:
  ◦ Which part of foot strikes floor
  ◦ Right and left leg movements
  ◦ Symmetry
  ◦ Position of rest of body

Inspection
- Muscle wasting
- Muscle hypertrophy
- Asymmetry
- Limb shortening
- Scars (e.g. lumbosacral, lengthening of TAs)

Tone
- Assess tone at hips, knees, and ankles
- Don't forget hip adductors and plantarflexors
- Clonus

Power
- What does gait and movement tell you?
- Power at hip, knee and ankle

Reflexes
- Knee jerks — if absent try reinforcement
- Ankle jerks
- Plantar response

Beth has difficulty walking. She is 4 years old. Please examine her legs for tone and power walks with:
- Flexed knees and hips
- Inturned feet
- Toe stepping
- No heel strike

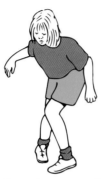

No marks or scars on back

tone ↑ in legs especially:
- Hip adductors
- → scissoring
- Plantar flexors
- → Toe pointing

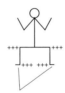

Sustained clonus

Beth has spastic cerebral palsy. When legs are affected more than arms, this is a diplegia.

Never forget:

- Say hello and introduce yourself
- General health
- Colour — ?pale/?cyanosed
- Quickly assess growth, nutrition and development
- Mention the obvious (e.g. drip, leg in plaster)

Look around for:

- Shoes — Piedro boots
- Look at soles of shoes for pattern of wear
- Ankle–foot orthoses
- Walking aids
- Evidence of urinary or faecal problems

Special points

- If the child is willing/able, begin by asking the child to walk, and then to sit on the floor and get up, **then** use the tendon hammer
- Use MRC classification of power if you wish but you do not need to
- Show children what you want them to do or give simple explanations

18

Ear, nose and throat

Chapter map

ENT problems are very common in children. The upper respiratory tract is the most common site of infection in the young child, and assessment of acute illness is not complete without examination of the ears, nose and throat (Section 3.5.2). Chronic disorders are important causes of long-term morbidity. The early diagnosis of sensorineural and conductive hearing loss is essential if educational and social effects are to be minimized (Section 10.4.5). Often more serious or chronic disorders are managed together with a paediatric ENT surgeon.

> Children are now vaccinated against *Streptococcus pneumoniae* and *Haemophilus influenzae*: two important causes of ENT infection.

18.1   Ear problems

18.1.1   Otitis media

Acute otitis media is common throughout the first 8 years. In the older child, the cardinal symptom, ear ache, makes detection easy; in infants it may not be so obvious. They usually have high fever and are irritable, rolling their heads from side to side, or rubbing their ears. Initially there is mild inflammation of the pars flaccida (the superior part of the tympanic membrane) with dilated vessels running down the handle of the malleus, and an absent light reflex. This progresses to a red, bulging, painful tympanic membrane, perforation and discharge of pus. A mildly pink dull drum may be present in any URTI.

A majority of otitis media is viral, but distinction from bacterial infection is difficult. The evidence indicates that simple analgesia is all that is needed in most cases, but antibiotics (amoxicillin) should be given if the child is very unwell, vulnerable (e.g. through immunosuppression or prematurity) or if symptoms persist for more than 4 days. Paracetamol is invaluable for the fever and pain. Persistent aural discharge (chronic suppurative otitis media) is a potential complication. To prevent further episodes, ensure pneumococcal immunizations are up to date, and avoid passive smoking, dummies (pacifiers), and supine feeding.

> **Rare important complications**
>
> - Mastoiditis
> - Lateral sinus thrombosis
> - Meningitis
> - Cerebral abscess.

Paediatrics Lecture Notes, Ninth edition. Simon J. Newell and Jonathan C. Darling. © 2014 John Wiley & Sons, Ltd. Published 2014 by John Wiley & Sons, Ltd.

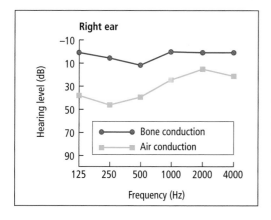

Figure 18.1 Audiogram: this child has right, moderate, conductive hearing loss.

Figure 18.3 The drum is dull and retracted in otitis media with effusion.

18.1.2 Otitis media with effusion (glue ear, secretory otitis media)

Glue ear is the most common cause of conductive hearing loss below the age of 10 years (Figures 18.1, 18.2 and 18.3). Sticky, serous material accumulates in the middle ear insidiously or after acute otitis media. The symptoms are deafness, speech delay, and older children may report a feeling of fullness or popping in the ear. It is especially common in children who have atopy, frequent upper respiratory infections or cleft palate. The eardrum is usually dull and retracted, and a fluid level may be seen. The malleus handle is more horizontal and appears shorter, broader and whiter. Antibiotics, antihistamines and decongestants may be tried. If there is significant deafness, an indwelling tube (*grommet*) is inserted through the eardrum to aerate the middle ear and is left for 6–12 months.

Hearing impairment is covered in Section 10.4.5.

18.2 Nose and sinuses

18.2.1 Sinusitis

The frontal and sphenoidal sinuses do not develop until 5 and 9 years, respectively. The maxillary and ethmoidal sinuses are small in these years and sinusitis is uncommon before the age of 5.

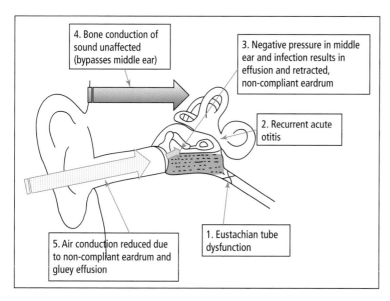

4. Bone conduction of sound unaffected (bypasses middle ear)

3. Negative pressure in middle ear and infection results in effusion and retracted, non-compliant eardrum

2. Recurrent acute otitis

1. Eustachian tube dysfunction

5. Air conduction reduced due to non-compliant eardrum and gluey effusion

Figure 18.2 Otitis media with effusion.

18.2.2 Allergic rhinitis

Recurrent bouts of sneezing, a persistent watery nasal discharge and watering eyes are typically worse outside in bright sunshine. The nasal mucosa is pale and oedematous. Hay fever is allergic rhinitis in late spring and early summer in response to grass pollen.

> **TREATMENT**
>
> If you are giving antihistamines, use non-sedating medication. You may need to warn teenagers about alcohol and sedation.

Other allergens include dust, animal dander and moulds. A careful history is more likely to identify the allergen than allergy tests. Nose and eye drops are useful. Therapeutic success with antihistamines and topical steroids is variable.

18.2.3 Epistaxis

Nose bleeds usually originate from the anterior inferior corner of the nasal septum (Little's area). Common causes are minor injury and URTIs. Children may alarm everyone by vomiting blood which they have swallowed. First aid consists of sitting the child up and squeezing the nose firmly, whilst the child is comforted and told to breathe through the mouth.

18.3 Throat

18.3.1 Tonsils and adenoids

Lymphoid tissue grows rapidly in the first 5 years of life. Tonsils and adenoids are usually small in infants and reach their greatest relative size between 4 and 7 years.

> Examine a young child's neck carefully, and you will find palpable lymph glands. Learn what normal glands feel like (Section 3.5.1, p. 32), so you will recognize enlargement due to infection.

18.3.1.1 Acute tonsillitis

This is very common in the age group 2–8 years but uncommon in infants. There is sudden onset of fever, sore throat and dysphagia. Vomiting and abdominal pains are common. The tonsils are enlarged and fiery red; white exudate appears in the tonsillar glands.

> **Rare important complications**
>
> **Immediate**
> - *Peritonsillar abscess (quinsy)*: severe symptoms of tonsillitis and dysphagia. The tonsil is displaced towards the midline. If suspected, refer to ENT that day.
> - *Cervical abscess*: infection localizes in a cervical lymph gland
>
> **Delayed**
> - *Acute nephritis* (Section 22.4.2): 2–3 weeks later
> - *Rheumatic fever* (Section 23.3.6): 1–2 weeks later.

Tender cervical lymphadenopathy is usual. Viral and bacterial tonsillitis cannot be distinguished clinically. The most common bacterial pathogen (30–40%) is β-haemolytic streptococcus. Infectious mononucleosis is associated with nasty tonsillitis in older children.

Paracetamol, cool drinks, and local anaesthetic throat spray can provide symptomatic relief. Don't routinely prescribe antibiotics. For persistent or severe symptoms, penicillin may be used to eradicate streptococci and reduce the risk of complications.

> **Cervical lymphadenopathy: differential diagnosis**
>
> - Reactive (e.g. tonsillitis) – vastly more common than any other cause
> - TB
> - Malignancy (lymphoma, leukaemia) – glands craggy, hard, tethered
> - Other infections (e.g. glandular fever, rubella, atypical mycobacteria, toxoplasma).

Cervical glands with recurrent tonsillitis are usually bilateral, fairly soft and mobile, and only rarely form a localized abscess. In most school-age children, some cervical nodes are palpable.

18.3.1.2 Obstructive sleep apnoea

In rare cases, enlargement of the tonsils or adenoidal tissue causes upper airway obstruction. This leads to difficulty in breathing, with loud snoring and a disturbed abnormal pattern of breathing during sleep. The result of disturbed sleep is tiredness during the day and behavioural problems. In severe cases, poor growth and development and a wide variety of symptoms are seen, and occasionally the nocturnal hypoxia may lead to pulmonary hypertension. Recognition is important: ask about snoring, and consider overnight pulse oximetry. Tonsillectomy/adenoidectomy gives good results.

18.3.1.3 Adenotonsillectomy

Indications

- Mastoiditis
- Recurrent/persistent tonsillitis (>3 attacks a year)
- Obstructive sleep apnoea
- Recurrent otitis media.

Tonsillectomy is not performed to prevent children catching colds, sore throats or bronchitis: it does not improve the child's appetite or growth. In the right children, results are very good.

18.3.2 Stridor

In young children, the larynx is small with walls that are flabby compared with the firm, cartilaginous adult larynx. It is a voice bag, not a voice box, and it collapses and obstructs easily.

 Stridor is mainly inspiratory, and is the noise made with upper airway obstruction, usually in the larynx.

18.3.2.1 Congenital stridor

Stridor caused by abnormalities of the pharynx, larynx or trachea may be audible from birth. The least rare form, 'congenital laryngeal stridor' (laryngomalacia), is due to floppy aryepiglottic folds. It does not cause serious obstruction and gradually disappears as the laryngeal cartilage becomes firmer during the first year of life. If it is severe enough to cause intercostal and suprasternal recession, or feeding problems, or if there is no improvement in the first weeks, laryngoscopy is advisable.

18.3.2.2 Acute stridor

In young children, especially infants and toddlers, stridor can progress to serious respiratory obstruction with alarming rapidity. If in doubt, admit. The main causes of acute stridor are:

1. Acute laryngotracheitis
2. Foreign body in the larynx (Section 19.5.4)
3. Epiglottitis.

 PRACTICE POINT

In acute stridor with respiratory distress, do not examine the throat: you may precipitate complete airway obstruction.

18.3.2.3 Acute laryngotracheitis (croup)

This is common, often mild, but sometimes alarming and potentially dangerous. Onset is sudden, often at night, with stridor, harsh cry and a barking cough (croup). Mild cases, with no stridor at rest, can be managed at home. Admit more severe cases, and those under 6 months, or distant from hospital. If obstruction is marked, there may be intercostal and suprasternal recession in addition to stridor. Children are treated with oral or nebulized steroids (unless symptoms are very mild). If there are more severe symptoms, nebulized adrenaline provides temporary relief.

Croup

- Age 1–4 years
- Mild/moderate systemic illness
- Viral infection
- Associated URTI
- Intubation rarely needed.

Antibiotics are not needed. Cold humidity gives symptomatic relief. Intravenous fluids may be needed; inhaled steroids may help. In severe cases, children should be monitored carefully. Fewer than 5% of children in hospital require intubation. If you think airway obstruction may be imminent, experts who can intubate are needed.

18.3.2.4 Epiglottitis

This life-threatening disease is prevented by immunization against *Haemophilus influenzae* (Chapter 14). This child with stridor is acutely ill and feverish, with a muffled cough. In this serious emergency, the child's airway is in grave danger of complete obstruction: she sits up, drooling because swallowing is difficult. At intubation, the swollen epiglottis may be seen like a cherry. Associated septicaemia is common, and prompt antibiotic and supportive treatment are essential.

✔ Summary

Acute ENT infection is a common cause of presentation to primary care and hospital, so it is important to look for it in any child with a fever. Most infections are viral and do not need antibiotic treatment unless severe, persisting for several days or unusual. Beware of the child with stridor, especially if you suspect epi-glottitis.

OSCE TIP

• Examine ENT.
• Manikin: examine ears and make diagnosis of otitis media, etc.

See EMQ 18.1 at the end of the book.

FOR YOUR LOG

• Examine ears and throat in young children as far as you are able without causing upset. Remember correct positioning is important, and you can always practice this. You can also practice on a manikin.
• Palpate cervical lymph nodes routinely when you examine children.

19

Respiratory medicine

Chapter map

Respiratory infections and asthma are major causes of morbidity and are common reasons for a child being taken to a doctor or admitted to hospital. Certain problems are more common at certain ages, and the same organism may cause different illnesses at different ages (e.g. respiratory syncytial virus (RSV) causes bronchiolitis in infants, and a cold or a sore throat in older children). Cystic fibrosis is one of the commonest life threatening genetically inherited conditions in the Caucasian population. Early recognition and careful paediatric management greatly improves outcome.

19.1 Symptoms of respiratory tract disease

Cough in children is usually an upper respiratory tract infection (URTI) and less often lung disease. A barking cough suggests a laryngeal or tracheal disorder, usually croup (see Table 19.1). Young asthmatics may cough instead of wheeze, especially at night. Children usually swallow their sputum unless it is copious. Purulent and blood-stained sputum are rare. Ear ache (manifested by pulling at the ear in young children) suggests acute otitis media, although remember that pain from lower back teeth may be referred to the ear.

Paediatrics Lecture Notes, Ninth edition. Simon J. Newell and Jonathan C. Darling. © 2014 John Wiley & Sons, Ltd. Published 2014 by John Wiley & Sons, Ltd.

Table 19.1   **Respiratory symptoms and their causes**

Symptom	Causes	Character
Cough	Croup	Barking
	URTI	Throaty
	Asthma	Worse at night
	Pneumonia	Productive of phlegm (but children usually swallow this)
	Bronchiolitis	RSV cough unpleasant with characteristic 'wet' sound
	Pertussis	Paroyxysms of coughing, ending with inspiratory 'whoop', persists many days
Shortness of breath	Asthma	
	Pneumonia	
	Bronchiolitis	
Noisy breathing		
Stridor (*a monophonic noise arising from the upper airway, usually inspiratory*)	Croup	Accompanied by barking cough
	Foreign body	History of inhalation or choking?
	Epiglottitis	Muffled cough, drooling, high temperature
		Rare since Hib vaccine
		If suspected, don't examine throat
Wheeze (*a polyphonic musical noise arising from the bronchi/ bronchioles, usually more expiratory than inspiratory*)	Asthma	Widespread
	Pneumonia	Focal
	Inhaled foreign body	Focal
	Bronchiolitis	Widespread, with inspiratory crackles in under-2s
Snuffles/nasal obstruction	URTI	
Ruttles/rattles	Mucus 'rattling' in large airways	

Respiratory distress and failure

Recognition of severe respiratory disease is essential. Intervene before respiratory distress leads to respiratory failure.

Respiratory distress (increased work of breathing)

- Tachypnoea (>50/min infants; >40/min in children)
- Intercostal/subcostal recession
- Use of accessory muscles (arms and shoulders)
- Expiratory grunting, nasal flaring and 'head-bobbing' in infants

Respiratory failure (respiratory effort insufficient or unsustainable)

- Severe respiratory distress or
- Diminished respiratory effort, apnoea
- CNS signs of hypoxia: agitation; fatigue; drowsiness
- Cyanosis
- Collapse.

19.2   Upper respiratory tract

Most illnesses of childhood are infections; most childhood infections are respiratory; most are URTI (Table 19.2). The incidence and type of respiratory infections varies with age (Figure 19.1).

PRACTICE POINT

Don't forget to examine the ears, nose and throat in febrile children – unless you suspect epiglottitis (see Section 18.3.2.4)!

In the infant, nasal obstruction due to the common cold may lead to feeding difficulties. Saline drops and gentle suction can remove obstructing mucus plugs from the nostrils, but decongestant drops should be

Table 19.2 **Upper respiratory tract infection (URTI)**		
Infection	**Description**	**Causes**
	All may cause fever, vomiting and anorexia	*The great majority are viral*
Common cold	Cough, rhinitis, sneeze	Viral
Tonsillitis	Enlarged, inflamed tonsils, +/- exudate	Viral or bacterial
Pharyngitis	Inflamed throat	Viral or bacterial
Acute otitis media	Ear ache, inflamed and bulging tympanic membrane	Viral or bacterial

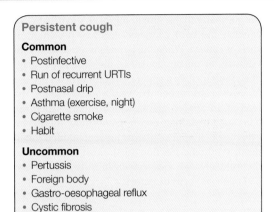

Persistent cough

Common
- Postinfective
- Run of recurrent URTIs
- Postnasal drip
- Asthma (exercise, night)
- Cigarette smoke
- Habit

Uncommon
- Pertussis
- Foreign body
- Gastro-oesophageal reflux
- Cystic fibrosis
- Tuberculosis
- Immune deficiency.

avoided. Eustachian tube obstruction often causes ear ache and the eardrums may appear congested. Antibiotics are not indicated. Paracetamol will reduce fever and relieve discomfort.

URTI may precipitate febrile convulsions (Section 17.1.1) and asthma attacks, and is sometimes the precursor of acute specific fevers, especially measles (Table 14.3) or bronchiolitis.

19.2.1 Recurrent coughs and colds

Recurrent coughs and colds, sometimes with sore throat and ear ache, are very common in young children, particularly if they have older school-age siblings, or mix with other children in a nursery. Some babies and toddlers are catarrhal much of the time. The first winter at school or nursery is frequently punctuated by upper respiratory infections.

Poor social circumstances and passive smoking predispose to catarrh. Some children will not blow their noses; some with severe nasal obstruction cannot. Aromatic inhalations and rubs can be useful in older children, but should be avoided in young infants, particularly under 3 months. Decongestants and cough suppressants are not recommended. The best healer is the passage of time.

19.3 Apnoea

Temporary cessation of breathing is a frightening occurrence. It can result from central respiratory depression or from mechanical obstruction (including the inhalation of food or vomit). It may occur during the first day or two of respiratory infections, particularly pertussis or RSV. However, many infants are rushed to hospital by their parents, who believe their child has stopped breathing. Often it is not clear whether anxious parents have merely misinterpreted

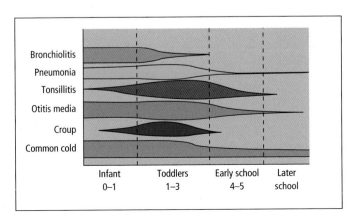

Figure 19.1 Incidence of respiratory infections.

the normal variable breathing of a small baby, or whether the baby genuinely has had a significant spell of apnoea. When the apnoea is associated with cyanosis, or unconsciousness, the differential diagnosis must include a seizure, congenital heart disease or airways obstruction. For very worried parents, the loan of an apnoea alarm, which sounds when the baby stops breathing, may be comforting. There is no evidence that apnoea alarms prevent sudden infant death syndrome (Section 15.3). Most children who die suddenly and unexpectedly in early life have not had previous spells of apnoea.

19.4 Influenza

Influenza tends to occur in epidemics, affecting particularly school children and young adults. The general symptoms of high fever, headache and malaise tend to overshadow the dry cough and sore throat, though there may be signs of pharyngitis, tracheitis or bronchitis. The main complications result from secondary bacterial infection of lungs, middle ear or sinuses. The brief incubation period and high infectivity favour massive outbreaks. Immunization against more common strains is given to children at risk of severe infection. Treatment is usually symptomatic. Antiviral agents may be considered in severe disease, or in at-risk children (e.g. chronic respiratory disease) presenting with milder illness during epidemics.

19.5 Lower respiratory tract

The bronchial tree and its blood supply are present by the 20th week of gestation, and thereafter only enlarge. In contrast, the alveoli increase in number from 20 million at birth to the adult complement of 300 million. Respiratory disease in early childhood may therefore interfere with future lung development as well as cause direct lung damage. Small airways obstruct or collapse early, leading to poor oxygenation or collapse of a lung segment.

19.5.1 Bronchitis

Acute bronchitis occurs at all ages and is characterized by cough, fever and often wheezing. It is a common feature of influenza and whooping cough. Persistent bacterial bronchitis is an occasional cause of chronic cough in children and may be confused with asthma. A cough swab may aid diagnosis, and a prolonged course of antibiotics (2 weeks or longer) is usually effective.

19.5.2 Bronchiolitis

Bronchiolitis is the most common cause of severe respiratory infection in infancy; 70% is due to RSV, 90% of children are immune to this virus by 2 years of age. Most children remain at home with this infection, but 1–2% of all infants are admitted each year, usually during the winter epidemics.

Younger infants and those with marked respiratory distress are more likely to need hospital admission. Supportive management includes skilled nursing, intravenous fluids, nasogastric feeding and oxygen, usually monitored with pulse oximetry. Nasogastric feeding is needed frequently to maintain fluid and calorie intake. Antibiotics are usually not indicated unless there is evidence of bacterial infection or severe disease. The RSV may be detected by fluorescent antibody test on nasopharyngeal secretions. Most infants recover within a few days. Up to half of infants with RSV bronchiolitis subsequently develop recurrent wheezing.

19.5.3 Pneumonia

19.5.3.1 Bronchopneumonia

This is most common in young children and in older children with a chronic condition affecting respiratory function (e.g. cystic fibrosis, severe cerebral palsy). A wide variety of organisms can be responsible. It commonly follows bronchiolitis, viral infection and whooping cough. Clinical features include rapid breathing, dry cough, fever and fretfulness. Generalized crepitations and rhonchi are usually present. Cyanosis occurs in severe cases and infants may develop cardiac failure. Chest X-ray often shows small patches of consolidation. Hospitalization is usually needed. Oxygen and a broad-spectrum antibiotic are given. Gentle physiotherapy helps to mobilize secretions. Infants may need tube feeding.

19.5.3.2 Lobar pneumonia

Pneumonia presents with sudden illness and high fever. The child is sick, looks flushed, breathes fast and has respiratory distress (Section 3.5.3). There may be no cough. Pleuritic pain may cause the child to lean towards the affected side, or may be referred to the abdomen or neck. The clinical signs of consolidation may not be present at first, but repeated examination will usually reveal them. A transient pleural rub is common. Lobar consolidation, with or without pleural effusion, is usually evident on X-ray (Figure 19.2).

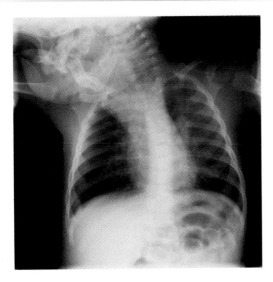

Figure 19.2 Chest X-ray showing right upper lobe collapse and consolidation.

> **Pneumonia: causative agents**
>
> - **Common**
>   - Viral (especially RSV)
>   - *Streptococcus pneumoniae*
> - **Uncommon**
>   - *Mycoplasma pneumoniae*
>   - *Staphylococcus aureus*
>   - *Mycobacterium tuberculosis*
>   - *Haemophilus influenzae* (rare since the introduction of Hib vaccine).

Lobar pneumonia is usually caused by *Streptococcus pneumoniae*, and penicillin achieves dramatic improvement within 24 h. In the ill child, the causative organism is not known initially and broad-spectrum antibiotics are used. At least the initial dose of antibiotics is given by injection, as an ill child is likely to vomit medicine. Not all children are severely ill and some can be treated at home. Fluid intake is more important than food. Paracetamol and tepid sponging will help reduce fever.

> **PRACTICE POINT**
>
> Remember that pneumonia may present with few respiratory symptoms or signs, and with 'non-respiratory' symptoms such as abdominal pain or vomiting. Therefore, a chest X-ray is often performed as part of the work-up for a young, febrile, ill child where there is no obvious focus of infection.

If improvement does not occur, or if signs or symptoms are still present after a week, careful examination including chest X-ray should be repeated to exclude complications such as pleural effusion or lobar collapse. In the older child particularly, mycoplasma should be considered. The possibility of *tuberculosis* should never be forgotten.

Staphylococcal pneumonia is a severe form of lung infection which usually affects young children and those with chronic predisposing disease. It is characterized by lung cysts on X-ray and the sudden appearance of empyema or pneumothorax. Prolonged treatment is required with an anti-staphylococcal antibiotic.

19.5.4 Inhaled foreign bodies

Toddlers are most at risk because they tend to put everything into their mouths. Older children sometimes accidentally inhale objects during games or whilst stuffing their mouths too full of peanuts or sweets. A foreign body may lodge at any level. At the time, the child will cough, splutter or make choking noises, but the episode is quickly forgotten and may not come out in the history without specific questioning.

> **PRACTICE POINT**
>
> Ask about foreign body inhalation when persistent cough, or chest infection not resolving.

In the larynx an object is likely to cause a croupy cough and stridor. If it passes through the larynx, it will lodge in a bronchus (right middle lobe or a lower lobe most often) and there will be no symptoms for a few days until infection, collapse or obstructive emphysema develop.

If a foreign body is suspected, radiography may demonstrate it (if it is radio-opaque) or show associated changes. Diagnosis may require direct laryngoscopy and bronchoscopy, which will be required to remove the object.

19.6 The wheezy child

Wheezing is an obstructive respiratory sound arising in the smaller branches of the bronchial tree: on auscultation, rhonchi can be heard. They are most marked in expiration because the bronchial tree dilates in inspiration.

Wheezing is most common in young infants. Some children have recurrent episodes limited to the first 2 years. In others, recurrent bouts of wheezing lead to the diagnosis of asthma.

Recurrent wheeze occurs in over 10% of children. The prevalence of mild and moderate asthma has increased.

19.7 Asthma

Asthma is one of the family of conditions grouped together under the term 'atopy'. The others include eczema and hayfever. All have raised IgE levels as part of the underlying pathology. It has a strong genetic basis, and it is unusual to make a diagnosis of asthma where there is no history of atopic conditions in either the child or the family.

> **Asthma**
>
> Recurrent, reversible obstruction of the small airways
> Clinical triad:
> - Cough
> - Shortness of breath
> - Wheeze.

It is important to try to understand the underlying factors in each wheezy child if the best help is to be given. In young children, URTIs appear to be the most common precipitating factor, but as the child grows up others may become apparent: specific allergens, exercise, emotional upsets and changes of weather or environment (Figure 19.3).

> **RESOURCE**
>
> The Scottish Intercollegiate Guideline Network (SIGN) website (**www.sign.ac.uk**) has a joint asthma guideline written with the British Thoracic Society (SIGN guideline 101, **www.sign.ac.uk/guidelines/fulltext/101**), along with details of a free smartphone app for all SIGN guidelines.

19.7.1 Asthma diagnosis

Diagnosis can be difficult in young children. After thorough assessment you should record the

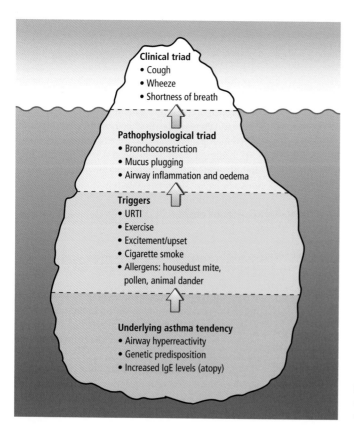

Figure 19.3 The pathogenesis of asthma. The clinical symptoms are the visible tip of an aetiological iceberg.

probability as high, intermediate or low, based on the following factors:

of home or school life. Precipitating factors should be sought. In all cases, it is worth reducing the child's exposure to common allergens.

Increased probability of asthma	Decreased probability of asthma
• Recurrent cough, shortness of breath (including chest tightness) and wheeze • Nocturnal symptoms • Worse following exposure to asthma triggers (see table) • Personal or family history of atopy • Widespread wheeze on auscultation • Improvement with asthma treatment	• Symptoms with colds only, no interval symptoms • Isolated cough • Symptoms suggesting hyperventilation (e.g. peripheral tingling) • Chest examination repeatedly normal when symptomatic • Normal PEFR or spirometry when symptomatic • No response to trial of asthma treatment • Clinical features pointing to alternative diagnosis

19.7.2 Assessing severity of asthma (Table 19.3)

19.7.3 Management

The aim is to reduce the frequency and severity of attacks and to give the child and family confidence that they can cope with attacks without disruption

Common asthma triggers

Infection
Viral infection is a common precipitant of asthma: infection is likely to be important in children who have most trouble in winter.

Allergy
Allergens can be best identified from the history (e.g. after specific exposure or in the pollen season). A family history of allergies is common. Specific antibody tests add little to management.

Emotions
Exceptionally, a severe emotional upset may precipitate a first attack of wheezing. Commonly, excitement or anxiety can precipitate or aggravate attacks.

Exercise
Exercise-induced wheezing occurs most readily when running in a cold atmosphere. Beware the child who can begin a game of football but not last longer than 20 min. Many asthmatics become wheezy on exertion, especially if it involves running.

Atmosphere
Dusty air, 'stuffy' and smoke-filled rooms, or changes in air temperature may precipitate wheezing.

Table 19.3 History, examination and investigation of asthma

History	Examination	Investigation
Acute		
What do child/parents think?	Level of respiratory distress	Oxygen saturation
Therapy received	Tachycardia	Blood gas — abnormalities occur late
Can child run/walk/drink/ talk?	Altered conscious level (drowsy or irritable)	Chest X-ray — if severe
	Beware silent chest (↓ air entry in severe attack)	PEFR — unreliable in acute attack
Chronic		
Child/parent opinion	Growth	Serial PEFR
Current therapy	Chest shape	Spirometry
Hospital admission	– ↑ AP diameter	

Lifestyle changes
    Sport
    School attendance
	– Harrison's sulci	

PEFR, peak expiratory flow rate.

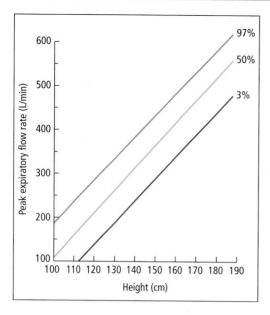

Figure 19.4 Normal peak expiratory flow rate and height.

Normal peak expiratory flow rate is related to height, not age.

PEFR = {(height above 100 cm) × 5 + 100} ± 100 L/min (Figure 19.4)

You will find charts in outpatient clinics and wards.

Those at home are advised not to smoke in the house, particularly in the child's bedroom. Emotional problems at home or school can often be helped, but asthma can generate its own emotional problems for the family. It can be a frightening condition. Some children react to animal fur or dander, and occasionally it is necessary for the family pet to be removed. House dust mite reduction measures can help.

In some children, the history of asthma is obvious. In others, colds 'go to the chest', cough persists and the parents may not notice the wheezing. Typically, the asthmatic child will have recurrent respiratory infections which last longer than those of her siblings. Night-time symptoms of poor sleeping or cough should raise suspicions. It is so common that it should always be sought on direct inquiry in every paediatric history.

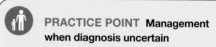

PRACTICE POINT **Management when diagnosis uncertain**

(intermediate or low probability)
Consider:
- PEFR/spirometry before and after bronchodilators
- Trial of asthma treatment
- Further investigation
- Specialist referral.

19.7.3.1 Administration of therapy
(Figure 19.5)

Whenever possible, asthma therapy should be given by inhalation (Figure 19.6). In children of school age, dry powder inhalers or metered dose aerosol inhalers (MDI) with a spacer device may be used. All aerosol agents are more effective through a spacer device, avoiding the need to synchronize inhalation with the aerosol and improving distribution of the drug in the bronchial tree. In infants, a metered dose inhaler with spacer device fitted with a face mask may be used with instruction. Nebulized therapy can be given with a little cooperation on the part of the child. It is always best to ask the parent or child to hold the face mask. This is particularly valuable during acute attacks requiring oxygen to deliver bronchodilators (see also Figure 28.2a).

Oral therapy with salbutamol or terbutaline is not effective and side effects are more likely. Leukotriene receptor antagonists can be given orally as granules sprinkled on food or as chewable tablets, and so can be useful in younger children. Occasionally, oral steroids and xanthines (e.g. theophylline) are necessary in children with severe chronic disease. Oral prednisolone may be given in a short course over a few days to bring about resolution of an acute severe attack.

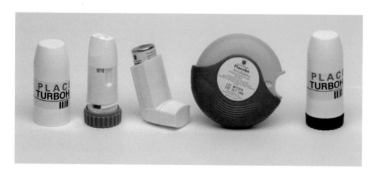

Figure 19.5 Inhalers used for asthma. The central one is a metered dose aerosol inhaler; the round one is an Accuhaler (a dry powder device); the others are Turbohalers (also dry powder devices).

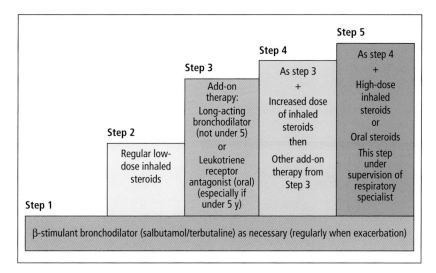

Figure 19.6 Stepwise approach to chronic asthma. Step up if control is poor and back down when good control is maintained. Have a low threshold to refer young children (< 5y) to a respiratory paediatrician where control is poor despite treatment.

The most common reason for poor control in chronic asthma is poor compliance. If control deteriorates abruptly, make sure the family have not just acquired a pet.

Early, adequate prophylaxis may reduce the likelihood of later, severe disease.

> Annual deaths from childhood asthma have gradually fallen from a peak in the 1960s, but 20–30 children die each year in the UK. This compares to over 1300 deaths annually in adults, the vast majority in over-65s.

19.7.3.2 Acute severe attacks

 TREATMENT **Treatment of acute asthma**

Bronchodilators – start with salbutamol, but consider adding ipratropium if not responding
Antibiotics are not given routinely.

Mild/moderate
- Bronchodilators via spacer (up to 10 puffs at a time)
- Oral prednisolone (3-day course)

Severe
- Oxygen by face mask
- Nebulized bronchodilators with oxygen
- Oral prednisolone (3-day course)

Severe attack not responding
- Admit to ICU or high dependency area
- Intravenous β bronchodilator.
- Intravenous hydrocortisone
- Intravenous aminophylline (caution!).

Children and their families should be taught to recognize acute severe attacks. Worrying features include failure to respond to usual therapy, exhaustion, severe respiratory distress (Table 19.3) and persistent symptoms.

 PRACTICE POINT **Pointers to severe or life-threatening asthma**

- Too breathless to talk or feed
- Any change in conscious level
- Any history of colour change or cyanosis
- Exhaustion or poor respiratory effort
- Tachycardia or hypotension
- Silent chest
- Peak expiratory flow less than 50% of best

Start treatment and transfer to hospital urgently.

Anyone who has had an asthma attack knows how frightening this can be: calm reassurance to the child and her parents is important. This should not replace the need for urgent assessment and therapy (Figure 19.7). Most respond to inhaled β bronchodilation, and in mild or moderate asthma this can be given as a metered dose inhaler via a spacer. Increase the dose by two puffs every two minutes up to ten puffs according to response, and transfer to hospital if not responding. In more severe asthma, a nebulizer should be used to deliver the bronchodilator.

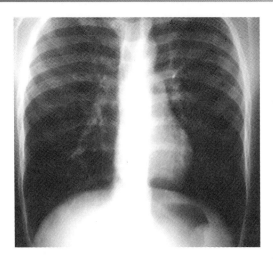

Figure 19.7 Chest X-ray showing hyperinflation in acute asthma.

 TREATMENT

Give oral prednisolone early in acute asthma.

Intravenous therapy with a β-stimulant, hydrocortisone or aminophylline is reserved for children with severe signs. Aminophylline infusion must always be given slowly in a high-dependency or intensive care setting, and great care should be used if a child is on maintenance theophylline therapy. Supportive therapy with fluids is important. Primary bacterial infections are uncommon, but antibiotics may be considered in severe attacks. Acute sudden deterioration should raise the suspicion of pneumothorax. Every admission to hospital or visit to out-patients should be used as an opportunity to review longer-term therapy. No child should be given inhaled therapy without being taught how to use it by an expert. It is important to watch a child using their inhalers and to examine their technique from time to time.

19.8 Cystic fibrosis

Cystic fibrosis (CF) is the most common, lethal inherited condition amongst Europeans. It is an autosomal recessive condition due to mutations of the gene on the seventh chromosome which codes for the cystic fibrosis transmembrane regulator – a protein which controls chloride transport across the cell membrane. Hundreds of mutations have now been found. In the UK, around 80% of mutations are a single amino acid abnormality

known as ΔF508. One in 25 of the population are asymptomatic carriers. CF affects 1 : 2500 children in the UK.

19.8.1 Clinical features and presentation

The common presentations of CF are:
- Fetal screening (mutation analysis)
- Neonatal screening (genetic or immunoreactive trypsin)
- Neonatal meconium ileus
- Recurrent respiratory infections
- Failure to thrive with fatty diarrhoea.

In the newborn baby, meconium may be so glutinous with viscid mucus that normal peristaltic waves cannot shift it (*meconium ileus*). Small amounts of meconium may be passed: generalized abdominal distension and vomiting develop over 24–48 h. Abdominal X-ray shows obstruction. Obstruction may be relieved by careful administration of a water-soluble hyperosmolar enema. Often surgery is necessary. Obviously, all children with meconium ileus must be tested for CF. '*Meconium ileus equivalent*' sometimes occurs in the older child.

 PRACTICE POINT
Cardinal symptoms of CF

- Recurrent chest infection
- Loose, offensive stools
- Failure to thrive.

Most of the unscreened children with CF present in childhood. CF should be considered with any combination of the cardinal symptoms. Malabsorption is due to deficiency of pancreatic enzymes and may start any time from birth. Abdominal distension and weight loss resemble coeliac disease. *Staphylococcus aureus*, *Haemophilus influenzae* and later *Pseudomonas* and other chest infections lead to lung damage and bronchiectasis (Figures 19.8 and 19.9). Untreated children have persistent productive cough, wheeze, hyperexpanded chest deformity and clubbing (Figure 19.10). Unusual presentations of CF include sinusitis, nasal polyposis and rectal prolapse.

 PRACTICE POINT

Infection control is very important in CF, and requires that children carrying different organisms are segregated in clinical areas.

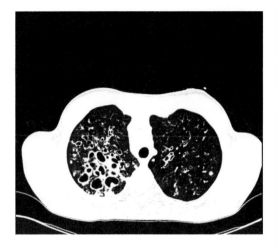

Figure 19.8 This chest CT in a 15 year old boy with CF shows severe bronchietasis in the right lung. The dilated bronchi are the black circular structures.

19.8.2 Investigation

The diagnosis rests on at least two abnormal sweat tests performed by people skilled in the procedure. Localized sweating is induced by iontophoresis with pilocarpine, and sweat is absorbed onto filter paper. In 99% of homozygotes, sweat sodium and chloride levels are raised over 70 mmol/L.

Mutation analysis is extremely helpful but cannot exclude CF as not all mutations are known.

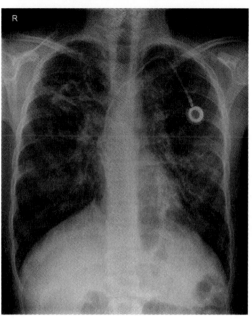

Figure 19.9 Chest X-ray in cystic fibrosis. There is hyperinflation and hilar enlargement, with linear 'tram lines' and ring shadows suggestive of bronchiectasis, and some patchy infective change in the right upper zone.

In affected families it forms a reliable test for fetal and neonatal screening. Pancreatic damage results in raised serum immunoreactive trypsin in

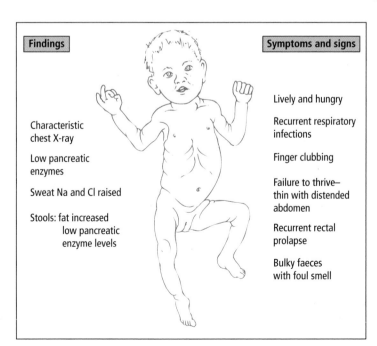

Findings	Symptoms and signs

Lively and hungry

Recurrent respiratory infections

Characteristic chest X-ray

Finger clubbing

Low pancreatic enzymes

Failure to thrive– thin with distended abdomen

Sweat Na and Cl raised

Stools: fat increased
low pancreatic
enzyme levels

Recurrent rectal prolapse

Bulky faeces
with foul smell

Figure 19.10 The young child presenting with cystic fibrosis.

the first 6 weeks of life. This can be detected in the blood spots collected for routine neonatal screening, and is now part of the national UK neonatal screeing programme. High sensitivity but relatively low specificity means that the test will pick up children without the disesase, leaving parents worried until they discover that their child does not have CF. Pre-symptomatic diagnosis, however, allows early introduction of the modern aggressive therapy which has transformed the prognosis.

19.8.3 Treatment and prognosis

The respiratory problems of CF are progressive. In the 1960s, babies survived for only a few months or years. Modern aggressive therapy, started at an early age, has transformed the prognosis for CF (Table 19.4). About 80% of today's children with cystic fibrosis should live into their mid 40s or 50s, and most can live reasonably normal and productive lives. Treatment is best provided by multidisciplinary teams working in specialist centres. Adherence to the demanding treatment regime can difficult. Gene therapy is an exciting future possibility.

19.8.3.1 Long-term complications of CF

- Respiratory failure
- Psychological/emotional problems
- Diabetes mellitus
- Portal hypertension
- Hepatic cirrhosis
- Cor pulmonale
- Distal intestinal obstruction syndrome
- Male infertility.

 # Summary

Respiratory problems, particularly bronchiolitis, croup, pneumonia and asthma, are common reasons for admission, and you need to know these conditions well. Make sure that you are familiar with asthma treatment. Cystic fibrosis, although rarer, illustrates the challenges of managing a chronic condition in childhood. The transformation in prognosis over recent decades is gratifying, but treatment is not easy.

 FOR YOUR LOG

- Observe a naso-pharyngeal aspirate being taken (for RSV in bronchiolitis)
- Watch a child's inhaler technique being checked.
- Measure a child's peak expiratory flow and know how to interpret it.
- Be familiar with asthma treatment devices (inhalers, aerochambers, nebulisers)
- Observe a sweat test.

 OSCE TIP

- Child with chronic respiratory problem, e.g. CF, asthma (see OSCE station 19.2).
- Acute respiratory illness – so common a child may have some wheeze.
- Assessment of acute or long-term respiratory status.
- Chest X-ray, e.g. pneumonia, pneumothorax.
- Video of severe asthma attack.
- Explain use of inhalers, peak flow meter and chart.

See EMQ 19.1, EMQ 19.2 and EMQ 19.3 at the end of the book.

Table 19.4 Treatment of cystic fibrosis

Respiratory	Nutritional	Family
Physiotherapy at least twice every day	Constant monitoring	Education
	Dietetic supervision	Teach parents/child to do physiotherapy
Early antistaphylococcal prophylaxis	High energy/protein 150% of average requirements	Recognition of relapse
Aggressive high-dose intravenous antibiotics for exacerbations	High-fat diet	Home intravenous antibiotics
	Pancreatic enzyme replacement therapy	Genetic counselling
Bronchodilators		Financial help (e.g. Disability Living Allowance)
		Emotional support

OSCE station 19.1: Examination of the respiratory system

Clinical approach:

Check hands
- Clubbing
- Colour
- Perfusion

Check face
- Colour
- Anaemia
- Respiratory distress

Chest

Inspection
Acute signs
- Respiratory rate
- Recession/increased work of breathing
- Added noises (cough, wheeze, etc.)

Chronic signs
- Chest shape
- Pectus carinatum/AP diameter
- Harrison's sulci

Percussion
- Percuss upper, mid and lower zones, anteriorly and posteriorly
- Dullness over the heart is normal

Auscultation
- Added noises
  ◇ Stridor
  ◇ Wheeze
  ◇ Crackles
  ◇ Crepitation
  ◇ Rub

James is 14 years old. Please examine his respiratory system

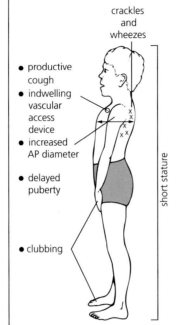

crackles and wheezes

- productive cough
- indwelling vascular access device
- increased AP diameter
- delayed puberty

- clubbing

short stature

James has cystic fibrosis with signs of chronic lung infection and asthma. He has poor growth, and no signs of puberty.

Never forget:
- Say hello and introduce yourself
- General health
- Colour — ?pale/?cyanosed
- Quickly assess growth, nutrition and development
- Mention the obvious (e.g. drip, leg in plaster)

Look around for:
- Inhalers
- Sputum pot
- Nasogastric tube, gastrostomy
- Vascular access device
- Oxygen — mask, nasal prongs
- Medications

Special points
- Evidence of atopic disease (e.g. eczema)
- Beware transmitted noises; listen again after asking the child to cough
- Percussion is usually unhelpful in children under 2 years, and they don't like it; omit it and explain why
- Percuss onto your finger, not direct onto clavicle
- Downward displacement of the liver occurs if the chest is overexpanded

---

OSCE station 19.2: Prescribing and explaining asthma treatment

This station assesses the candidate's ability to prescribe, explain and demonstrate appropriate asthma treatment.

'You are an FY1 doctor attached to a paediatric ward. Abigail is a 4 year-old girl admitted with asthma, who needs medications to be prescribed before going home. You have been asked to prescribe them and explain their use to the parent. You have been told by the registrar that she needs to be on a regular preventer inhaler at a standard dose, and a reliever inhaler. She needs two more days of oral steroids at a dose of 2mg per kg per day. Her weight is 15 kg.'

You have been asked to

- Prescribe the medication
- Explain to the parent how and when to use it.

You have 10 minutes for this station.
(A standard discharge prescription sheet, and demonstration inhalers etc would be provided.)

(continued on next page)

(continued)

Simulated patient script

You are Jane/Richard Riley and you are the parent of 4 year-old Abigail who has about to go home from the paediatric ward. You have been told she has asthma and this has been explained to you. Now one of the junior doctors is going to come and explain about the asthma treatment Abigail will be starting.

- Abigail was diagnosed with asthma on this admission having had 4 episodes of being wheezy and short of breath in the past 2 months. She had not been admitted until this episode.
- If asked what you know about asthma/ say that someone has explained to you about what asthma is, and you just need to know how to use the medications.
- If asked what you know about using an inhaler, say 'Well I have been told that the inhaler will help Abigail's breathing but that's all.'
- The candidate should give you details of drugs to be used but, if he/she does not ask, say 'What do I use it with?'
- Follow the candidate's instructions as you understand them.

This is a 10-minute station. The candidate is a junior doctor (FY1), who is asked to explain how and when to use the medication and demonstrate the use of a metered dose inhaler (MDI) and spacer – the standard device for the treatment of asthma.

You will be asked to mark the candidate on 2 points:

- I understood how to use the inhalers
- I understood when to use each inhaler

Marksheet

Prescription
- Beclomethosone MDI 200 micrograms bd inh via aerochamber (100 bd acceptable)
- Salbutamol MDI 200 to 600 micrograms (2–6 puffs) prn inh via aerochamber
- Prednisolone 30 mg (6 tablets) daily for 2 days
- One aerochamber
- Clearly written, signed and dated

Introduction
- Introduction and orientation (name and role, explains purpose of interview, confirms patient's agreement)
- Elicits parent's knowledge of device
- Names the device
- Explains purpose of device
- Explains clinical situation when it is used

Inhaler technique: teaches/shows
- Shake canister
- Correctly attach to aerochamber
- Ensure mask is over nose and mouth and make a seal with the face
- Breathe out fully
- Spray 1 puff
- Hold mask on and allow the child to breathe normally for 10 seconds
- Wait 30 seconds to see if repeat dose is needed (for bronchodilators)
- Shake canister and repeat dose

Use of inhaler:
- Explains which drugs should be used
- Explains how the drugs should be used
- Rapport (shows interest, respect and concern, appropriate body language
- Information giving and explaining (clear, unambiguous explanation, jargon-free, well paced, checks understanding, invites questions
- Fluency and organization (systemic and logical flow)
- Closure (summarizes main points, thanks parent)

SP to mark:
- I understood how to use the inhalers
- I understood when to use each inhaler.

20

Cardiology

Chapter map

Most cardiac conditions present as a heart murmur, heart failure or the presence of cyanosis. Congenital heart disease is the most common cause of cardiac problems in children (Table 20.1). Primary myocardial disease and endocarditis are rare. Rheumatic fever (Section 23.3.6) and heart disease are still prevalent in developing countries, but are now rarely seen in Europe.

Doctors who look after children need to be able to recognize the possibility of heart disease, distinguish it from normal, and assess the urgency of the need for cardiological assessment. This can be difficult.

20.1   Innocent murmurs

These murmurs (also called benign, functional and physiological) occur in children without any cardiac abnormality and are especially common in the newborn. Three main types of innocent murmur are recognized.

 KEY POINTS

- Cardiac murmurs do not always mean heart disease.
- Severe heart disease may occur without a murmur.

PRACTICE POINT Clinical features of an innocent murmur

- Asymptomatic
- Accentuated by fever/exercise
- Varies with respiration/posture
- Systolic/continuous
- Quiet (grade 1 or 2)
- Never harsh in character.

RESOURCE

Try Auscultation Assistant at **www.med.ucla.edu/wilkes/index.htm** to listen to the murmurs below.

20.1.1 Vibratory murmur

This is like the quiet buzzing of a bee. It is very short, mid-systolic and less obvious when the child sits up. It usually disappears by puberty.

20.1.2 Pulmonary systolic murmur

This is a soft, blowing ejection systolic murmur, heard at the upper left sternal edge. The differential diagnosis is a mild pulmonary stenosis.

20.1.3 Venous hum

This is due to blood cascading into the great veins. It is a blowing continuous murmur best heard above or below the clavicles. The hum is greatly diminished when the ipsilateral internal jugular vein is compressed, or when the child lies down flat.

20.2 Changes in circulation at birth

The changes that take place in the circulation at birth explain why symptoms of congenital heart disease may not occur until a few weeks after birth (Figure 7.1 and Figure 20.1). In the fetus, only 15% of the right ventricular blood enters the lungs, the rest passes through the ductus arteriosus to the descending aorta; the ductus is as large as the aorta.

After birth, the ductus closes within 10–15 h and the pulmonary artery pressure falls over the first 3 days of life. In lesions with a left-to-right shunt, the volume of blood shunted increases over the first weeks as pulmonary blood pressure falls.

RESOURCE

Search YouTube for 'fetal heart circulation amariekaleidoscope02' to find a useful video summarizing these changes (and including some embryology) (**www.youtube.com/watch?v=uwswhoKfkmM**).

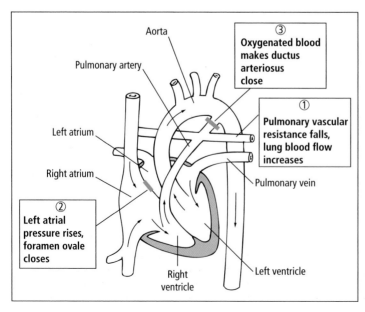

Figure 20.1 Fetal anatomy changes at birth.

PRACTICE POINT Paediatric ECGs

These changes explain why ECGs are different in children. In fetal life, the right ventricle is relatively large because it is helping to support the high-pressure systemic circulation. Over early childhood, its relative size reduces, and so the QRS axis slowly swings from right-sided to its adult left-sided position. This means that paediatric ECGs cannot be interpreted using adult criteria.

Table 20.1 **Congenital heart abnormalities**

Condition	Typical heart abnormality
Down syndrome	Atrioseptal defect
Trisomy 13 or 18	Complex septal defects
Turner's syndrome	Coarctation of the aorta
Marfan's syndrome	Aortic aneurysm

20.3 Congenital heart disease

Congenital abnormalities of the heart (Table 20.1) are the most common important group of congenital anomalies. In Europe, most heart disease in children is congenital. There is a spectrum of severity in each defect from mild to severe, and in every lesion changes take place as a child grows, sometimes for better and sometimes for worse. Most severe symptoms occur in the first year of life, particularly in the newborn infant, and urgent investigation and treatment are required. Mild lesions cause no symptoms, are compatible with a normal life and require no treatment. Full initial assessment and follow up is important to prevent secondary changes in the myocardium.

In children with isolated congenital heart disease, recurrence risk for subsequent siblings is about 3%. The risk to offspring of a parent with congenital heart disease is 5–10%; 10–20% of children with congenital heart disease have other abnormalities.

Heart defects occur in nearly 1% of live born infants. An abnormal heart may be found in around 10% of spontaneously aborted fetuses. Routine examination of the heart antenatally has led to an increased rate of fetal diagnosis.

Causes of congenital heart disease

Genetic
- Extra chromosomes (e.g. trisomy 21, Down syndrome)
- Missing chromosome (e.g. 46 XO, Turner syndrome)
- Chromosome mutations (e.g. 22q mutation)

Maternal illness
- Congenital viral infections (e.g. rubella, toxoplasmosis)
- Maternal disease (e.g. diabetes mellitus, systemic lupus erythematosus)

Maternal exposure to drugs/chemicals during pregnancy
- Therapeutic (e.g. warfarin, phenytoin)
- Toxins (e.g. excessive alcohol, illicit drugs)
Idiopathic (common).

20.3.1 Risk of endocarditis

Children with structural congenital heart disease are at increased risk of infective endocarditis. Antibiotic prophylaxis is no longer advised for procedures that might cause a bacteraemia (e.g. dental work). Evidence indicates: bacteraemias are commonly caused by everyday activities such as toothbrushing; a lack of association between endocarditis and prior interventional procedures; lack of efficacy of antibiotic prophylaxis. Instead, patients and families are given general advice about good oral health, when to suspect endocarditis and that there may be increased risk after invasive procedures (including body piercing).

 RESOURCE

The British Heart Foundation publishes a series of parent information leaflets on congenital heart disease. Go to **www.bhf.org.uk** and search for 'congenital heart disease'.

 RESOURCE

Prophylaxis against endocarditis
See NICE guideline CG64 at **www.nice.or.uk (http://guidance.nice.org.uk/CG64)**.

20.4 Neonatal presentations

> **PRACTICE POINT**
>
> If a newborn with a heart murmur is fit to go home, tell the parents what symptoms may occur. Their baby needs to come back early if they are concerned.

20.4.1 Heart murmur

The most common clinical presentation is the discovery of a heart murmur during routine examination in the first days of life (Section 7.4.1). Perform a full clinical assessment and a careful search for other congenital abnormalities. If any cardiac symptoms are present, arrange urgent cardiological assessment. If the infant remains well, but the murmur persists beyond 24–48 h, assessment by an experienced paediatrician or cardiologist is justified. In most paediatric practice, if a murmur is present over the first weeks of life, even if it is thought to be innocent, echocardiography is performed.

20.4.2 Cyanosis

Distinguish between central and peripheral cyanosis.

> **PRACTICE POINT**
>
> **Central**
> - Tongue and peripheries blue
> - Concentration of deoxygenated haemoglobin >5 g/dL
> - Indicates significant disease
>
> **Peripheral**
> - Hands and feet blue
> - Common and normal in the first days of life.

In some infants, cyanosis becomes gradually more apparent, while the infant remains otherwise well. This presentation is typical of Fallot tetralogy (see Section 20.5.4.1). In some infants, the presentation is dramatic. The infant is hypoxic, and may be collapsed and acidotic, with a clinical picture which is hard to distinguish from severe infection. A nitrogen washout test may be helpful.

The infant is placed in 100% oxygen for 10–20 min. In severe lung disease, persistent fetal circulation and cyanotic congenital heart disease, the blood oxygen does not rise.

In some conditions, blood flow to the lungs is dependent on the patent ductus arteriosus. The infant becomes very ill when the ductus closes. The emergency treatment aims to maintain duct patency with prostaglandin. Neonatal intensive care and ventilation is often required. Definitive treatment depends upon diagnosis.

20.4.3 Heart failure

Acute heart failure may occur in left-sided obstructive lesions (e.g. coarctation of the aorta). In such infants, systemic blood flow may depend upon the ductus, and prostaglandin may be used. Over the first weeks of life, increasing left-to-right shunting may produce right heart failure of insidious onset with a characteristic set of signs and symptoms (see Section 20.7). In mild failure, these are hard to recognize.

20.5 Classification of congenital heart disease

Eight lesions represent 80% of congenital heart disease (Figure 20.2). Obstructive lesions reduce flow in the outflow tracts or aorta. If the lesion produces a connection between the systemic and pulmonary

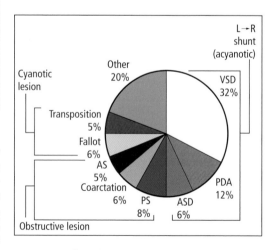

Figure 20.2 Classification of congenital heart disease.

circulations, a left-to-right shunt occurs. In the cyanotic lesions, there is obstruction to the pulmonary circulation (e.g. Fallot) or abnormal circulation (e.g. transposition of the great arteries).

20.5.1 Diagnosis

Initially assessment is by clinical examination. Chest X-ray and ECG are helpful, but the most important diagnostic tool is echocardiography with Doppler assessment, which allows estimation of flow. Only rarely is cardiac catheterization required. Full assessment of non-cardiac problems can be critically important if major surgery is being considered.

20.5.2 Left-to-right shunts

20.5.2.1 Ventricular septal defect (VSD) (Figure 20.3)

The natural history of VSD depends upon the size of the defect, the changes that occur with growth and the pulmonary vascular resistance.

Small defects

Patients have no symptoms and the heart murmur is heard during routine examination. Seventy-five per cent close in the first 10 years of life (the majority by 2 years) but closure goes on occurring in adult life. The only risk is of bacterial endocarditis.

Medium-sized defects

These cause symptoms in infancy. Heart failure results in poor feeding and slow weight gain. Symptoms appear in the first months of life, often precipitated by a chest infection. Improvement occurs following medical treatment. As the child grows, the defect becomes relatively smaller, symptoms lessen and weight gain improves. Spontaneous closure usually occurs.

Large defects

Symptoms begin in the first weeks of life. Heart failure is difficult to control and tube feeding is necessary. A small number close, but most need surgery. In infancy, persistent high pulmonary blood flow leads to increased pulmonary vascular resistance. The volume of the left-to-right shunt diminishes and heart failure improves. It is important not to be misled by this apparent improvement because, if the defect is not closed before the age of 2 years, changes in the lung vessels become permanent. Without surgery, pulmonary vascular disease worsens, the shunt reverses, the patient becomes cyanosed and breathless and life expectancy is markedly reduced (Eisenmenger syndrome). The only management of pulmonary vascular disease is prevention with early surgery.

Signs

- Pan-systolic murmur at the left sternal edge (turbulent L→R blood flow)
- Maximal in the third and fourth left interspaces
- Loud murmurs cause a systolic thrill

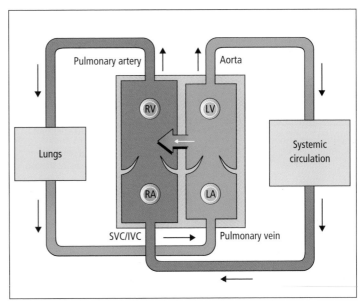

Figure 20.3 Ventricular septal defect. Note that the diagrams in this section are schematic rather than anatomical, and provide a simple approach to understanding the various lesions. Oxygenated blood is shown in red, dexoygentated blood in purple.

- Murmur is harsh, like the sound of wood being sawn
- Murmur may become louder as the lesion closes, because of greater turbulence.

Treatment

- Control the heart failure with medical treatment (e.g. diuretics, ACE inhibitors)
- Surgical closure (cardiopulmonary bypass) if symptoms cannot be controlled or danger of pulmonary vascular disease.

20.5.2.2 Patent ductus arteriosus (PDA) (see Figure 8.4)

PDA is most common in the preterm infant. Murmur and heart failure are noted in the first weeks during intensive care, and it may be difficult to reduce the infant's ventilation requirements. Control of heart failure may be sufficient. Some preterm infants require duct closure medically, using indomethacin as a prostaglandin inhibitor, or by surgical ligation. Spontaneous closure occurs up to 3 months after birth.

In the term infant, if the ductus is patent during the first 2 weeks of life, spontaneous closure is rare. A large PDA leads to heart failure, and in others the persisting risk of bacterial endocarditis is an indication for surgical closure.

Signs

- Collapsing pulses due to sudden leak of blood from the aorta to the pulmonary artery
- Preterm infant may have tachycardia and bounding pulses
- Continuous, 'machinery' (systolic and diastolic) murmur

- Maximal under left clavicle (Figure 20.4)
- May be a thrill.

Treatment

- Treat heart failure medically
- If duct persists, close by surgical ligation or using small 'double umbrella' device placed in the ductus through a cardiac catheter.

20.5.2.3 Atrial septal defect (ASD)
(Figure 20.5)

ASD does not usually cause symptoms in childhood because the left-to-right shunt is small. In the majority a heart murmur is discovered during routine examination and the child has few or no symptoms. Symptoms occur in the second and third decades, pulmonary hypertension develops secondary to the large blood flow into the lungs, and heart failure and atrial dysrhythmias result.

Signs

- Right ventricular heave – increased blood volume
- Ejection systolic murmur in pulmonary area – excessive blood flow through a normal pulmonary valve
- Second heart sound widely split – takes longer for volume-overloaded right ventricle to empty, pulmonary valve closure is delayed
- Wide splitting does not vary with respiration and is described as 'fixed' (Section 3.5.3, p. 35).
- Chest X-ray shows pulmonary plethora.

Treatment

Close surgically by school age to prevent late pulmonary hypertension.

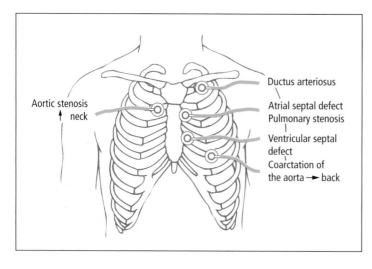

Aortic stenosis ↑ neck

Ductus arteriosus
Atrial septal defect
Pulmonary stenosis
Ventricular septal defect
Coarctation of the aorta → back

Figure 20.4 The murmur is heard loudest at the point shown. Some loud murmurs can be heard over the whole precordium. Some murmurs radiate in a characteristic direction.

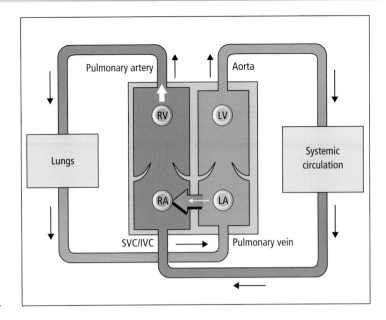

Figure 20.5 Atrial septal defect.

20.5.3 Obstructive lesions

20.5.3.1 Coarctation of aorta (Figure 20.6)

This describes narrowing of the aorta around the site of the ductus, impairing blood flow to the lower half of the body.

Severe coarctation

If severe, acute symptoms occur in the neonatal period. Blood flows through the patent ductus arteriosus from the pulmonary artery to the lower half of the body. When the duct closes, the left ventricle cannot maintain the flow of blood to the aorta, and left and right ventricular failure results. Unless treatment is given urgently, the child dies.

Signs
- Baby breathless, grey and collapsed
- Hepatomegaly
- Pulses are better in the arms than the legs but may be difficult to feel everywhere
- Blood pressure lower in the legs than the arms
- No murmurs.

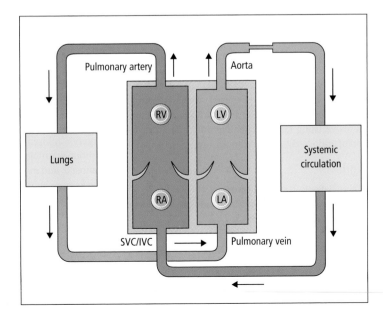

Figure 20.6 Coarctation of the aorta.

Treatment
- Prostaglandin E to re-open the ductus
- Control heart failure prior to urgent surgery
- Ductus is ligated and coarctation repaired.

Mild coarctation

These children often have no symptoms, and gradually a collateral circulation develops. Hypertension occurs in the head and arms. Without surgery, most would die in their 30s and 40s.

Signs
- Pulses in the arms and neck normal
- Femoral and leg pulses delayed, weak or absent
- Blood pressure is raised in the arms, lower in the legs
- Systolic murmur may be present, best heard between the shoulder blades.

 PRACTICE POINT

Routine examination of the femoral pulses is key to detection of coarctation.

Treatment
Surgery is advised in all patients as soon as the diagnosis is made.

20.5.3.2 Aortic stenosis (AS)

Most children with mild stenosis have no symptoms and no restriction of exercise is necessary. In adult life, valve calcification occurs and the stenosis becomes more severe. In severe stenosis, syncope and dizziness are the first symptoms, and the risk of sudden death is 1%. In the severe group, stressful exercise may cause symptoms or even angina, and is avoided. In critical (very severe) stenosis, heart failure occurs in the first weeks of life, and if AS is not recognized 50% die. The severity of the stenosis is assessed by measuring the pressure gradient across the valve using Doppler echocardiography. Prevention of endocarditis is very important.

Signs
- Harsh ejection systolic murmur
- Maximal in the aortic area (second right interspace) and conducted to the neck
- Ejection click may be heard
- Systolic thrills occur in the suprasternal notch and over the right carotid artery
- ECG shows left ventricular hypertrophy.

Treatment
- Valve replacement eventually needed for most children with significant AS
- Balloon dilatation is used to relieve stenosis and delay valve replacement.

20.5.3.3 Pulmonary stenosis (PS)

Most pulmonary stenosis is mild, will not affect a child's health and is unlikely to worsen during the patient's lifetime. In more severe stenosis, although there may be no symptoms, the stenosis becomes relatively greater as the patient grows and progressive hypertrophy of the right ventricular muscle occurs. Eventually there is a limitation of cardiac output, and breathlessness, dysrhythmias and heart failure occur. Critical pulmonary stenosis in infancy will cause early death unless recognized, and may present dramatically when the ductus arteriosus closes.

Signs
- Loud ejection systolic murmur maximal in the pulmonary area (second left interspace)
- May be a thrill
- Murmur radiates backwards
- Right ventricle heave
- Wide splitting of the second sound
- ECG shows right ventricular hypertrophy.

Treatment

Balloon dilatation or surgery to relieve severe stenosis.

20.5.4 Cyanotic lesions

20.5.4.1 Tetralogy of Fallot (Figure 20.7 and Figure 20.8)

This is usually diagnosed antenatally, but otherwise tends to present in the first month of life with a murmur and the gradual onset of cyanosis. Surprisingly, cyanosis may not be obvious. The classical picture of cyanosis at rest and on exertion, in the child who squats in order to increase pulmonary blood flow, is now avoided by surgery. Children with Fallot develop cyanotic attacks. Without warning, the child becomes breathless and cyanosed, and may lose consciousness fleetingly. Such attacks may be dangerous, and recognition of a typical history is important. Children with Fallot are at risk of myocardial infarction, cerebral vascular accidents, endocarditis, embolus and cerebral abscess.

Signs
- Without surgery, children are cyanosed with clubbing
- Right ventricle heave

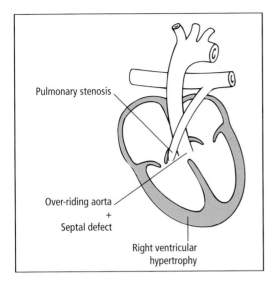

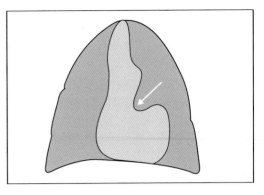

Figure 20.9 Boot-shaped heart on chest X-ray in tetralogy of Fallot.

Figure 20.7 Tetralogy of Fallot. The four features that make up the tetralogy are: (1) VSD; (2) over-riding aorta; (3) pulmonary artery stenosis; and (4) right ventricular hypertrophy.

- Systolic murmur at the upper left sternal edge due to the narrowed right ventricular outflow tract
- Cardiac failure does not occur.

X-ray

Right ventricular hypertrophy: boot-shaped heart, with pulmonary artery bay (arrowed) due to small pulmonary artery (Figure 20.9).

Treatment

- Treat cyanotic attacks with oxygen, β-blockers and analgesia
- Corrective surgery usually performed within the first year
- When severe early symptoms, a temporary anastomosis is created between the subclavian artery and the pulmonary artery to increase pulmonary blood flow.

20.5.4.2 Transposition of the great arteries (TGA) (Figure 20.10)

- Two independent parallel circulations
- Oxygenated pulmonary venous blood→pulmonary artery
- Deoxygenated systemic venous blood→aorta

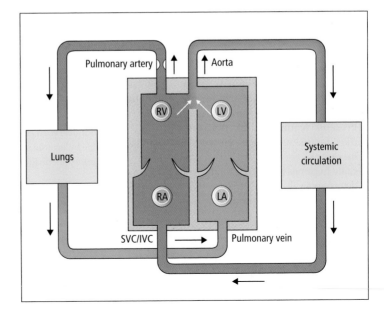

Figure 20.8 Tetralogy of Fallot.

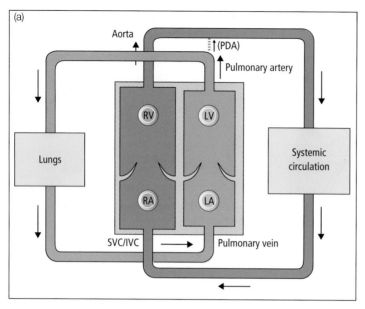

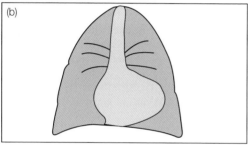

Figure 20.10 Transposition of the great arteries. (a) Once the patent ductus closes, there is no connection between the systemic and pulmonary circulations. (b) The chest X-ray is an 'egg on its side'.

- Mixing of two circulations depends on one of:
  - Atrial septum
  - Ductus arteriosus
  - VSD.

Signs

- There must be a connection between the two parallel circulations to allow some mixing, or the condition is incompatible with life
- Presents acutely in the first days of life, as the ductus arteriosus closes and cyanosis increases
- Child becomes breathless, unable to feed and may be extremely ill
- May or may not be a murmur.

X-ray

The heart has a narrow pedicle and is like an egg, with the pointed part of the egg forming the apex of the heart ('egg on its side').

Treatment

- Without urgent treatment these children die.
- Prostaglandin is given to maintain patency of the ductus arteriosus.
- Emergency treatment is balloon septostomy. A cardiac catheter is passed through the atrial septum. A balloon on the end is then inflated and pulled back sharply into the right atrium in order to tear the atrial septum. This allows mixing of blood between the two atria.
- Surgical correction is performed in the first months of life by 'arterial switch', when the aorta and pulmonary artery are divided above the valves and switched over.

20.6 Surgical treatment of congenital heart disease

As cardiac surgery advances, there is a tendency to operate on the common lesions earlier in life. This often means operating before the child has any symptoms. Surgery is generally safe, with operative mortality less than 5%. In a large majority, long-term myocardial function is normal.

PRACTICE POINT **Informing parents about heart disease**

- Parents are shocked to hear their child has heart disease
- Cause is usually unknown – it is not their fault
- Congenital heart disease is not like ischaemic heart disease
- Exercise restriction is hardly ever necessary (except in severe aortic stenosis)
- Try to provide written information and a diagram
- Echocardiography (cardiac ultrasound) is the important early investigation
- Not all congenital heart disease requires surgery
- Advice about endocarditis is important.

20.7 Cardiac failure

Heart failure is a medical emergency. It occurs more commonly in the first 3 months of life than in any other period of childhood and is usually due to congenital heart disease (Figure 20.11). Earlier onset implies a more severe heart lesion. It is also caused by myocarditis, endocarditis and dysrhythmias.

Clinical features
- Poor feeding
- Breathless on exertion
- Sweating
- Poor weight gain
- Excess weight gain (oedema).

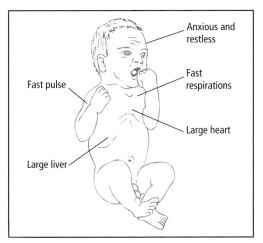

Anxious and restless

Fast pulse

Fast respirations

Large heart

Large liver

Figure 20.11 Cardiac failure in infancy.

20.7.1 Treatment

- Prompt treatment is essential
- Cardiac assessment (echo, chest X-ray, ECG) and treatment of cause
- Prop the child up and give oxygen
- Correct acidosis, hypoglycaemia, hypocalcaemia or anaemia
- Treat respiratory infection with antibiotics
- Feed by nasogastric tube
- Medication: diuretics are important; furosemide is often combined with spironolactone to prevent potassium loss. Systemic vascular resistance and the work of the left ventricle can be reduced with a vasodilator (e.g. ACE inhibitor).

20.8 Dysrhythmias

Abnormalities of sinus rhythm are not usually of cardiac origin. Bradycardia means hypoxia. A tachycardia is often seen in association with fever, dehydration or any acute illness. If episodic dysrhythmia is suspected from the history, ambulatory 24 h ECG monitoring can be extremely helpful.

20.8.1 Supraventricular tachycardia (SVT)

SVT is the most common symptomatic dysrhythmia in childhood. It may rarely occur in utero and is controlled by treating the mother. Infants with SVT become acutely ill, collapsed and grey, and need urgent help. The pulse is very fast, too fast to count. ECG shows a narrow complex tachycardia (greater than 250 bpm).

20.8.1.1 Treatment

- Oxygen
- Vagal stimulation (facial immersion in iced water or the application of an ice bag) if well
- Rapid intravenous injection of adenosine is usually successful
- If unstable with depressed conscious level, perform synchronized cardioversion
- Intensive care may be required
- Some children require long-term treatment to prevent recurrence.

20.8.2 Ventricular extrasystoles

In childhood, extrasystoles are not uncommon and usually of no significance. If there are symptoms or multiple extrasystoles, investigation and treatment are required.

20.8.3 Congenital heart block

Heart block may lead to stillbirth. It is usually associated with maternal lupus antibody. Most infants are asymptomatic, but occasionally a pacemaker is necessary.

20.9 Hypertension

Measuring blood pressure is not difficult in children. The correct size cuff must be used (see Section 3.5.4, p. 35 and Figure 28.2c), and in all but the smallest infants reliable measurements may be obtained using automated auscultation methods (e.g. Dinamap). A child's blood pressure must be considered against age-related reference values.

In general those children who have a blood pressure about the 90th centile in early life tend to remain at that end of the distribution curve in later childhood and probably also in adult life. The blood pressure of any child has a close correlation with that of the parents and siblings. In children, hypertension usually has a cause.

20.9.1 Causes of hypertension

- Renal disease
  - Glomerulonephritis
  - Pyelonephritis
  - Congenital defect
  - Renal artery stenosis
- Endocrine
  - Steroid therapy
  - Phaeochromocytoma
  - Congenital adrenal hyperplasia
- Coarctation of the aorta
- Essential.

Compared with adults, a primary cause is found more often and, if treated surgically (e.g. unilateral kidney disease or coarctation), may abolish hypertension. Some 10–15% have essential hypertension and a cause is not found.

Hypertension may be asymptomatic, or may present in a wide variety of ways: failure to thrive, fits, encephalopathy, retinopathy, heart failure or, in the older child, headaches and malaise. Diuretics and hypotensive drugs are used as for adults – and tolerated rather better by most children.

Summary

You should now be able to describe the difference between innocent and pathological murmurs, and know the main types of congenital heart disease. Don't forget that cardiac problems can sometimes present with vague symptoms, such as poor feeding in heart failure. In young babies who collapse a few days after birth, consider whether the ductus arteriosus could have closed. If you can't feel the femoral pulses when doing a baby check, think of coarctation.

 FOR YOUR LOG

- Listen to an innocent murmur
- Listen to pathological murmurs (either real or recorded)

 OSCE TIP

- Child with murmur, e.g. VSD, PS, ASD (see OSCE station 20.1)
- Child without murmur, e.g. normal, postoperative, coarctation
- Sound/video recording of murmur
- Assessment of child's cardiac status – are they well? exercise tolerance
- Is this child in heart failure?
- Take and interpret BP with correct cuff and correct chart.

See EMQ 20.1, EMQ 20.2 and EMQ 20.3 at the end of the book.

OSCE station 20.1: Examination of the cardiovascular system

Clinical approach:

Check hands
• Clubbing
• Colour
• Perfusion

Check face
• Colour
• Anaemia
• Respiratory distress

Pulses
• Rate
• Rhythm
• Both radials, and a brachial
• Femorals? brachio-femoral delay
• Is character of pulses clearly abnormal?

Chest

Inspection
• Scars
  ◇ Remember under arms and on back

Palpable
• Localize apex
• Parasternal heave
• Palapable thrill

Auscultation
• Is heart louder on left?
• Two heart sounds
• ?loud P2 ?split second sound

Murmurs
• Loudness/quality
• Localization
• Radiation
• Timing

George is 4 years old. Please examine his cardiovascular system
• Normal inspection.
  ◇ No scars + no symptoms (this narrows it down!)
  ◇ Not cyanosed (so, no R→L shunt)
• Pulses normal, femorals ✓✓ normal blood pressure (e.g. 85/55)

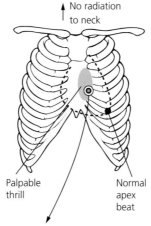

No radiation to neck

Palpable thrill

Normal apex beat

• lower left sternal edge
• 3rd–4th intercostal space
• loud, harsh murmur
• pansystolic

George has an asymptomatic ventricular septal defect.

Never forget:

• Say hello and introduce yourself
• General health — is the child breathless?
• Colour — ?pale/?cyanosed
• Quickly assess growth, nutrition and development
• Mention the obvious (e.g. drip, leg in plaster)

Look around for:

• Nasogastric tube
• Pulse oximeter

Special points

• Blood pressure and pulse vary with age
• Use correct BP cuff size and tell the child what you are doing
• Timing a murmur is difficult in young children — most are systolic
• Do not suggest Fallot's in a pink 13-year-old with no scars
• Cardiovascular malformations are more common in some syndromes (e.g. Down)

21

Gastroenterology

Chapter map

Intestinal disorders are usually acute and infective. They are most serious in infancy, when fluid and electrolyte balance can become dangerously disturbed within a matter of hours and cause death or brain damage. Assessment of chronic disorders can be difficult. In most children, recurrent abdominal pain, gastro-oesophageal reflux, constipation and persistent diarrhoea are benign and self-limiting. Less common but equally important are intestinal obstruction, and malabsorption states including coeliac disease and cystic fibrosis. In children, ulcerative colitis and Crohn disease are uncommon, while peptic ulcers and neoplasm are rare.

This chapter will first review major gastrointestinal presenting symptoms, and then key pathologies.

> **PRACTICE POINT**
>
> If symptoms are not acute, remember to plot growth. Normal growth is always reassuring, even if it does not exclude chronic gastrointestinal disease.

21.1 Symptoms

21.1.1 Vomiting

Acute-onset vomiting is a common symptom. It is highly non-specific and commonly not due to gastro-enterological disease. Projectile (forceful) vomiting in the first weeks of infancy may mean pyloric stenosis. Consider intestinal obstruction or ileus if vomiting is persistent or bile stained.

Persistent mild symptoms are very common in babies, who bring up small amounts of food when breaking wind after a feed. This is *possetting*, a normal process, and the baby is happy and gains weight well. Significant vomiting will be accompanied by weight loss, or at least inadequate weight gain.

Causes of vomiting

Feeding errors
- Infants: faulty feeding technique (especially overfeeding)
- Older children: dietary indiscretions

Infection
- Gastritis (with or without enteritis)
- Parenteral infections (e.g. tonsillitis, meningitis, pneumonia, urinary infection)
- Appendicitis

Mechanical
- Intestinal obstruction, congenital or acquired
- Gastro-oesophageal reflux

Dietary protein intolerance
Raised intracranial pressure
- Meningitis, encephalitis
- Space-occupying lesions (tumour, abscess, haematoma)

Psychological problems
- Rumination
- Bulimia

Miscellaneous
- Periodic syndrome (cyclical vomiting – part of migraine spectrum)
- Travel sickness
- Poisoning.

 PRACTICE POINT

Remember the '3 B's' in a vomiting baby: **B**ile? **B**lood? **B**onny (i.e. gaining weight)?

21.1.1.1 Gastro-oesophageal reflux

Asymptomatic, infrequent reflux of gastric contents is physiological. Reflux is most common in young infants, who effortlessly regurgitate milk over parents, furniture and carpets. The vast majority remain well; reassurance and growth monitoring is all that is justified, and symptoms resolve in infancy with maturation of lower oesophageal sphincter function. Beware if any of the following are present, since they indicate more serious reflux and the need for expert assessment and management: suboptimal weight gain, feeding problems, haematemesis, anaemia and recurrent respiratory symptoms. Reflux is most common and more often severe in infants with cerebral palsy or neurodevelopmental problems, and in preterm infants and young children with chronic respiratory disorders. Investigations include barium studies, 24 h monitoring of oesophageal pH and endoscopy.

In most infants, parents are reassured, and no treatment is given. Surgical treatment with fundoplication (see Figure 21.1), is rarely needed.

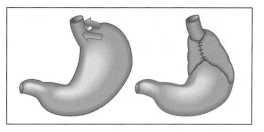

Figure 21.1 Nissen's fundoplication involves wrapping the fundus of the stomach around the lower oesophagus, so that it is occluded by increased intra-abdominal pressure.

 TREATMENT
Gastro-oesophageal reflux

- Reassurance
- Feeding technique – avoid overfeeding, smaller more frequent feeds
- Positioning
  - Raise head of cot (brick under each leg)
  - Avoid semi-supine position (e.g. in infant seat) after feeds
- Milk thickeners
- Antacids
- Gastric acid secretion (H_2 blockers, proton pump inhibitors)
- Fundoplication (rare).

21.1.1.2 Haematemesis

This is not common. Fresh or altered blood may have been swallowed (e.g. epistaxis, tonsillectomy, cracked nipple in the breast-fed infant). Acute gastritis, oesophagitis (typically with reflux), oesophageal varices and peptic ulcer should be considered. Exclude bleeding diathesis. If recent haematemesis is suspected, check the stools for occult blood.

21.1.2 Abdominal pain

21.1.2.1 Acute abdominal pain

Abdominal pain

Condition	Site of pain and tenderness
Non-organic pain	Central
URTI/tonsillitis	Central/RIF
Pyelonephritis	Loins
Lower lobe pneumonia	Upper abdomen
Constipation	Lower abdomen
Mesenteric adenitis	Lower abdomen, often RIF

RIF, right iliac fossa; URTI, upper respiratory tract infection.

This important symptom is highly non-specific. Acute central abdominal pain and vomiting are, for example, common symptoms of tonsillitis. In infants, abdominal pain may be inferred from spasms of crying, restlessness and drawing up the knees. Children can indicate the site of a pain from about the age of 2 years. If there is generalized illness, vomiting, bowel disturbance or fever, assess carefully and re-examine after a few hours. Intussusception, complicated hernia and appendicitis are amongst the important surgical causes. Acute abdominal pain is a typical presenting feature in diabetic ketoacidosis (Section 27.1), Henoch–Schönlein syndrome (Section 23.3.5) and sickle cell disease (Section 25.2.2.3).

Appendicitis

Acute appendicitis occurs at all ages but is uncommon under the age of 2 years. The classical history of central abdominal pain, moving to the right iliac fossa, aggravated by movement and associated with fever and acute phase response, raises suspicion, which may be confirmed by the finding of localized tenderness in the right iliac fossa. Unfortunately, it is not always that easy.

Diagnostic difficulties may be caused by an appendix in an unusual position. Diagnosis of appendicitis is particularly difficult in younger children. The doctor who diagnoses appendicitis before perforation in a 2-year-old deserves praise. Consider imaging (ultrasound/CT) in difficult cases.

21.1.2.2 Chronic abdominal pain

 PRACTICE POINT

Protracted gastrointestinal symptoms: if examination and growth are normal, serious pathology is unlikely.

Recurrent abdominal pain is common throughout childhood and usually of no serious significance when the child is otherwise healthy (Figure 21.2). History, examination, growth assessment and urine microscopy and culture are always justified. The idea that one should exclude all organic causes is naive and usually not possible. Constipation is a common cause and is usually, but not always, apparent on history and examination.

In some children, recurrent abdominal pain betrays emotional disorders. It has often persisted for a year or more by the time medical advice is sought. The child may complain of pain several times in a week and then not at all for a month or two. As children with recurrent abdominal pain are usually of school age, the parents often suspect some stress

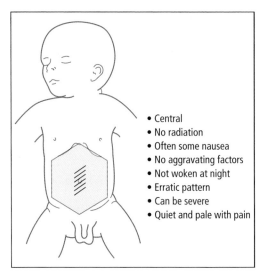

- Central
- No radiation
- Often some nausea
- No aggravating factors
- Not woken at night
- Erratic pattern
- Can be severe
- Quiet and pale with pain

Figure 21.2 Recurrent abdominal pain.

at school. In many there is a family history of irritable bowel syndrome or migraine, and the childhood equivalent of irritable bowel syndrome is increasingly well recognized. Irritable bowel syndrome, non-ulcer dyspepsia and abdominal migraine may be helped by specific treatments for these conditions.

Recurrent abdominal pain

Features implying organic disease:

Pain
- Not central
- Wakes at night
- Related to food

Associated symptoms
- Vomiting/diarrhoea
- Generalized illness
- Dysuria, daytime enuresis

Growth failure.

21.1.3 Abdominal distension

Abdominal distension can be difficult to assess because of the great, normal variation. Fat babies appear to have bigger tummies than thin, muscular babies. Toddlers are normally rather pot-bellied in comparison with older children. Causes include fat, faeces, flatus and fluid: do not forget to test for ascites (Section 3.5.5, p. 36).

 PRACTICE POINT

The best test for abdominal distension – ask the mother 'Is it distended?'!

21.1.4 Diarrhoea

Diarrhoea or constipation requires detailed enquiry. The number and consistency of stools passed by children, especially infants, is very variable. Breast-fed babies pass loose, bright yellow, odourless stools, between seven times a day and once every 7 days. Bottle-fed babies pass paler, firmer stools which may cause straining during defaecation. Unless this straining causes pain or rectal bleeding, it should not be called constipation. Chronic or severe constipation may lead to abdominal pain, abdominal distension, rectal bleeding and feeding problems, and may be associated with emotional and behaviour disorders (Section 11.5.2.1, p. 104).

Causes of diarrhoea

Feeding errors
- In infants, too much, too little or the wrong kind
- In older children, dietary indiscretion

Inflammatory
- Bacterial or viral infection
- Postenteritic syndrome
- Ulcerative colitis/Crohn disease
- Giardiasis
- Parenteral infections

Malabsorption states
- Steatorrhoea (e.g. coeliac disease, cystic fibrosis)
- Disaccharide intolerance

Food intolerance/allergy
Protein-losing enteropathy.

Many toddlers and some older children continue to have three or four bowel actions a day, after meals. 'Toddler diarrhoea' describes the occurrence of frequent loose stools at this age without any pathology, and is due to a rapid bowel transit time. Undigested food is seen in the stool within a few hours of being eaten (our personal best was carrots at 20 min).

Chronic constipation in infants or children may lead to faecal impaction and overflow soiling. This may be mistaken for diarrhoea.

21.1.4.1 Dehydration

Early recognition of shock (suboptimal peripheral perfusion) and hypovolaemia is very important in the acute illness. No one sign diagnoses dehydration (Table 21.1).

Urine output is reduced as dehydration becomes more severe. Children are very efficient at maintaining central blood pressure in the face of hypovolaemia. Hypotension is a late sign, and BP is normal in most children with shock.

In every acutely ill child, check for hypovolaemic shock: the pale, mottled, floppy infant with cold sweaty hands and feet is in shock. Emergency treatment is needed to restore circulation.

21.1.5 Constipation and soiling

This is most common at 5–10 years. Often there is no obvious trigger, or there has been minor change in diet or bowel habit (for example with illness or travel). Constipation leads to faecal retention (Figure 21.3). Hard stool causes pain or anal fissure which inhibits defaecation and increases constipation. At other times, poor toilet training has resulted in infrequent and incomplete bowel actions. The rectum becomes distended with impacted faeces. In extreme cases, only liquid matter can escape, causing overflow diarrhoea with faecal soiling. The child is often unaware of this. His school companions, in contrast, are only too well aware of it, and the child with soiling may become a social outcast.

The abdomen contains hard, faecal masses, often filling the lower half of the abdomen. There is unlikely to be confusion with the rare Hirschsprung disease

Table 21.1 Dehydration

	Mild	Moderate	Severe
% Bodyweight loss	<5	5–10	>10
Appearance	Normal/unwell	Anxious/agitated, restless or sleepy	Drowsy/floppy, lethargic
Eyes/fontanelle	Normal	Sunken	Very sunken
Mucous membranes	Normal/dry	Dry	Very dry
Capillary refill	Normal (<2 s)	Normal/prolonged	Prolonged
Peripheral perfusion	Normal	↓ Peripheral perfusion	Cold hands and feet
Blood pressure	Normal	Normal	Low

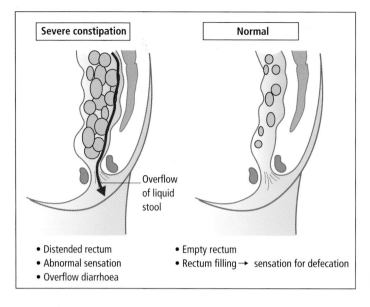

• Distended rectum
• Abnormal sensation
• Overflow diarrhoea

• Empty rectum
• Rectum filling → sensation for defecation

Figure 21.3 Constipation and overflow.

(see Section 21.2.2.1, p. 211), which usually presents at a much earlier age with failure to thrive.

TREATMENT Management of constipation

General advice
• Increased dietary fibre (e.g. bran)
• Ideally the whole family should adopt a high-fibre diet
• Increased fluid and exercise
• Instant success is not to be expected – rectum takes time to resume its normal calibre and sensation.

Bowel training
• Regular toileting (1–2 times daily, 20 minutes after meal – to benefit from the gastrocolic reflex)
• Can combine with star chart)

Laxatives
• Consider disimpaction – thorough emptying of accumulated faeces with laxatives (rarely enemas)
• Faecal softening agents (e.g. Macrogols – polyethylene glycol 3350 with electrolytes; lactulose)
• Stimulant laxative may be added later
• May be needed for many months.

RESOURCE

Go to **www.nice.org.uk** and search for 'constipation in children' to review the latest UK NICE guidance. Also see OSCE station 21.2: Constipation.

Encopresis (deliberate deposition of stool in inappropriate places) is a symptom of serious psychological upset, and the advice of a child psychiatrist should be sought.

21.1.6 Rectal bleeding

Blood in the stools is an alarming symptom, although the cause is often trivial. The most common cause is anal fissure. Bleeding from the duodenum or above will usually cause melaena, although copious bleeding (e.g. swallowed blood after epistaxis or tonsillectomy) may cause red blood to appear with the stool. Blood from the ileum or colon is freely mixed with faecal matter; that from the rectum or anus is only on the surface of the stool. Examination of the perineum, anus and rectal examination (Section 3.5.5, p. 36) may reveal the site of bleeding, or confirm the presence of blood in the stool (Table 21.2).

Piles and rectal carcinoma are very rare in children, and children with more than one episode without known cause should be seen in hospital. Colonoscopy is helpful. *Meckel's diverticulum* is an embryological remnant of the vitelline duct on the ileum and is present in 2% of the population, although in most it causes no symptoms. It often contains gastric mucosa which may ulcerate and bleed, causing rectal bleeding and anaemia. Radioactive technetium is selectively taken up by gastric mucosa and this provides the basis for an elegant diagnostic test.

Table 21.2 **Causes of bleeding per rectum**

Site	Condition	Clinical picture
Ileum	Intussusception	Colicky pain; redcurrant jelly stool; palpable mass
	Meckel's diverticulum	Intermittent abdominal pain and bleeding (red or melaena)
Colon	Dysentery (*Shigella, Salmonella*)	Acute mucoid diarrhoea and pain
	Ulcerative colitis	Chronic mucoid diarrhoea and pain
	Crohn's disease	Abdominal pain, diarrhoea and growth failure
	Intussusception	As above
Rectum	Polyp	Recurrent bleeding: no pain
	Prolapse	Prolapse visible
Anus	Fissure/constipation	On defaecation, much pain and little blood
	Sexual abuse	Dilated/sore anus

21.2 Pathologies

21.2.1 The mouth

21.2.1.1 The teeth

There is considerable normal variation in the time of eruption of teeth, which may lead to unnecessary worry (Section 3.3). Preventative dental health is important for all children. Frequent sugary food should be avoided; we should not forget iatrogenic problems with medicines or vitamin drops. The bottle to suck while falling asleep or the dummy soaked in sweet fluid should be banned. Severe dental problems are more common in children with neurodevelopmental problems and in association with acid reflux.

Include the teeth in the examination of the mouth. It gives an opportunity for congratulation or health education.

Prevention of caries

↓**Plaque-forming organisms**
- Brushing and flossing

↓**Carbohydrates**
- Between meals
- At night

Adequate fluoride
- Supplemented drinking water
- Fluoride toothpaste

Regular dental supervision.

21.2.1.2 Cleft lip and palate

Cleft lip may be unilateral or bilateral (see Figure 7.6). It results from failure of fusion of the maxillary and frontonasal processes. In bilateral cases, the premaxilla (section of the upper lip just below the nose) is anteverted. There is always an associated nasal deformity (Section 7.4).

Cleft palate may occur alone or with cleft lip. It results from failure of fusion of the palatine processes and the nasal septum. Clefting causes nasal regurgitation of feeds, and later 'cleft palate speech' because of nasal escape. Otitis media and sensorineural deafness are more common with clefts. Special feeding techniques are often necessary. Submucous cleft palate, in which the muscle of the soft palate is cleft but the overlying mucosa is intact, is much less common. Always look for other congenital abnormalities.

Early referral to a multidisciplinary team (including orthodontists, plastic surgery, speech therapy) is needed. Most surgical repairs are done within the first 3 months.

21.2.1.3 Micrognathia and retrognathia

Some babies are born with a receding jaw, the mandible being either underdeveloped or displaced backward (Figure 21.4). In severe cases, the tongue (which is also abnormally far back) obstructs breathing from birth. In combination with cleft palate, this is known as *Pierre–Robin syndrome*. Problems with airway and feeding are most severe in early infancy. In most, mandibular growth and improved coordination lead to resolution.

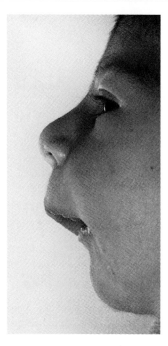

Figure 21.4 An infant with micrognathia and retrognathia.

21.2.1.4 Stomatitis

> **Risk factors for candidiasis**
>
> • Extreme prematurity
> • Poor hygiene
> • Broad-spectrum antibiotics
> • Chronic illness
> • Malnutrition
> • Immunodeficiency
> • HIV.

Stomatitis due to *Candida albicans* (monilia: thrush) is common in infancy. It appears as tiny white flecks inside the cheeks, on the tongue and on the roof of the mouth (Figure 21.5). Milk curds are a little similar but are larger and can easily be detached with a spatula. *Candida albicans* can be cultured from a swab, but treatment is often given on clinical grounds. *Candida albicans* may also infect the skin of the napkin area (Figure 24.4).

> **TREATMENT Oral candidiasis**
>
> • Deal with risk factors
> • Topical antifungal (e.g. nystatin, miconazole)
> • Treat for a few days after apparent cure.

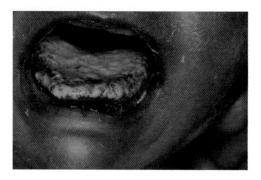

Figure 21.5 Oral thrush

After infancy, stomatitis is usually due to a first infection with herpes simplex type 1 or coxsackie A virus (Section 14.4.3.2, p. 132). Treatment is mainly supportive, with maintenance of hydration, but oral acyclovir may be used for more severe cases if started within 3–4 days.

In *Stevens–Johnson syndrome*, severe mouth ulceration is associated with conjunctivitis, erythema multiforme and severe systemic illness.

21.2.2 Intestinal obstruction

> Bile-stained vomiting is obstruction until proven otherwise.

The causes of intestinal obstruction vary with age. In the younger child, fluid and electrolyte losses rapidly lead to dehydration and circulatory failure.

> **Cardinal symptoms**
>
> • Vomiting ± bile
> • Pain
> • Abdominal distension
> • Constipation.

> **TREATMENT Essential management**
>
> • Early diagnosis
> • Correction of fluid and electrolyte losses
> • Skilled surgery and anaesthesia.

> **PRACTICE POINT**
>
> Gastrointestinal malformations present in the fetus or newborn. After infancy, inguinal hernia is the most common cause of bowel obstruction.

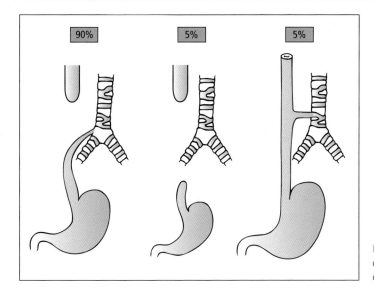

90%   5%   5%

Figure 21.6 Three forms of oesophageal atresia ± tracheo-oesophageal fistula.

21.2.2.1 In the newborn

Fetal swallowing is essential for control of amniotic fluid volume. Obstruction high in the gastrointestinal tract leads to accumulation of fluid (polyhydramnios). No newborn infant with a history of polyhydramnios should be fed milk without ruling out oesophageal atresia (Figure 21.6).

> **PRACTICE POINT**
> **Definitions**
> • Atresia: passage not formed
> • Stenosis: passage narrowed.

Oesophageal atresia is usually associated with *tracheo-oesophageal fistula*. Typically, there is poly-hydramnios, and after birth the infant is 'bubbly' because saliva cannot be swallowed. Diagnosis must be made before milk is given as feeding will lead to choking, cyanosis and aspiration. This is a disastrous start in life for an infant who needs urgent surgery. If there is any suspicion of oesophageal atresia, a wide-bore nasogastric tube should be passed to demon-strate patency of the oesophagus. Early diagnosis and skilled surgery offer the best chance of cure. Other severe congenital abnormalities are present in about half the cases.

Atresias at lower levels cause vomiting and dis-tension. In high obstruction, vomiting occurs early.

Vomit contains bile if the obstruction is below the ampulla of Vater. *Duodenal atresia* and stenosis are particularly common in Down syndrome. *Rectal atresia* (imperforate anus) should not be missed on newborn examination. Infants with low, complete obstruction do not pass meconium, but those with high obstruction do.

Other congenital gut abnormalities

Hirschsprung disease is due to absence of the myen-teric plexus in a segment of bowel, most commonly in the rectosigmoid region. Delayed passage of meconium is followed by constipation and disten-sion. Rectal biopsy yields the diagnosis. Treatment is surgical.

In the embryo, the developing gut herni-ates from the abdominal cavity, returning with a twist so that the caecum ends up in the right iliac fossa. *Malrotation* occurs when this process is incomplete. It may result in obstruction from peri-toneal bands compressing the intestine or volvulus. *Meconium ileus* is pathognomonic of cystic fibrosis (Section 19.8).

In *exomphalos*, the normal embryonic herniation development has become permanent. Bowel and other abdominal viscera protrude from the umbili-cus, often enclosed in a membrane. *Gastroschisis* describes a serious congenital defect of the abdomi-nal wall with herniation of peritoneal contents. Prior to surgical repair, a nasogastric tube is passed, fluid replacement is given and herniated intestine is wrapped in plastic.

21.2.2.2 Infancy and childhood

Intestinal obstruction at later ages may be caused by pyloric stenosis, intussusception, volvulus, strangulated inguinal hernia or other rare causes. Plain abdominal film may assist diagnosis (Figure 21.7).

Intussusception

> **Intussusception**
>
> - Paroxysms of colicky pain
> - Quiet and pale between attacks
> - Cardinal features of obstruction (see box above)
> - Redcurrant jelly stool (blood and mucus)
> - Sausage-shaped mass (often right upper quadrant).

Intussusception occurs most commonly in infancy. Change in diet and intestinal flora or viral infection cause hypertrophy of Peyer's patches, which may form the apex of the intussusception. The intestine folds inside itself, leading to obstruction and local intestinal ischaemia. Once established, spasms of pain become more frequent and severe. Dehydration and hypovolaemia are common. The intussusception can be felt in the abdomen, but this is difficult. Ultrasound may be helpful in diagnosis (Figure 21.8). Air contrast enema is the diagnostic and therapeutic method of choice. Air is insufflated per rectum and will hopefully reduce the intussusception. Contrast medium can be used in the same way. If reduction is unsuccessful or there is perforation or gangrenous bowel, operation and possibly resection is needed.

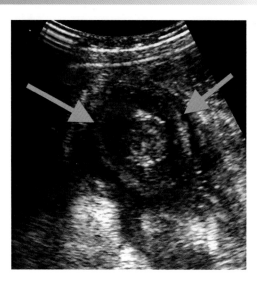

Figure 21.8 Tranverse ultrasound scan through the intussusception shows a 'target' (arrowed) – the intussuscepted bowel in the centre with a sleeve of more distal bowel around it.

 PRACTICE POINT

If air enema is performed within 12 h of intussusception, successful reduction is achieved in over 90%. Diagnostic delay makes surgery more likely.

Pyloric stenosis

Hypertrophic pyloric stenosis occurs in 1 : 150 boys and 1 : 750 girls. Increased incidence in monozygotic twins and close relatives indicates a genetic contribution. It is not congenital (present at birth) and has never been found in stillborn infants. Hypertrophy of the circular muscle of the pylorus leads to progressive obstruction (Figure 21.9).

Symptoms usually begin gradually in the second or third week of life. Vomiting becomes projectile (forms a forceful jet across the room) and is frequent and copious. Weight gain stops and is followed by weight loss. Despite vomiting, the baby remains ravenous. A *test feed* is performed to make the diagnosis. Watch the infant feed. As the stomach fills, waves of peristalsis become visible, crossing the epigastrium from left to right. Gastric peristalsis increases until the infant vomits, when the vomitus may shoot out several feet. The hypertrophic pylorus is felt in the right hypochondrium around the time of vomiting. It is the shape and size of a large olive and very firm.

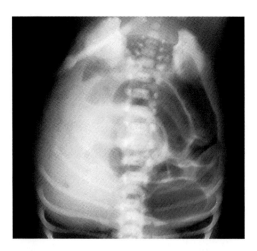

Figure 21.7 Plain abdominal X-ray showing dilated loops of small bowel.

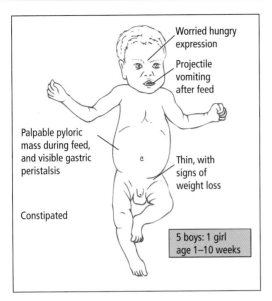

Worried hungry expression

Projectile vomiting after feed

Palpable pyloric mass during feed, and visible gastric peristalsis

Thin, with signs of weight loss

Constipated

5 boys: 1 girl
age 1–10 weeks

Figure 21.9 Pyloric stenosis.

Diagnosis is often confirmed by ultrasound, demonstrating a large pylorus and a narrow elongated canal.

Repeated vomiting leads to dehydration and large losses of hydrochloric acid. The result is a hypochloraemic alkalosis. It is important to correct dehydration and electrolyte abnormalities before surgery. In Ramstedt's operation (pyloromyotomy), the pylorus is exposed through a horizontal skin incision and the hypertrophic muscle divided along its length until the mucosa bulges up. This can be performed laparoscopically. Postoperatively most infants will tolerate milk a few hours later, and the prognosis is excellent.

 PRACTICE POINT

Blood gas in pyloric stenosis
pH 7.50 PCO_2 4.6 kPa   Bicarbonate 36 mmol/L
Alkalosis because pH > 7.40; high bicarbonate + normal CO_2, therefore: metabolic alkalosis.

21.2.3 Hernia

Hernias in children may involve the umbilicus, the diaphragm, or the inguinal or femoral regions. They differ in some important ways from hernias in adults.

21.2.3.1 Umbilical hernia

This is common and harmless. There is a well defined, circular defect centred on the umbilicus. Umbilical hernias are always easily reducible and virtually never strangulate. When babies with an umbilical hernia cry, the hernia protrudes. Spontaneous resolution is usual before the first birthday though it may take up to 5 years. Treatment is reserved for large non-resolving lesions.

21.2.3.2 Diaphragmatic hernia

This congenital abnormality occurs when one side of the diaphragm is not formed. Usually this is detected on fetal ultrasound before birth. Abdominal contents herniate into the chest early in fetal life and prevent normal lung growth. Most diaphragmatic hernias are left sided: at birth the abdomen appears scaphoid (empty – literally boat shaped); the apex beat is displaced to the right; pulmonary hypoplasia leads to respiratory failure within hours of birth. Chest X-ray makes the diagnosis clear. Early intubation and positive pressure ventilation are usually necessary, and survival depends on lung size and surgery.

21.2.3.3 Inguinal hernia

This is common in boys, rare in girls. It is often bilateral. It is very common in extremely preterm infants. A big hernia will form a large swelling in the scrotum, which can be reduced quite easily if the baby is quiet.

A small hernia will cause a swelling in the groin which may be visible intermittently. The smaller hernia is more likely to strangulate. Complications are common and spontaneous resolution does not occur. Surgical repair should be undertaken within days. The hernial sac is resected and the defect repaired (herniotomy).

21.2.4 Gastrointestinal infections

21.2.4.1 Infective diarrhoea

 PRACTICE POINT

In infants with gastroenteritis:
- Breast feeding should not stop
- Formula milk can be reintroduced as soon as rehydration is achieved.

Acute, infective diarrhoea is common. It spreads rapidly through a closed community such as a household or a hospital ward. It is potentially lethal, especially in the very young or malnourished. The cause is viral or bacterial, although a similar illness may result from ingestion of bacterial exotoxins or chemical poisons. Causative organisms may be found in 70%. Rotavirus is found in over 50% of cases (this will fall with the advent of immunization Tables 14.1, 14.2), and more common bacterial infections include *Campylobacter*, *Salmonella*, *E. coli* and *Shigella*. *Cryptosporidium* is particularly important in immunodeficient children.

The main danger is that diarrhoea and vomiting quickly upset the fluid and electrolyte balance. Dehydration must be recognized early (see Section 21.1.4.1). The basis of treatment is rehydration and correction of electrolyte balance. The answer is a beautiful example of applied physiology. The combination of sodium and glucose provides accelerated uptake of salt and water through glucose-coupled sodium co-transport. *Oral rehydration solutions* (ORS) are conveniently made up from pre-packed sachets of dry powder. After careful reconstitution, small volumes are given at frequent intervals in order to rehydrate and then maintain hydration. Only a minority require intravenous rehydration. When hospital admission is needed, there must be strict barrier nursing to prevent the spread of infection to others.

TREATMENT ORS	
Na	60 (mmol/L)
K	20 (mmol/L)
Cl	60 (mmol/L)
Citrate	10 (mmol/L)
Glucose	90 (mmol/L)

The introduction of ORS has made a major contribution to reduction in worldwide childhood mortality.

Hypernatraemic dehydration (serum sodium > 150 mmol/L) is now rare but remains a dangerous condition where the electrolyte disorder must be corrected slowly (not more than 1 mmol/L/h). Antibiotics should be reserved for systemic infection. In *Salmonella* and *Shigella* infections, antibiotics may delay clearance of the pathogens.

21.2.4.2 Postenteritic syndrome

In less than 5% of gastroenteritis, a combination of lactose intolerance and/or acquired dietary protein intolerance occurs. This results in the return of watery diarrhoea each time milk is reintroduced, together with continued weight loss. Careful dietetic appraisal and management usually results in resolution within 2 months.

21.2.4.3 Helicobacter pylori

The discovery of this organism has revolutionized the treatment of peptic ulceration in adults. Its association with peptic ulcers, which are rare in children, is strong. Colonization appears to occur in childhood, is usually asymptomatic and prevalence is declining in developed countries (<10%). Indiscriminate testing and treatment is not appropriate. Diagnosis may be made by one or more of the following three methods: (1) stool antigen test; (2) a 'breath test' which exploits *Helicobacter*'s ability to split urea (given orally) and produce carbon dioxide (measured in the breath); and (3) positive culture from endoscopic biopsy. If *Helicobacter* is found, eradication therapy is sometimes appropriate.

21.2.4.4 Giardiasis and worms

Giardia lamblia is a protozoon which may live in the child's intestine without disturbing their health. Occasionally it causes chronic diarrhoea and malabsorption (Section 21.2.5). Stools may contain cysts, or the organism is found in duodenal aspirate or biopsy. Treatment is with metronidazole.

Threadworms (*Enterobius vermicularis*) are relatively common. They cause no symptoms apart from perianal itching which may disturb sleep. Diagnosis is usually made by seeing the worms on the perianal skin or stool. Ova may be found on the perianal region, using cellophane swabs or Sellotape. Mebendazole is the drug of choice for children over 2 years. Success is achieved by treating the whole family, including parents. Apparent failure is usually due to re-infection.

The *roundworm* (*Ascaris lumbricoides*) is uncommon in Europe. There are usually no symptoms before a worm is passed with the stools. *Tapeworms* (*Taenia saginata* and *T. solium*) present with the passage of segments. Treatment may be difficult. *Hookworm* (*Ancylostoma*) is an important cause of iron-deficient anaemia in developing countries.

21.2.5 Malabsorption states

Malabsorption

- Abnormal stools
- Poor growth
- Nutrient deficiency.

Poor absorption may be specific to one nutrient or generalized. Malabsorption with steatorrhoea is usually due to coeliac disease or cystic fibrosis. Fatty stools are offensive, pale and bulky, and frequent. They are difficult to flush down the toilet because of their tendency to float. Abdominal distension due to gas and fluid is accompanied by weight loss and muscle wasting.

> **Special investigation of malabsorption**
>
> - Dietary assessment
> - Growth assessment
> - Stool for fat content and culture
> - Laboratory assessment of nutrition
> - Sweat test
> - Coeliac disease antibodies
> - Jejunal biopsy.

21.2.5.1 Coeliac disease

Coeliac disease is an immune-mediated sensitivity to gluten in wheat, rye or other cereals. It occurs in individuals with HLA-DQ2 or 8 haplotype, who are genetically susceptible. Symptoms can only occur after the introduction of cereals into the diet during weaning. Early introduction of cereals before 4 months of age may increase the risk of coeliac disease. The classical presentation (Figure 21.10) is now less common. Children present at a later age with a variety of gastrointestinal symptoms, variable growth failure and iron-deficient anaemia. The diagnosis is suggested by coeliac disease antibodies (anti-tissue transglutaminase or anti-endomysial), but a clear diagnosis of coeliac disease may require a jejunal biopsy, which shows subtotal villous atrophy (Figure 21.11a and b). Always exclude cystic fibrosis and infection with *Giardia lamblia*.

(a)

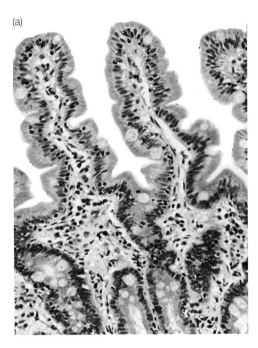

(b)

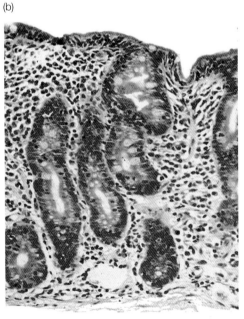

Figure 21.11 (a) In the normal small intestine, the long villi are easily seen. (b) In coeliac disease, there is villous atrophy, and the crypts are hyper plastic.

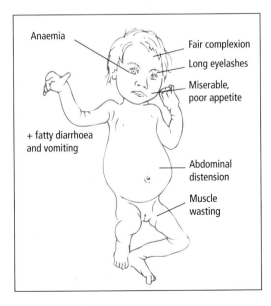

Anaemia

Fair complexion

Long eyelashes

Miserable, poor appetite

+ fatty diarrhoea and vomiting

Abdominal distension

Muscle wasting

Figure 21.10 Classical coeliac disease.

Treatment is lifetime exclusion of all foods containing wheat, rye and barley. The response is rapid and dramatic over a few weeks, with recovery of the villi to normal and rapid catch-up growth. Specific nutrient deficits (e.g. iron, fat-soluble vitamins) must be addressed. Regular follow up of compliance with support from a dietician is essential. Before committing someone to a life-long gluten-free diet, it is vital to be sure of the diagnosis. Some people with coeliac disease 'tolerate' gluten without acute symptoms, but taking gluten will increase the risk of lymphoma. Occasionally gluten intolerance in early life is temporary, so a gluten challenge may help at a later date.

21.2.5.2 Cystic fibrosis

Cystic fibrosis (CF) is the most common cause of pancreatic malabsorption. Advances in nutritional management have been central to the improvements in the prognosis of CF. CF is dealt with in Section 19.8.

21.2.6 Food allergy and intolerance

21.2.6.1 Food intolerance

Food intolerance is an unwanted abnormal response to food. All studies using double blind challenges have shown that symptoms are too often ascribed to reaction to foods. Food intolerance may be allergic, metabolic (e.g. lactase deficiency), toxic (e.g. food colourings) or irritant (e.g. chilli). Food intolerance including allergy can be secondary to gut disorders (e.g. postenteritic syndrome and Crohn disease).

21.2.6.2 Food allergy

 PRACTICE POINT

Most common food antigens leading to allergy
- Cow's milk protein
- Soya
- Eggs
- Wheat
- Peanut
- Others: fish, crustacea, nuts, strawberry, additives.

Food allergy is a reproducible clinical reaction to specific foods accompanied by an abnormal immune response. It occurs in 1–2% of children and is more common in the young. The reaction may be an acute emergency, for instance with anaphylaxis, angioneurotic oedema and urticaria. A more gradual reaction is usual, with vomiting, diarrhoea (and even colitis), failure to thrive or eczema.

Allergy tests are of limited value in diagnosis, although raised levels of IgE specific to individual food proteins are suggestive of allergy. Skin prick tests may also be used. Some believe that food additives (e.g. artificial colourings and flavourings) cause hyperactive behaviour. Challenge with food antigen is done for diagnosis and to establish remission.

 PRACTICE POINT

Diagnosis of food allergy
Remove antigen → symptom resolves
Challenge → symptom recurs.

Increasing numbers of children have acute severe reactions to food antigens, especially in those with asthma. Peanut and cow's milk are the most common. The family need to be trained in resuscitation, and some are given adrenaline to use in an emergency (see Section 14.3). If there is risk of severe reaction, challenges are performed in hospital.

21.2.6.3 Disaccharide intolerance

Disaccharide intolerance usually involves lactose, and occurs in:

- Postenteritic syndrome (temporary complication of gastroenteritis)
- Coeliac disease or cystic fibrosis (not common)
- Permanent hereditary lactase deficiency (rare).

Hydrolysis of disaccharides
Lactose → glucose + galactose
Sucrose → glucose + fructose.

The condition causes a fermentative diarrhoea with frothy explosive stools. A good clinical response to the exclusion of the offending sugar suggests the diagnosis. If the intolerance is temporary, lactose may be cautiously reintroduced once recovery from the underlying cause is complete. Formal diagnosis depends on finding acid disaccharides in the stools, a positive hydrogen breath test after ingestion of the suspect sugar, and deficiency of disaccharidases on jejunal biopsy specimens.

21.2.7 Chronic inflammatory bowel disease

 Inflammatory bowel disease
- Abdominal pain
- Diarrhoea
- Rectal bleeding
- Growth failure.

Ulcerative colitis and *Crohn disease* are not common. However, over a quarter of inflammatory bowel disease presents in childhood, and the incidence of Crohn disease is increasing. The two conditions do not differ in essentials from the adult pattern. Children with the classic symptoms are diagnosed early. Crohn diease particularly presents with non-specific features, notably growth failure and weight loss. Occasionally there may be no gut symptoms. Specific clues to Crohn diease include oral disease and perianal sepsis, fissures and skin tags. An acute phase response (e.g. raised C-reactive protein) is found on investigation. Contrast studies and isotope-labelled white cell scans are helpful. The diagnosis rests on histology of biopsy specimens obtained at endoscopy.

Treatment is empirical and not very satisfactory. Remission may be induced by steroids and maintained with salicylates. Crohn disease may be controlled with a period on a liquid feed diet. Immunosuppressive agents are helpful, and monoclonal antibody to tumour necrosis factor is used in refractory cases. Surgery is usually avoided in childhood.

In infancy, colitis is usually due to cow's milk intolerance and responds to the exclusion of cow's milk.

21.2.8 Hepatic failure

Hepatic failure is rare. It occurs in fulminating viral infections (e.g. hepatitis, Epstein–Barr (Section 14.4.3.2, p.131), severe obstructive jaundice, metabolic disorders (Section 27.7) and with a variety of different poisons including paracetamol. Early referral to a specialist centre for investigation and consideration for liver transplant is essential.

Reye syndrome is the name given to a devastating illness of young children in which there is an acute encephalitis together with acute liver failure. There is a high mortality. The cause is unknown but, because of a possible association with salicylate therapy, aspirin should not be used in children under 12 years.

 Summary

Vomiting is an important but non-specific symptom in childhood. Know the list of causes. In the infant, consider reflux, pyloric stenosis and overfeeding,

but don't forget less obvious causes like urinary tract infection. Abdominal pain is a common reason for emergency and outpatient presentation, and again has many causes. Many young children have recurrent benign abdominal pain (which may have a psychological root), but worry when the pain is not central, growth is poor, or if the child is missing lots of school. Chronic constipation is a common outpatient problem, which responds well to sustained laxatives and a behavioural programme, underpinned by careful explanation and support.

We have covered the 'surgical' pathologies of hernias and intestinal obstruction. Intussusception can be difficult to spot, but early diagnosis avoids need for surgery. Infective diarrhoea is usually easy to diagnose because it has gone round the family. Coeliac and Crohn diease are both notorious for their varied and subtle presentations. Finally, don't forget to assess growth in the evaluation of gastrointestinal problems.

 FOR YOUR LOG

- History in a vomiting infant.
- Consultation for gastro-oesphageal reflux.
- Consultation for constipation.

? OSCE TIP

- Examination of the abdomen (see OSCE station 21.1).
- Video of infant vomiting, growth chart and lab results, e.g. pyloric stenosis.
- Inguinal hernia.
- Abdominal X-ray of intestinal obstruction.
- Non-gastroenterological abdomen, e.g. spherocytosis.

See EMQ 21.1, EMQ 21.2, EMQ 21.3 and EMQ 21.4 at the end of the book.

OSCE station 21.1: Persistent diarrhoea

Task: You are to take a history from Kirsty's parent. Kirsty is 18 months of age, and has had frequent loose stools for 3–4 months. The stools fill her nappy and overflow. She has no significant past medical history. The examiner will observe your history-taking, and at the end ask you what you think.

Don't forget, take a full history but note:

Kirsty's history: key points

What are the stools like?	*Frequency, consistency and contents*	**Loose, pale and bulky stools.**
Any abnormal contents?	*Blood, mucus, parasites, undigested food, vegetables*	**Her stools are very offensive stools, but no blood.**
Associated symptoms?	*Vomiting, abdominal distension, mouth/ perinanal disease*	**Stools do not flush away easily. Abdomen is always swollen.**
How is Kirsty?	*Is she her normal self otherwise? Is she energetic and playing and developing normally?*	**Always tired and moaning, and will not play for long.**
Dietary history?	*Is diet reasonable on quick assessment? Is there excessive fluid intake? What is fibre intake?*	**Diet is normal and her appetite is generally good.**
Growth?	*Parent-held record (red book): interpret growth chart*	**Weight and height have fallen from the 50–75th centiles. Weight now around 10th and height is 10–25th centile.**

Kirsty's history has important pointers to malabsorption and steatorrhoea. You cannot tell the cause from this history. It could be coeliac disease, cystic fibrosis or giardiasis. Many young children with persistent loose stools have toddler diarrhoea (Chapter 21) but would be growing normally.

OSCE station 21.2: Constipation

You are working in primary care as a junior trainee. Mrs McTaggart has brought her 7 year old son James who has been soiling 3 times a week for a month. The GP, Dr Black, has diagnosed constipation, because James has been passing hard stools once a week for 4 months, and has significant faecal loading palpable in the abdomen. There is no history to suggest any other organic cause or any psychological upset. School are calling Mrs McTaggart in to help change James every time he soils, although when it occurs at home he usually sorts himself out without help. She has asked that you explain the diagnosis and agree a management plan with Mrs McTaggart. James is not present.

Introduction

Introduce yourself and your role, explain what you have been asked to do, and confirm with Mrs McTaggart that she is happy with that. Brief clarifying questions will help to confirm key points in the history and set the scene for your explanation. check **I**deas, **C**oncerns and **E**xpectations (ICE).

Mrs McTaggart heard the GP mention constipation but is very sceptical. 'James' main problem is loose stools – how can that be constipation?' The GP mentioned laxatives, but 'Surely that will only make matters worse?' She will only be persuaded to agree to appropriate treatment if you give a clear and sympathetic explanation.

Explain the diagnosis

Explain that constipation is common, can build up gradually and does not need to have an obvious trigger. Explain the concept of overflow, and 'baggy' bowel (see Section 21.1.5). A diagram may be useful. Take time to address her concerns about the diagnosis, and be clear why this is constipation. Ask if she has any other questions regarding diagnosis – *'Surely some investigations are needed?'* – explain that investigations are not necessary.

Management plan

* *General advice* – increased fibre, fluid and exercise. Deal with it in a low-key supportive way at school – talk to teacher about whether she could facilitate discreet access to a toilet, and James to take in clean pants and wipes.
* *Laxative disimpaction* – a stool softening osmotic agent (polyethylene glycol 3350 with electrolytes) to be taken in escalating daily doses until clearout (warn that soiling may get worse).
* *Laxative maintenance* – continue the stool softener regularly (1 paediatric sachet twice daily would be a reasonable dose), adjust up or down to achieve soft, formed daily stools. Continue for many months – if stopped too soon, the constipation will recur. A stimulant laxative (like senokot or picosulphate) is sometimes added after 2–3 weeks.
* *Sitting exercises and star chart* – James to get a star for sitting on the toilet and pushing for 3–5 minutes once or twice a day, 20 minutes after a meal. Another star for any stool passed in the toilet. Don't give stars for clean pants (could encourage with-holding). No withdrawal of stars or punishment for soiling – low-key, matter of fact approach.
* *Follow-up* – offer an early appointment in 2 weeks to review how things are going with the disimpaction.

Summarize and ask if any other questions

Summarize key points. Offer a leaflet. Ask if any questions.
What about side effects of the medication? Could he become addicted?
Reassure that the medication is safe, stays within the bowel and helps to hold water which softens, and is not addictive. The main problem is initial worsening of the soiling and/or diarrhoea, but this is a necessary stage of treatment. Also see OSCE station 4.1: 'Shock'.

22

Urinary Tract and Genitalia

Chapter map

The commonest problems seen in primary and secondary care are urine infections, wetting problems and various concerns about the genitalia. Congenital problems are mainly picked up antenatally – posterior urethral valves is one of the most important. You should be able to recognize the classic paediatric presentations of acute nephritis and nephrotic syndrome, and know an approach to presentations of haematuria and vaginal discharge. After a review of urinary tract development and urine examination, this chapter covers congenital abnormalities, then renal diseases, followed by urine infection and enuresis, and finishes with a section on genital problems.

22.1 Development

The fetus passes urine from the 12th week of intrauterine life, and by term swallows and passes 500 mL/day. Most of the amniotic fluid is fetal urine. Excretion of waste products occurs as the fetus is being effectively haemodialysed by the placenta.

Birth demands a rapid drop in urine output. Limited excretory function is needed because body growth is rapid and milk contains exactly the right substances required for growth with little excess. When this situation is altered, the limitations of the immature kidney are seen. If the neonate has excess intravenous fluid, she becomes oedematous. If she has diarrhoea, the

Paediatrics Lecture Notes, Ninth edition. Simon J. Newell and Jonathan C. Darling. © 2014 John Wiley & Sons, Ltd. Published 2014 by John Wiley & Sons, Ltd.

kidneys fail to conserve fluid adequately. Compared with the adult, a relatively small decrease in renal perfusion, e.g. from mild dehydration or cardiac failure, may result in a raised plasma urea level.

Renal growth continues throughout childhood by means of increase in nephron size and not by the production of new nephrons.

22.2 Urine examination

22.2.1 Collection

Urine examination is a useful window into the urinary tract and beyond (Table 22.1). Proper collection in infants requires patience and care and is best done by 'clean catch'. Alternative methods include adhesive urine-bags, or urine collection pads. Catheter sampling or suprapubic aspiration with ultrasound guidance are sometimes performed when there is a pressing need to reach a diagnosis (e.g. suspected sepsis (Figure 22.1).

22.2.1.1 Clean catch method

- Have sterile container ready.
- Ensure baby has been fed.
- Wait patiently!

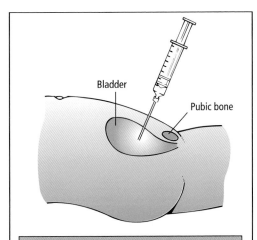

- Ensure urine has not been passed recently
- Use a portable ultrasound (if available) to check for full bladder
- Ask assistant to hold infant's legs down
- Clean skin
- Insert 21–23 g needle, 1 cm above symphisis pubis, angled as shown
- Aspirate gently during insertion
- Keep to midline, not more than 3 cm deep

Figure 22.1 Suprapubic aspiration.

- When baby starts to void, collect into the container.
- Don't collect until a second or so after voiding has started.
- Try gently tapping the suprapubic region to encourage micturition.

22.2.1.2 Urine-bag method

- Wash genitalia and perineum with water (not antiseptics) and dry.
- Apply bag, ensuring a seal all the way round the genitalia.
- Do not replace a nappy over the bag.
- Remove the bag as soon as the baby has voided.
- Cut a hole in a corner of the bag and allow urine to drain into a sterile container.

PRACTICE POINT Haematuria

- Microscopic – detectable only with dipstick and microscopy
- Macroscopic ('gross') – visible to the naked eye – urine looks red or smoky brown.

22.3 Congenital anomalies

Fetal ultrasound provides warning of many renal abnormalities. Renal agenesis, urethral valves and other obstructive lesions are detected (Figure 22.2).

22.3.1 Renal

22.3.1.1 Agenesis

The ureteric bud fails to develop so that the ureter and kidney are absent. If unilateral, the child may live a healthy life provided the other kidney is normal. Bilateral agenesis is lethal; oligohydramnios is noted during pregnancy, and affected infants have pulmonary hypoplasia and characteristic facial appearance (*Potter syndrome*).

22.3.1.2 Hypoplastic kidneys

The small kidneys are deficient in renal parenchyma. They are not usually associated with other abnormalities.

22.3.1.3 Dysplastic kidneys

These contain abnormally differentiated parenchyma. They are commonly associated with obstruction and other abnormalities of the urinary tract.

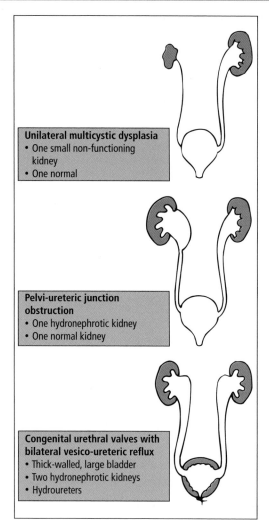

Unilateral multicystic dysplasia
• One small non-functioning kidney
• One normal

Pelvi-ureteric junction obstruction
• One hydronephrotic kidney
• One normal kidney

Congenital urethral valves with bilateral vesico-ureteric reflux
• Thick-walled, large bladder
• Two hydronephrotic kidneys
• Hydroureters

Figure 22.2 Congenital urinary tract abnormalities.

Polycystic kidney disease

A form of renal dysplasia.
Infantile polycystic disease
• Massive kidneys
• Renal failure early in life
• Autosomal recessive
Adult polycystic disease
• Autosomal dominant
Not usually detected in early life
• Kidneys not enlarged, function well during childhood.

22.3.2 Ureteric abnormalities

The most common problem is pelvi-ureteric junction obstruction (PUJO) (Figure 22.2) which may cause hydronephrosis and permanent renal damage. Duplication of the ureter and pelvis may occur on one or both sides. If it only affects the upper half of the ureter, it is not important. If there are two ureters extending down to the bladder with two separate ureteric openings, abnormalities of the lower ureter are common. A *ureterocele* is a cystic enlargement of the ureter within the bladder which may cause obstruction.

22.3.3 Bladder and urethral abnormalities

22.3.3.1 Posterior urethral valves

These are an important cause of obstruction to urine flow and occur almost exclusively in boys. They are usually detected antenatally, or present in early infancy, as acute obstruction or chronic partial obstruction with dribbling micturition.

Obstruction may cause direct damage by back pressure or predispose to urinary tract infection, which may cause further damage. Most obstructive abnormalities can be corrected by surgery. Obstruction of the lower urinary tract is frequently associated with renal dysplasia.

 PRACTICE POINT

Ask about urinary stream and feel for the bladder in boys with suspected urine infections, or failure to thrive.

22.3.3.2 Hypospadias (Figure 22.3)

The urethral opening is on the ventral surface of the penis. If it is at the junction of the glans and shaft, no treatment is needed, but if it is on the shaft of the penis plastic surgery is required. In all but the mildest cases, there is ventral flexion (*chordee*) of the penis. There may be associated meatal stenosis.

 PRACTICE POINT

Avoid circumcision in hypospadias, because the foreskin is used in reconstruction.

Table 22.1 Evaluation of urine

Inspection

Translucency – cloudy appearance usually due to chemical deposits (especially in cold, stale urine). Infected urine is usually hazy, and can be cloudy.

Colour – Blood may make the urine appear red, pink, reddish-brown, or 'smoky'. Other reasons for unusual colours include ingested foods (e.g. beetroot), sweets and drugs (e.g. rifampicin). Orange-pink stains in the nappy are normal and due to urate crystals.

Frothiness – suggests presence of protein or bile.

Smell – may be altered by infection (foul, fishy due to urea-splitting organisms), drugs (e.g. penicillin), or chemicals produced by body metabolism (e.g. ketones or due to rare inborn errors of metabolism (see Chapter 27)).

Dipstick testing

Chemically impregnated test strips (OSCE station 22.1) test for the following:

- **Protein** – trace is normal, often due to concentrated urine, but if more than one sample has ≥1+, measure the protein:creatinine ratio. Transient proteinuria may occur with fever or hard exercise. Persistent proteinuria is a feature of nephritis and kidney damage.
- **Glucose** – either due to a low renal threshold or hyperglycaemia (check blood glucose for diabetes mellitus).
- **Haemoglobin** – though extremely sensitive, positive reactions are abnormal and usually due to haematuria. Haemoglobinuria and myoglobinuria also produce a positive test, so send for microscopy to identify red cells.
- **pH** – usually 5 or 6, but is alkaline in infants with pyloric stenosis (see Chapter 21) and sometimes due to urine infection or alkaline medicines.
- **Ketones** – common with illness, anorexia or vomiting, and in the many school children who have had no breakfast.
- **Nitrites and leucocytes** – nitrites indicate infection because most urinary pathogens reduce nitrate to nitrite. Excess leucocytes (+ or more) may be the result of any inflammation, including infection. The presence of both leucocytes and nitrites is strongly suggestive of infection, and their absence is reassuring, but a sample should always be sent for microscopy and culture when infection is suspected in a young child.

Microscopy

- **Cells** – Normal urine should not contain more than 2 *red cells* $\times$ 10^6/L and 5 (boys) to 50 (girls) *white cells* $\times$ 10^6/L. The most common causes of haematuria are urinary tract infection and glomerulonephritis.
- **Casts** are formed in the renal tubules. They may be due to glomerulonephritis when they are made up of red cells (these become granular as cells disintegrate). Hyaline casts devoid of cells are seen in proteinuria.
- **Bacteria** – *Escherichia coli* bacteria (the commonest cause of urine infection) appear as gram negative motile rods.

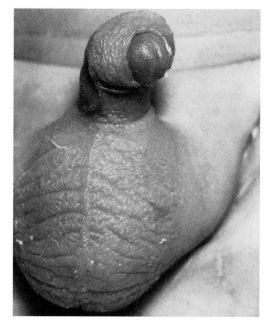

Figure 22.3 Hypospadias. The meatus is at the junction of the glans and shaft.

22.4 Renal disease

22.4.1 Terminology

Note that several different pathologies may be associated with one syndrome, and vice versa. For instance, proliferative glomerulonephritis may be found in several different clinical syndromes. One syndrome may be associated with several different morphological pictures, and have several different aetiologies.

> **Classification system**
>
> - SYNDROMES: collection of symptoms and signs, e.g. acute nephritic syndrome, nephrotic syndrome
> - PATHOLOGY: results of biopsy, e.g. proliferative glomerulonephritis, minimal changes
> - AETIOLOGY: e.g. diabetic, poststreptococcal.

The most important syndromes of renal disease in childhood are:

- Acute nephritic syndrome
- Recurrent haematuria

- Nephrotic syndrome
- Symptomless proteinuria
- Renal calculi
- Renal insufficiency.

22.4.2 Acute nephritic syndrome

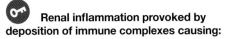 **Renal inflammation provoked by deposition of immune complexes causing:**

- Haematuria
- Oliguria
- Hypertension
- Raised serum creatinine.

22.4.2.1 Aetiology

The best-known form is *poststreptococcal glo-merulonephritis*, which usually occurs 2–3 weeks after a β-haemolytic streptococcal throat infection. Immune complexes composed of streptococci, antibody and complement are deposited in the glomeruli. This provokes proliferation of the endothelial cells (proliferative glomerulonephritis). Although now rare in developed countries, it is common worldwide.

An acute nephritic syndrome may also occur at the time of pneumococcal pneumonia, septicaemia, glandular fever and other viral infections. It is sometimes seen in Henoch–Schönlein syndrome (Section 23.3.5) and the collagen diseases.

22.4.2.2 Features

- Age 3+ (peak 7 years)
- Sudden onset of illness 2–3 weeks after pharyngitis
- Coca-cola coloured urine
- Facial oedema (especially eyelids)
- Abdominal or loin pain
- ↑ blood pressure.

22.4.2.3 Investigations

A small volume of blood-stained urine is passed. In addition to copious red blood cells there is an excess of white cells and proteinuria. Red cell and granular casts are present. The serum creatinine is raised in two-thirds of children. If the cause is streptococcal, ASO titre is raised and serum complement is reduced. Blood pressure is raised.

22.4.2.4 Course and treatment

Oliguria lasts for only a few days. Diuresis usually occurs within a week and is accompanied by return of serum creatinine and blood pressure to normal.

The haematuria and proteinuria gradually subside over the next year. During the oliguric phase, fluid and protein are restricted, but it is rarely necessary to start a strict renal failure regime. Other treatment is symptomatic. Over 80% make a full recovery, but a few develop progressive renal disease.

22.4.3 Recurrent haematuria syndrome

 KEY POINTS

- Episodes of haematuria
- Association with exercise, or systemic infection
- Red cell and granular casts in the urine.

The bouts of haematuria usually occur at the time of a systemic infection or exertion. The haematuria results from nephritis of unknown cause. The child may feel unwell but more often has no symptoms. The urine contains red cell and granular casts.

Between attacks the urine is normal or shows microscopic haematuria. Proteinuria is less common and may indicate more serious renal disease. Investigations are done to exclude other causes of haematuria: urine culture, ultrasound scan and intravenous pyelogram for a tumour or stone, and screening tests for bleeding disorders.

Clinical approach to haematuria

Source
- **Renal** – brown colour, glomerular casts, features of nephritis
- **Lower tract** – red, may vary with phase of micturition (e.g. terminal haematuria)

Differential diagnosis
- Urine infection (UTI symptoms? – positive microscopy and culture)
- Glomerulonephritis (check BP, do U&Es, ASOT, complement)
- Recurrent haematuria syndrome
- Tumour (abdominal mass? – renal USS)
- Bleeding diathesis (other bleeding or easy bruising? – clotting screen)
- Trauma
- Urinary stones and hypercalcuria (family history?)
- Drugs.

22.4.3.1 Nephrotic syndrome

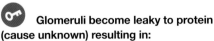 **Glomeruli become leaky to protein (cause unknown) resulting in:**

- Heavy proteinuria
- Hypo-albuminaemia
- Oedema.

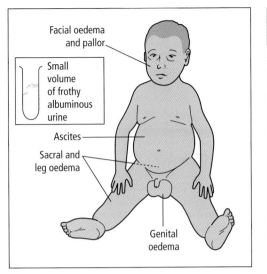

Facial oedema and pallor

Small volume of frothy albuminous urine

Ascites

Sacral and leg oedema

Genital oedema

Figure 22.4 Nephrotic syndrome.

Table 22.2 **Acute nephritic and nephrotic syndromes**

	Acute nephritic syndrome	Nephrotic syndrome
Child		
Oedema	Mild facial	Gross
Blood pressure	Raised	Normal
Urine		
Albumin	+ +	+ + + +
RBC	+ + + +	0 or +
WBC	+ +	0
Casts	Cellular/granular	Hyaline
Bacteria	0	0
Serum		
Albumin	Normal	Low

22.4.3.2 Features

Peak onset is between the ages of 2 and 5 years. Apart from the gradual onset of generalized oedema, the child may be only mildly off colour. Other symptoms are directly related to oedema, for instance discomfort from ascites or breathlessness from pleural effusion (Figure 22.4).

22.4.3.3 Aetiology

Over 90% of childhood nephrotic syndrome is the result of primary renal disease of unknown cause. Nephrotic syndrome secondary to systemic illness is less common than in adults, the least rare cause being Henoch–Schönlein syndrome (Section 23.3.5). In Africa, malaria is an important cause.

22.4.3.4 Pathology

Up to the age of 5 years, over 80% of affected children show no significant abnormality on renal biopsy, hence the term 'minimal change disease', which has a good prognosis. After the age of 10, more serious pathology becomes likely.

22.4.3.5 Investigations

The urine is frothy and there is heavy albuminuria. Highly selective proteinuria, i.e. urine containing a high proportion of small molecular weight proteins, is a good prognostic feature suggesting minimal change histology. Hyaline casts are abundant. Serum albumin is below 25 g/L and the serum cholesterol is usually raised. Serum creatinine is usually normal (Table 22.2).

22.4.3.6 Treatment and prognosis

Corticosteroids are given in large doses for 4 weeks. While there is oedema, fluid and salt are restricted: diuretics may be needed if the oedema is causing symptoms. Most children go into remission within 2 weeks of starting steroids. Diuresis occurs and the oedema and albuminuria disappear rapidly. A large proportion relapse within the next year. They can be given further courses of steroids, but if the relapses are frequent, cyclophosphamide will usually produce a longer remission.

The long-term prognosis is good. Although frequent relapses can be most troublesome during childhood, with increasing age they become less frequent and most children grow out of the condition by the time they are adults and thereafter have normal renal function and good health. A few (mainly those initially unresponsive to steroids) develop renal insufficiency.

22.4.4 Symptomless proteinuria

PRACTICE POINT

Persistent proteinuria is a sign of renal disease and requires investigation.

Before embarking on elaborate tests of renal function or a biopsy, it is important to exclude *postural proteinuria* (orthostatic), since this is most common between 10 and 15 years. Such children have proteinuria when up and active but not when lying in bed. Postural proteinuria is generally considered a benign condition which does not progress.

22.4.5 Renal calculi

Stones in the urinary tract of children are less common than in adults. Occasionally they cause pain or renal colic, but more often are detected by chance on X-ray. Most stones are of infective origin, especially in boys with a proteus infection. A 'urinary stone screen' should be sent to test for chemicals that predispose to stone formation (e.g. calcium, oxalate, cystine), and blood to check serum calcium and phosphate.

22.4.6 Renal insufficiency (renal failure)

22.4.6.1 Acute renal failure

Acute renal failure (acute kidney injury) describes the situation in which previously healthy kidneys suddenly stop working. It is a rewarding condition to treat in childhood because many children who present acutely will recover, for example from acute tubular necrosis due to hypovolaemic shock. A particularly notorious example is haemolytic–uraemic syndrome.

> **Haemolytic–uraemic syndrome (HUS)**
> - Affects mainly older infants and toddlers
> - Due to verotoxin-producing *E. coli* 0157
> - Follows a brief gastroenteritis-like illness
> - Clinical triad: haemolytic anaemia, thrombocytopenia and acute renal failure
> - Management – early peritoneal dialysis in a paediatric renal unit
> - 80% recover completely.

22.4.6.2 Chronic renal failure

Progressive renal insufficiency or *chronic kidney disease* is uncommon. In early life, congenital abnormalities, particularly renal dysplasia, are the main cause. Thereafter, various forms of glomerulonephritis are the most common cause. Children with end-stage renal disease have the same features as adults, e.g. anaemia, hypertension and renal rickets: in addition, they fail to grow.

Successful transplantation is the aim, and results for children are better than for adults. Until transplantation is possible, the child is maintained on dialysis: continuous/intermittent ambulatory peritoneal dialysis is frequently used despite the common complication of peritonitis. Erythropoietin is used to treat the anaemia. The child's complex medical and nutritional needs demand a multidisciplinary team.

22.5 Urinary tract infection (UTI)

> 🔑 In young and ill children, give intravenous antibiotics without waiting for microscopy results. Look for other infections (meningitis, septicaemia, pneumonia).

> UTI is more likely to cause renal damage in pre-school children if:
> - Infant (under 1 year)
> - Upper tract infection
> - Vesico-ureteric reflux present ('backfiring' of urine up to the kidneys on micturition)
> - Delay in treatment.

22.5.1 Incidence

From birth to adolescence the prevalence of UTI is just over 1%. In the neonatal period, boys are more often infected, but thereafter girls predominate (25 times more likely). By the age of 2 years, 5% of girls have had a urinary tract infection.

22.5.2 Pathology

The most common pathogen is *Escherichia coli*. Bacteria of the same strain are usually present in the child's gut and it is assumed that the organism enters the urethra via the perineum.

22.5.3 Features

In the infant, symptoms are usually non-specific – vomiting, fever, irritability, lethargy. There may be prolonged jaundice in the neonate. Most children will have an infection confined to the lower urinary tract (*cystitis*) which merely causes dysuria, urgency or wetting without significant systemic illness. However, with upper tract involvement (*pyelonephritis*), illness with fever and loin pain is common.

> Check urine in a child with an unexplained fever.

Risk factors for UTI or underlying pathology

- Poor urine flow
- History of previous UTI
- Recurrent fever of uncertain origin
- Antenatally-diagnosed renal abnormality
- Family history of vesicoureteric reflux (VUR) or renal disease
- Constipation
- Dysfunctional voiding
- Enlarged bladder
- Abdominal mass
- Evidence of spinal lesion
- Poor growth
- High blood pressure.

22.5.4 Investigations

Dipstick tests are usually positive for nitrite and leucocytes, and there may be haematuria and proteinuria. Motile bacteria are visible on microscopy in addition to excess white cells. Send a sample for culture if one or more of these tests is positive, there are risk factors (see table), or the child is under 3 years (Table 22.3).

 PRACTICE POINT

If the urine looks crystal clear and is negative for blood, nitrite and leucocytes, infection is most unlikely.

 Diagnosis of urine infection on microscopy and culture

- Pure growth of one species of bacteria
- >10^5 organisms/mL (or any growth from a suprapubic sample)
- Pyuria usually present (>50 WBC × 10^6/L).

If these criteria not met, send repeat sample – contamination may be the cause.

Table 22.3 Interpreting urine cultures

Culture result	Interpretation
<10 000 organisms/mL	Normal
10 000–100 000 organisms/mL	Unsure, therefore repeat
>100 000 organisms/mL	Urinary tract infection
Mixed growth	Contamination

22.5.5 Initial management of UTI

 TREATMENT

- ↑ fluid intake
- Encourage micturition
- Prompt chemotherapy:
  - Oral trimethoprim if child quite well
  - Broad-spectrum systemic antibiotic in infants, and for complicated or presumed *upper* tract infection
  - May need to change when antibiotic sensitivities available
- Check urine after antibiotics completed.

22.5.6 Further investigation and management

 PRACTICE POINT

The aim is to identify structural problems, scars and vesico-ureteric reflux, and to prevent or minimize future problems.

Younger children and those with atypical or recurrent infections (see Box) are investigated more thoroughly because of higher risk of problems. Older children with single, typical infections do not need investigation, but it is worth giving general advice about prevention. Recurrent infections that are a nuisance may be treated with prophylactic antibiotics.

Atypical and recurrent urine infections

Atypical UTI
- Seriously ill or sepsis
- Red flags (poor urine flow, abdominal mass, raised creatinine)
- Slow response to treatment (>48h)
- Unusual organism (not *E.coli*)

Recurrent UTI
- ≥ 3 UTIs (or ≥ 2 if any upper tract infection)

 Prevention of UTIs

Regular water-drinking

Regular micturition

Avoid constipation

For girls:
- **Check wiping from front to back (avoids gut flora reaching urethra)**
- **Avoid perineal irritation sometimes caused by bubble baths or strong soaps**
- **Regular washing and thorough drying of perineum**
- **Wear loose-fitting clothes (not tight trousers).**

22.5.6.1 Renal ultrasound scan

- In children under 6 months, or those with recurrent or atypical infections
- Identifies obstructive abnormalities and structural problems
- Assists diagnosis of acute pyelonephritis
- Discrepancies in renal size may indicate scarring.

22.5.6.2 Abdominal X-ray

Consider if there is suspicion of renal stones or spinal abnormalities.

22.5.6.3 Isotope scan (e.g. DMSA, MAG3)

- Perform in young children with atypical or recurrent infection
- Wait until 4-6 months after infection (otherwise hard to interpret)
- Inject i.v. radiolabelled isotope and visualize on scintigraphy
- Identifies renal scars and differential renal function
- Working renal tissue picks up the isotope and so a renal image is seen
- Scars show as blank areas
- Rate of excretion is seen as the kidney clears the isotope.

22.5.6.4 Micturating cystourethrogram (MCUG)

- Perform in infants < 6 months with atypical or recurrent UTIs, or when vesico-ureteric reflux is suspected (e.g. other tests abnormal, or family history)
- Catheterize bladder, fill with radio-opaque dye, watch on X-ray while child micturates
- Defines urethral abnormalities and vesico-ureteric reflux.

Table 22.4 **Investigation protocol for confirmed UTI**

Age	Typical infection (not atypical or recurrent)	Atypical or recurrent infection
< 6 months	USS	USS, DMSA, MCUG
6 months–3 years	None	USS, DMSA
Over 3 years	None	USS (+DMSA if recurrent)

This table is based on the 2007 UK national guideline by the National Institute for Clinical Excellence (see CG54 at www.nice.org.uk).

These are initial investigations. For young and ill children, the ultrasound should be done during the acute episode, otherwise within a few weeks. If any are abnormal, more investigations may be needed.

22.5.7 Vesico-ureteric reflux

Present in 1/4 children with urine infection

Minor degrees unimportant

When mild tends to resolve spontaneously

Major reflux is a set-up for infection (Figure 22.5):
- During micturition, urine refluxes up the ureter, filling and distending the calyces
- At end of micturition urine falls back to form a stagnant pool.

22.5.7.1 Management

- Prophylactic antibiotics to prevent infection
- Surgical correction is possible for severe or problematic reflux

Follow up important
- One-third have a recurrence of infection within a year
- Culture urine a few days after completing initial therapy
- Re-culture at least once in the next 3 months, *even though the child is symptomless*
- One of the causes of end-stage renal failure.

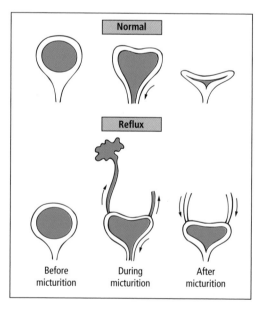

Figure 22.5 Vesico-ureteric reflux (shown by micturating cystogram). At the end of micturition a puddle of stagnant urine remains in the bladder.

22.5.7.2 Prognosis

Infection of the renal parenchyma may cause permanent or progressive damage, leading to renal scarring, insufficiency and hypertension. Most children with UTI do not incur renal damage. Renal damage is most likely in those with associated obstruction of the urinary tract, and in those who have severe infection and gross reflux early in life – under the age of 2.

22.6 Enuresis

Children learn to be dry by day at about 2 years, and by night at about 3 years. By 4 years, 75% of children are dry by day and night. Most children who wet have 'intermittent' enuresis: it is rare to encounter children of school age who have never had a dry night. Bed wetting (*nocturnal enuresis*) is a more common problem than daytime wetting (*diurnal enuresis*).

22.6.1 Nocturnal enuresis

> **Causes of nocturnal enuresis**
>
> - Lack of release of arginine vasopressin (ADH) during sleep with excess urine production
> - Low functional bladder capacity
> - Inability to wake to full bladder sensation
> - Interference with learning (low IQ, delay, anxiety, unclear social approval/disapproval)
> - Psychological distress: family dysfunction; bullying; abuse
> - Medical conditions: urinary tract infection; constipation; diabetes mellitus; diabetes insipidus
> - Inadvertent behaviour reinforcement (e.g. child comes into parents' bed when wet)
> - Genetic factors (a positive family history is common).

Most enuretic children do not suffer from either a psychological illness or an organic illness.

 KEY POINTS

- Boys are slower at acquiring dryness than girls
- Proportions of children wetting the bed by age:

Age	%
5 years	15
9 years	9
15 years	1

Examine the child to exclude physical problems and to reassure the family. Where there is normal daytime bladder function or there have been a few nights completely dry, then there can be no serious defect of the urinary tract such as ectopic ureter or neuropathic bladder.

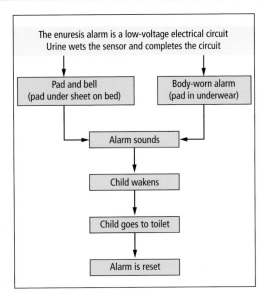

Figure 22.6 Enuresis alarms

Consider dipsticking the urine for glucose, and for signs of infection, particularly if the enuresis is secondary (i.e. has begun after more than 6 months of dryness).

Management is rewarding, since with success (which is usual) children grow in self-esteem. Stress and blame make things worse, and punishment has no place. Rewards and encouragement help and a star chart is a useful tool (see Section 11.4.1.1). It also helps assess progress. Conditioning therapy by enuresis alarm (Figures 28.2(d) and (i)) is used over the age of 7, and is successful in 2/3rds of children. Alarms need to be used for 3 or 4 months, require much effort by the child and family, and frequent follow-up. They should be avoided when the home situation is already fraught or parents are blaming the child.

22.6.2 Diurnal enuresis (daytime wetting)

Roughly 1% of healthy children over the age of 5 have troublesome daytime wetting; most of them are reliably dry at night. The problem is more common in girls and is usually the result of *urge incontinence* due to instability of the detrusor muscle of the bladder. Half of the girls who wet by day have recurrent bacteruria (Figure 22.7). This can lead to a vicious cycle of infection and wetting. There is an increased incidence of emotional disorder compared with children who merely wet the bed. With increase in age there is a natural tendency to become dry, and this is accelerated by eradication of bacteruria, alongside more frequent and regular voiding.

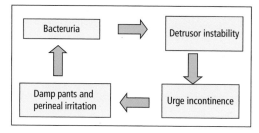

Figure 22.7 Wetting-infection cycle

TREATMENT Drugs used in enuresis

For most children with uncomplicated enuresis, alarms are best.

Drugs are usually reserved for children age 7 years and above.

Drugs reduce bed wetting whilst the drug is being taken.

Children tend to relapse when the drug is stopped, but a slow wean may help.

Useful for short trips, or longer term when alarms have failed or are inappropriate.

Desmopressin
- Analogue of AVP
- Drug of choice
- Tablets or sublingual (not nasal spray)
- Take at bedtime
- Reduces nocturnal urine output and therefore wetting
- Minimise fluid intake for 1h before and 8 h after dose

Oxybutinin
- Anticholinergic
- Used alone or with Desmopressin
- Used when symptoms of bladder instability (e.g. daytime wetting, urgency and frequency)

Imipramine
- Tricyclic antidepressant
- Used for anticholinergic effect
- Little used because:
  - Greater incidence of side effects
  - Dangerous if taken in overdose (e.g. by younger sibling).

RESOURCE

Enuresis
National Institute of Clinical Excellence Guidance can be found at **www.nice.org.uk/guidance/CG111**

22.7 Male genitalia

22.7.1 Undescended testicles

The testicles normally descend into the scrotum about the 36th week of gestation and are therefore usually fully descended in the newborn full-term infant. Spontaneous descent may occur later, but the older the child, the less likely is this to happen. If a testis remains undescended after puberty, it will not mature properly and will be sterile.

'Undescended' testicles are often incompletely descended and are palpable in the inguinal canal. If such a testis cannot be brought into the scrotum by sweeping warm, flat fingers down the inguinal region, or if the testis cannot be felt at all, orchidopexy (surgery to bring the testis down into the scrotum) is advised.

Incompletely descended testes need to be distinguished from retractile testes and ectopic testes. Ectopic testes are rare and may be located in the superficial inguinal pouch, near the femoral ring, or in the perineum.

PRACTICE POINT

Retractile testes are very common and normal. An active cremaster muscle withdraws the testis into the inguinal canal or higher, especially if examined with cold hands.

22.7.2 Hydrocele

At birth it is quite common to find fluid in the scrotal sac. It almost always clears up without treatment. In older infants and children, there may be a tense hydrocele on one or both sides. It does not cause symptoms but is often associated with inguinal hernia. Surgery is therefore advised.

22.7.3 Circumcision

The normal foreskin

- The foreskin is still in the process of developing at birth and is often non-retractable in early childhood. By age 3 it retracts in 90%.
- The process of separation of the foreskin from the glans is spontaneous and does not require manipulation.
- In a small proportion of boys, this natural process of separation continues to occur well into childhood.

In *paraphimosis*, the tight foreskin is retracted behind the glans penis and cannot be returned. If reduction is not possible with anaesthesia, an emergency dorsal slit followed later by circumcision may be needed.

Inflammation of the foreskin is common in babies while they are still in nappies. It requires treating as for nappy rash and is a contraindication to circumcision because of the risk of a meatal ulcer. Circumcision is performed for religious reasons in Jewish and Muslim boys.

> **PRACTICE POINT Clinical indications for circumcision**
>
> Pathological phimosis – scarring of the opening of the foreskin making it non-retractable (unusual before age 5)
>
> Recurrent balanitis (inflammation under the foreskin) is an occasional indication.

22.8 Female genitalia

22.8.1 Adherent labia minora

Mild inflammation of the vulva is quite common in young girls, and sometimes this can lead to development of firm adhesions between opposing surfaces of the labia minora. Urine is passed normally, but the appearance may suggest that there is no vaginal orifice. The labia separate with repeated application of oestrogen cream.

When having their perineum examined, young girls are likely to be happiest if lying supine on their mother's lap or on a couch with their legs up in the lithotomy position. They can see what the examiner is up to. The labia are gently pulled apart to check that they are not adherent and the vulva is inspected. Vaginal examination should only be performed by those with expertise.

22.8.2 Vaginal discharge

> **Causes of vaginal discharge**
>
> **White mucoid (leucorrhoea)**
> - In neonate, normal
> - At puberty, normal
>
> **Offensive yellow (vulvovaginitis)**
> - Aged 2–5 years, associated with poor hygiene
> - Infection
> - Sexual abuse
> - Foreign body
>
> **Bloody (vaginal bleeding)**
> - In neonate may be normal
> - Menstruation
> - Sexual abuse
> - Foreign body
> - Tumour
>
> **Menarche.**

Soreness and irritation of the vulva (vulvovaginitis) is common in young girls is usually due to poor local hygiene, irritants (tights, bubble baths) and lack of protective oestrogen. Micturition may be painful. Avoidance of irritants and oil in the bath usually help. Staining of the pants may result from normal heavy secretion of mucus particularly around puberty. Careful daily washing and drying of the perineum will relieve both conditions. A purulent vaginal discharge is uncommon. The possibility of sexual abuse or an underlying foreign body should be borne in mind, and pus should be cultured and examined for *Trichomonas* and other sexually transmitted diseases. Treat with antibiotics if there is a pure growth of a pathogen.

Summary

Know the main types of renal disease in childhood – especially post-streptococcal glomerulonephritis and nephrotic syndrome which are both classic paediatric conditions. Urinary tract infections are approached differently in young children because of the risk of underlying abnormality (including vesico-ureteric reflux) and renal damage. Nocturnal enuresis is common and usually responds well to treatment.

> **FOR YOUR LOG**
>
> - Clerk children with some of these conditions, e.g. nephrotic syndrome, urinary tract infection and enuresis.
> - Observe explanation of use of an enuresis alarm.
> - Sit in on consultation about urinary tract infection with advice about prevention (or read a patient information leaflet).
> - Watch renal investigations such as renal ultrasound, DMSA scan or MCUG.

> **OSCE TIP**
>
> - Dipstick a urine sample (see OSCE station 22.1).
> - Photo or video of nephrotic syndrome.
> - Descent of testes.
> - History or management of enuresis.
> - Approach to haematuria
> - History or management of UTI

See EMQ 22.1, EMQ 22.2 and EMQ 22.3 at the end of the book.

OSCE station 22.1: Urine testing

Clinical approach:

Check
- Name and date on sample
- Any clinical information given

Inspection
- Appearance
  - ◇ Clear/cloudy/hazy
  - ◇ Red: blood, dietary pigment, drugs
  - ◇ Frothy: high protein content
- Smell
  - ◇ Musty: infection, old specimen
  - ◇ Abnormal smell: dietary; inborn error of metabolism

Reagent strip urinalysis
- pH: usual range pH 5–7
- Blood: normally negative; trace maybe normal
- Protein: normal = negative or trace; scored: + to ++++
- Specific gravity: varies with hydration,and renal function; usually1.010–1.020
- Glucose: normally negative; scored:trace to ++++
- Ketones: found in starvation, diabetes etc.
- Nitrite: larger amounts associated with infection
- Leucocytes: larger amounts associated with infection

A 3-year-old girl presents with fever and vomiting. Please test her urine

- Shake gently, and hold up to light

The urine appears slightly hazy, and has a musty unpleasant smell

- Immerse a reagent stick in the urine and remove
- Tap excess urine from the stick
- Hold stick horizontally and start timing
- Read colour reaction at times indicated on label of bottle

This urine shows:
pH: 8
blood: trace
protein: +
nitrite: positive
leucocytes: large

The findings are typical of a urine infection.

Never forget:
- Find the container that the dipstix came in and read instructions on it
- The reagent stick must be lined up with the key printed on the container for interpretation
- Make sure the stick is the right way up!
- Reagents react at different times: it is important to time this test

Look around for:
- Clinical notes, growth charts

Special points
- Interpret your observations in the light of any clinical history
- Always consider urine infection in acutely ill children
- Consider whether any laboratory investigation is needed (e.g. urine culture)
- Urinalysis 'dipstix' vary in the number of reagents on each stick
- Do not do this for the first time in the undergraduate examination

OSCE station 22.2: Enuresis

Mrs Granger has come to see you in primary care clinic to ask for advice regarding her 7 year old son John, who wets the bed 6 nights per week. He has never been reliably dry at night. He has no daytime symptoms of urgency, frequency or wetting, and has never had any urinary infections. He has always worn pull-ups (nappies) at night. He is due to go on a cub camp in 3 weeks time. The rest of the history is unremarkable, and there is no suggestion of constipation. Assume that physical examination and dipstick testing of the urine is normal. The only action that Mrs Granger has tried is to wake John to go the toilet at about 11.30pm (lifting), but he seems half asleep. **Please advise about management.**

From this information, you can deduce that John has primary monosymptomatic enuresis, and there do not appear to be any obvious triggers such as (organic) urine infections, constipation or psychological upsets. The task is clearly about management, and although some initial brief clarification about history might be reasonable, it's important not to spend long on this.

Introduce yourself, use John's name, establish ideas, concerns and expectations (ICE). Clarify priorities, e.g. for him to be dry for the camp, or in the longer term, and if she has a particular treatment or questions in mind. Depending on answers, you could suggest the following, checking for understanding and further questions as you proceed:

General advice

Avoid constipation, good daytime habits of drinking water and regular micturition, positive non-punitive supportive approach, bedding protection, lifting generally not helpful unless John is waking up properly, easy access to toilet (e.g. avoid high bed, light on landing), come out of pull-ups for at least a week or so every few months.

(continued)

Star charts

When trying out of pull-ups, could award stars for dry nights, or for behaviours helping towards dryness (e.g. passing urine last thing at night, waking and helping change sheets if wet). See Chapter 11. Don't persist for too long if no progress.

Alarms

This is the best option for long-term success and can be arranged at a local clinic. Explain main types (body-worn and pad and buzzer) and this will help him learn to respond during the night to full bladder signals. Good chance of success (nearly 70%) over 2–3 months, will need regular follow up while using. Check practicalities (e.g. bedroom shared?) and that home/school situation steady (avoid if stressful events occurring).

Drugs

Explain that Desmopressin (melts or tablets) given at bedtime would be a good short-term option especially for the cub-camp and is effective in about two-thirds (half of whom will be completely dry). Warn about excessive fluid intake late evening and nights because of effect on reducing fluid output from kidneys: only one glass of fluid from the hour before to 8 hours after.

Summary and questions

Finish with a brief summary and check that you have answered questions and addressed concerns.

OSCE station 22.3: Urinary tract infection management and prevention

Mr Mojsa has brought his 3-year-old daughter Rose back to the GP surgery after she was diagnosed and treated for a urinary tract infection 3 days ago. She presented with low-grade fever, smelly urine, new onset of day-time wetting, and stinging on micturition. The urine dipstick strongly suggested infection and she was started on a 3 day course of Trimethoprim. You have the culture result now available (see below). Urine dipstick is now negative and Rose is back to normal. The rest of a complete history reveals only that has mild ongoing constipation and often gets some vulval erythema and soreness (no discharge). She has never had previous UTIs.

Urine result:

WBC 728/microlitre (normal range < 40)
RBC <140/microlitre (normal range < 140)
Culture: >10^5cfu/ml E.Coli
Sensitive to Trimethoprim, Nitrofurantoin, Resistant to Amoxil/Ampicillin.

Task: Mr Mojsa asks the following questions about management and prevention – your task to answer them.

Was this a definite urine infection, and does she need a different antibiotic?	*The result indicates a definite infection, and that the organism was sensitive to the antibiotic used. There is no need for a different antibiotic.*
Does Rose need any tests to check her kidneys?	*No, since she has responded quickly to the antibiotic treatment, has a typical organism and has not had previous infections, there is no need to do any investigations.*
Could the infection have damaged her kidneys?	*No, again because she has responded quickly, and everything suggests this was a lower tract infection which would not cause renal damage at this age.*
How can further infections be prevented?	*Go through the prevention advice (see Section 22.5), particularly emphasizing avoidance of constipation through fluid, fibre and laxatives (see Chapter 21).*
What is the vulval soreness likely to be and how can this be prevented?	*This is likely to be vulvovaginitis which is common at this age. Advise good hygiene (with thorough drying), avoidance of irritants (e.g. bubble baths and perfumed soaps), cotton pants or loose fitting clothes, and oil of oilatum in the bath. Simple emollient creams are often helpful, and occasionally oestrogen or steroid creams are used if things are not settling.*

23

Bones and joints

Chapter map

Concerns about bones and joints are common. This chapter reviews common variations in structure and posture, and the different causes of bone and joint pain or dysfunction (including infection, inflammation, and necrosis).

23.1 Structural variation and congenital abnormalities

The normal flat-footed baby becomes a bow-legged toddler and then a knock-kneed primary schoolchild before growing into a graceful adolescent. It is important to recognize normal variation and problems requiring investigation and treatment (Figure 23.1).

Examine the child:

- Standing and lying
- Walking and running
- Limb lengths
- Scars
- Muscle wasting
- Uneven wear of shoes.

23.1.1 Flat feet

At birth the feet look flat. A child's feet continue to look flat as a toddler. By the third year the feet begin to appear to have a normal plantar arch.

23.1.2 Bow legs (genu varum)

Bow legs are most common from 0 to 2 years. The knees may be 5 cm apart when the feet are together:

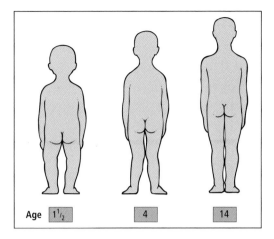

Figure 23.1 Normal variation of legs with age.

the toes point medially. Marked bowing may mean rickets (Section 12.4.2.4).

23.1.3 Knock knees (genu valgum)

This is most apparent at 3–4 years of age. When the knees are together, the medial tibial malleoli may be up to 5 cm apart. In obese children, the separation may be even greater but, by the age of 12, the legs should be straight. Separation of over 10 cm or unilateral knock knee requires an X-ray and, probably, a specialist opinion.

23.1.4 Intoeing

This is usually a normal variation and resolves by the age of 8 years.

23.1.5 Scoliosis

> **Causes of scoliosis**
> - Idiopathic (95%)
> - Vertebral anomalies, e.g. hemivertebrae
> - Muscle weakness, e.g. cerebral palsy.

Postural scoliosis is commonly seen in babies: it goes when the baby is suspended and has completely gone by the age of 2 years. Scoliosis is again common at adolescence, especially in girls. If it is postural, it disappears on bending forward. Structural scoliosis produces asymmetry on bending: a hump on flexion (Figure 23.2). Asymmetry of scapulae and shoulders may be more conspicuous than the spinal curve.

> **PRACTICE POINT**
>
> True (non-postural) scoliosis should be referred to orthopaedics promptly.

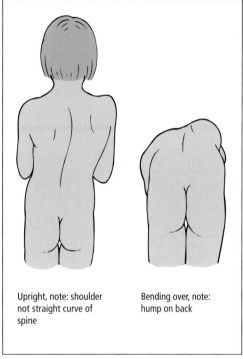

Upright, note: shoulder not straight curve of spine

Bending over, note: hump on back

Figure 23.2 Structural scoliosis becomes more obvious when she bends to touch her toes.

23.1.6 Talipes (club foot)

Postural talipes is common at birth, resulting from the fetal foot position in utero. If the foot with talipes equino-varus can be fully dorsiflexed and everted so that the little toe touches the outside of the leg without undue force, it is postural and will get better. Structural talipes cannot be corrected. Early orthopaedic referral is needed for splintage or surgery. The sooner treatment is begun the better the outcome. Talipes calcaneovalgus is usually easily corrected by simple exercises (Figure 23.3).

23.1.7 Developmental dysplasia of the hip (DDH)

DDH is also known as congenital dislocation of the hips. Acetabular dysplasia is important in causation.

> **Risk factors for DDH**
> - Breech
> - Positive family history
> - Girls > boys
> - Neuromuscular or joint problem (e.g. spina bifida, talipes).

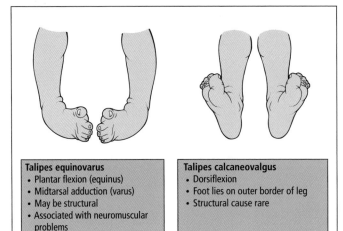

Talipes equinovarus
- Plantar flexion (equinus)
- Midtarsal adduction (varus)
- May be structural
- Associated with neuromuscular problems

Talipes calcaneovalgus
- Dorsiflexion
- Foot lies on outer border of leg
- Structural cause rare

Figure 23.3 Two forms of talipes.

All babies should be examined in the neonatal period for DDH (OCSE station 23.1). Examination is repeated at infant health checks. If there is clinical suspicion or the infant is high risk, hip ultrasound is more reliable than clinical examination. X-ray is unreliable in the first months because of poor ossification.

- 1% of babies have some developmental dysplasia or hip instability
- 1 in 1000 have severe congenital dislocation
- early treatment with splinting in full abduction is successful in most
- late presentation with a limp has a poor prognosis, needing surgery and predisposing to early osteoarthritis.

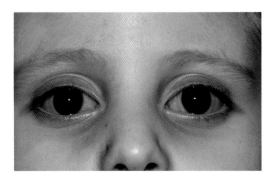

Figure 23.4 Osteogenesis imperfecta. The sclera are blue in colour.

 PRACTICE POINT

Screening tests for dislocated hips are not 100% sensitive (cases are missed) or 100% specific (the test may be abnormal in a normal infant).

23.1.8 Osteogenesis imperfecta

This is a group of rare genetic conditions due to mutations in the genes coding for collagen. They are characterized by brittle bones and lax ligaments. In the severe, lethal forms (dominant mutations or recessive inheritance), multiple fractures occur in utero. In less severe cases (usually dominant inheritance), children are prone to fractures, may have blue sclera and develop deafness in adult life (Figure 23.4).

23.1.9 Skeletal dysplasia

These congenital dysplasias are rare. Many are genetically determined. *Achondroplasia* is the most

common. It is due to an autosomal dominant gene. In 50% a new mutation occurs, both parents being normal. There is extreme short stature with disproportionate shortness of limbs, and a large skull vault. Intelligence is normal.

Some short-limbed dwarfism is incompatible with survival after birth (*thanatophoric*). Accurate diagnosis is important for genetic counselling.

23.2 Bone and joint infection

23.2.1 Osteomyelitis

Pyogenic infection of bone is more common in children than in adults, and in boys than in girls.

The usual site is the metaphysis of one of the long bones, particularly in the legs. *Staphylococcus aureus* is the most common pathogen.

Osteomyelitis

Symptoms
- Fever
- Variable pain, illness
- Pseudoparesis
- Local tenderness
- Redness, swelling

Investigations
- Blood count: neutrophilia
- C-reactive protein↑
- Blood culture
- Radioisotope scan
- X-ray.

Early diagnosis is difficult: an infant may merely refuse to use the affected limb (pseudoparesis). X-ray is normal at first. After 2 weeks, bone rarefaction and periosteal new bone formation may be seen. Radioisotope bone scan is usually abnormal from the start.

Osteomyelitis demands intensive antibiotic treatment in hospital to try to prevent long-term effects on bone and joints. With early treatment, complete resolution occurs in most cases. If diagnosis is delayed, surgical drainage is more likely to be needed.

Flucloxacillin is the best antibiotic for most infections due to *S. aureus*. MRSA needs treatment with vancomycin.

23.2.2 Septic arthritis

Bacterial joint infection can occur at any age from the newborn. The most common cause is haematogenous spread of *S. aureus*. Symptoms and signs may be very like osteomyelitis. The affected joint is hot, swollen and immobile.

Early diagnosis is important for a good outcome. It is a difficult diagnosis in toddlers and infants especially when there is hip involvement. Septic arthritis should be managed with the orthopaedic surgeons. Joint aspiration usually provides a diagnosis. Joint lavage and drainage may be needed.

23.3 Arthritis and arthralgia

23.3.1 Irritable hip (transient synovitis)

This commonly is associated with viral infection. Unlike septic arthritis, the child is not usually ill, or febrile. Pain is on walking and there is limited

abduction and rotation. Infection screen and joint aspiration may be needed to exclude bacterial infection. Treatment is symptom relief, and improvement occurs in days.

23.3.2 Arthritis

 PRACTICE POINT Arthritis

- Local pain
- Swelling
- Joint red and hot
- Limited movement.

Arthritis simply means inflammation in a joint, and there are many causes. If there is no history of joint swelling, arthritis is unlikely. Pain arising in the hip may be referred to the knee. It is common in viral infections in children. Chronic arthropathy causes serious disability.

Causes of arthritis

Those that may result in permanent joint damage
- Juvenile idiopathic arthritis
- Acute septic arthritis
- Haemarthrosis (joint bleeding in coagulation disorders)

Those that usually resolve completely
- Reactive arthritis: viral infections
  - Rubella
  - Immunization
  - Mumps
- Henoch–Schönlein syndrome
- Generalized allergic reactions
- Rheumatic fever.

23.3.2.1 Juvenile idiopathic arthritis (JIA, juvenile chronic arthritis)

JIA classification

- Systemic-onset (Still's)
- Polyarticular
- Pauciarticular
- Psoriatic
- Enthesitis-related

JIA is defined as a chronic arthritis before the age of 16 years, lasting at least 3 months, after exclusion of other primary diseases. Children do not always easily fit into one of the classifications.

Systemic disease (Still's)
- Pre-school children
- Generally unwell
- Swinging, high fever
- Splenomegaly
- Lymphadenopathy
- Erythematous (salmon pink) rash
- High CRP
- Polymorph leucocytosis
- Rheumatoid/antinuclear factors negative

Polyarticular JIA
- Any age
- Over four joints
- Symmetrical
- Hands, wrists, knees, ankles
- No systemic inflammation

Pauciarticular JIA
- Young children
- Up to four joints
- Knees, ankles, elbows
- Muscle wasting
- Antinuclear antibody positive
- Risk of uveitis.

Rarely children develop juvenile rheumatoid arthritis with a typical pattern of hand and even cervical spine involvement and with positive rheumatoid factor. Enthesitis means inflammation at the site of tendon insertion. In enthesitis, large joint arthritis and iritis also occur, mostly in older boys who are HLA type B27. Psoriatic arthritis may start well before the rash – suspect it if nail-pitting, or a first degree relative with the condition.

 TREATMENT Management of JIA

- Multidisciplinary team is key!
- Physiotherapy
- Non-steroidal anti-inflammatory drugs
- Local/systemic steroids
- Methotrexate
- Anti-cytokine antibodies.

Fifty per cent of children make a complete recovery. In 50% the disease is progressive and crippling. Iridocyclitis is an important complication.

23.3.3 Joint hypermobility syndrome

Children with very mobile joints may suffer pain after exercise, or after prolonged sitting. Symptoms are often worse around the adolescent growth spurt. When mild, reassurance and general advice about posture and pacing activity is all that is necessary.

More severe cases need evaluation for collagen disease and may benefit from physiotherapy.

23.3.4 Other collagen diseases

Systemic lupus erythematosus (SLE), polyarteritis nodosa, dermatomyositis and the other collagen disorders are rare in children. SLE tends to occur in adolescent girls, particularly in black races. It tends to present as a multisystem disorder and responds well to treatment with corticosteroids.

23.3.5 Henoch–Schönlein purpura (anaphylactoid purpura)

 HSP

- Most common in children aged 2–10 years
- Vasculitic process
- Involves the following four organ systems:
  - Skin - pathognomonic purpuric rash
  - Joints
  - Gut
  - Kidneys.

Skin

The rash is distributed over the extensor surfaces of the limbs, particularly the ankles and the buttocks (Figure 23.5). It begins as a maculopapular, red rash, which gradually becomes purpuric (resulting from the vasculitis, the platelet count is normal). Swelling of the face, hands and feet is common.

Joints

Pain (arthralgia) of medium-sized joints is common and may progress to an obvious arthritis with red, swollen, tender joints.

Alimentary system

Colicky abdominal pain occurs and may be severe enough to mimic an acute abdominal emergency. Vomiting and diarrhoea are common, haematemesis and melaena less common. Intussusception may occur (Section 21.2.2.2, p. 212). Perforation is very rare.

Kidneys

Renal injury is caused by deposition of IgA immune complexes. Haematuria is common but, when accompanied by persisting proteinuria, is of concern. With more severe involvement, the glomerulonephritis causes an acute nephritic syndrome or nephrotic syndrome. Acute or chronic renal failure may occur in a small minority. The renal complications are

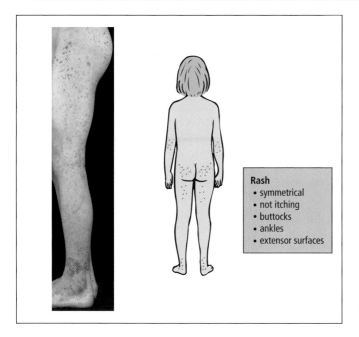

Figure 23.5 Henoch–Schönlein purpura.

responsible for the main morbidity and mortality of Henoch–Schönlein syndrome.

 PRACTICE POINT

In HSP, dipstick urine for blood and protein (parents are asked to do this at home for a few weeks), and measure BP.

HSP usually resolves after 1–3 weeks. The cause is unknown and treatment is symptomatic. Recurrence may occur for several months after onset.

23.3.6 Rheumatic fever

Rheumatic fever is still an important cause of acquired heart disease in children throughout the world, but in Europe it has become rare. It results from a sensitivity reaction to a group A β-haemolytic streptococcal infection usually after acute tonsillitis (Figure 23.6). Treatment includes antibiotics, anti-inflammatory agents and long-term penicillin prophylaxis against recurrence.

Figure 23.6 Rheumatic fever signs.

Rheumatic fever

- Transient arthritis
- Pancarditis
- Cardiac valve damage
- Rash (erythema marginatum)
- Erythema nodosum
- Chorea
- High ASO titre.

23.4 Osteochondritis and epiphysitis

These terms are applied to bone changes that occur, particularly in epiphyses of children, as a result of avascular necrosis. They present as bone pain, with local swelling and tenderness. There is limitation of movement, and adjacent muscles may waste. In weight-bearing joints, permanent damage may occur.

23.4.1 Perthes disease

This is avascular necrosis of the femoral head, often in boys (sex ratio 5 : 1) aged 5–8 years. It causes a limp and pain (which may be referred to the knee). The femoral head is softened and becomes misshapen, leading to osteoarthritis in early adult life. Treatment is controversial, but aims to restore the normal femoral head shape. Bedrest, traction, casts, calipers and surgery are all used. The condition usually resolves over 1–3 years.

23.4.2 Osgood–Schlatter disease

Traction epiphysitis of the tuberosity of the tibia occurs in children aged 10–15 years. There is local pain and tenderness at the top of the tibia over the tuberosity. This usually resolves satisfactorily without treatment. Occasionally judicious restriction of activity is needed.

23.5 Slipped upper femoral epiphysis

The epiphysis of the femoral head is displaced, often after minor trauma. This condition usually occurs during the adolescent growth spurt, and is more common in obesity. There is a pain, a limp and restricted movement. Diagnosis is made on X-ray. Treatment is surgical with fixation.

 Summary

Knowing the range of normal structure and posture helps to pick out those needing referral and treatment, and to reassure the rest. Early identification of unstable or dislocated hips greatly improves outcome. Bacterial bone and joint infection is serious and needs rapid diagnosis and treatment. The most common cause of acute arthritis is reactive following viral infections, but it is important to know about other acute causes, such as the classic childhood syndrome of Henoch Schonlein Purpura. Chronic arthritis can be very disabling and requires specialist multidisciplinary team management. Acute hip pain may be irritable hip (acute, quite well), or septic hip (ill, high fever). Chronic hip pain may be Perthes (5–8 yrs) or slipped femoral epiphysis (teenager).

 FOR YOUR LOG

- Observe hip examination and practice on a manikin
- Take a history of a child presenting with arthritis or arthralgia
- Practice pGALS examination (Section 3.5.7, p. 39).

 OSCE TIP

- Examination of a joint.
- Neonatal hip examination (see OSCE station 23.1).
- Observation and examination of child with juvenile idiopathic arthritis.
- Examine spine for scoliosis.

See EMQ 23.1 at the end of the book.

OSCE station 23.1: Testing for dislocation of the hips

Clinical approach:

Inspection
- Difference in leg length
- Skin creases or asymmetry
- Associated abnormalities

ABduct both hips
- They should ABduct fully
- There should be symmetry

Ortolani's sign
- The femoral head clunks back into the acetabulum at 45–60 degrees of ABduction

Barlow's manoeuvre
- Support the pelvis on a firm surface or your hand
- Flex and ADduct the hip
- Apply posterior and lateral pressure to attempt to dislocate the hip
- ABduct the hip, and see if the hip relocates

This model is used for teaching examination of the hips in the newborn. Please show me how this examination is done

ABduction

Ortolani's test: both hips are ABducted fully until they lie flat on the bed. A dislocated hip will not ABduct.

Barlow's manoeuvre

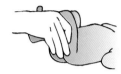

examiner's right hand holding thigh, with finger on greater tronchanter

examiner's left hand supporting pelvis

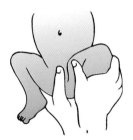

maintaining pressure the hip is ABducted

if right hip is dislocatable, the hip will 'clunk' back into place during ABduction.

In the exam, a teaching model with an abnormal hip is likely to be used

Never forget:
- Say hello and introduce yourself
- General inspection — has the infant any congenital abnormality?
- Quickly assess general health
- Mention the obvious (e.g. drip, leg in plaster)

Look around for:
- Hip splints — devices designed to hold the hips in ABduction
- Hip harness–similar device with straps that go over the shoulder
- Double nappies

Special points
- Ligamentous clicks (like you get in your fingers) are of dubious significance
- Describe tests as normal or abnormal — it is much more clear than positive/negative
- Barlow's is easier if you support the pelvis with one hand and test one hip at a time
- Make sure someone takes you through these specialized techniques

24

Skin

Chapter map

Skin disorders are common in children. The infant's skin with its thin epidermis and immature glands is particularly liable to infection and blistering. Birthmarks, rashes and eczema are common in pre-school children. The incidence of skin disease declines until adolescence when acne is common. Skin manifestations are seen in a number of systemic problems, which are covered elsewhere in this book, and pointers to the appropriate chapters are included.

24.1   Birthmarks

Birthmarks involve blood vessels (naevus, haemangioma) or an excess of pigment in the skin. Haemangiomas are malformations of blood vessels, not neoplasms.

24.1.1   Naevi

The main types of naevi are described below.

24.1.1.1   Stork marks

So named because their position fits with the idea that babies are brought by storks (now discredited!), these are flat, pinkish capillary haemangiomas between the eyebrows, on the forehead and eyelids and on the nape of the neck. They fade gradually over the first 2 years (Figure 24.1).

24.1.1.2   Port wine stain (naevus flammeus)

Port wine stain is a capillary haemangioma (Figure 24.1). In the infant, it is flat and pale pink

Paediatrics Lecture Notes, Ninth edition. Simon J. Newell and Jonathan C. Darling. © 2014 John Wiley & Sons, Ltd. Published 2014 by John Wiley & Sons, Ltd.

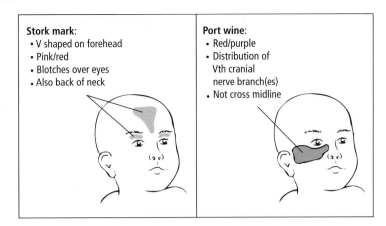

Stork mark:
- V shaped on forehead
- Pink/red
- Blotches over eyes
- Also back of neck

Port wine:
- Red/purple
- Distribution of Vth cranial nerve branch(es)
- Not cross midline

Figure 24.1 Stork mark and port wine stain.

and easily overlooked, but it then darkens to form a flat purple patch of skin which is unsightly. It does not fade. Treatment is difficult. Good results have been achieved using laser, but camouflage with cosmetics is often the best treatment. Sturge–Weber syndrome is a rare association of a unilateral port wine stain of the face (usually in the area of the first division of the trigeminal nerve) and an intracranial haemangioma of the pia-arachnoid on the same side (Figure 24.2). Affected children may present with seizures, hemiplegia, learning problems or glaucoma.

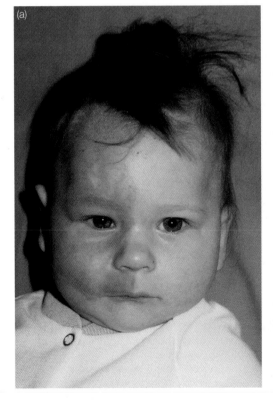

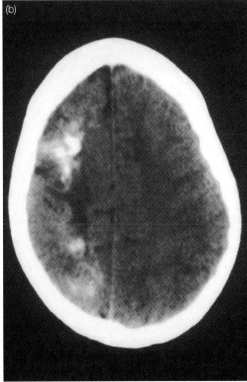

Figure 24.2 Sturge–Weber syndrome: (a) the naevus flammeus and (b) CT abnormality (the white areas in the cortex).

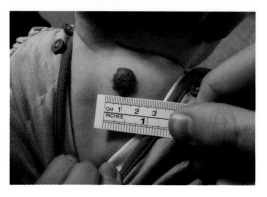

Figure 24.3 Strawberry naevus.

24.1.1.3 Strawberry mark

This is a soft, raised, bright red capillary haemangioma (Figure 24.3). Sometimes it involves deeper tissues and is combined with a cavernous haemangioma which gives it a blue tinge. Common sites are the head, neck and trunk. It appears in the days after birth, and enlarges in the first 6 months to form a raised red lesion. White areas develop in the lump (so that it looks like a strawberry) and it gradually becomes paler and flatter. They nearly all disappear completely before school age. Parents need reassurance. Some that block vision, interfere with feeding or are extremely unsightly may be treated medically or surgically. Spontaneous regression does not leave a noticeable scar, whilst treatment often does.

24.1.2 Abnormal pigmentation

Moles usually develop after the age of 2. They are common and rarely cause anxiety. Single café-au-lait spots are without significance, but six or more patches greater than 0.5 cm in diameter suggest neurofibromatosis (Section 17.4). Pigmented and de-pigmented lesions are seen in tuberous sclerosis (Section 17.4).

24.1.2.1 Albinism

Albinism is a group of genetically determined metabolic disorders with deficient pigmentation. In white people, autosomal recessive varieties affect the skin, hair and often the eyes. In black people, autosomal dominant, partial albinism is more common and does not affect the eyes.

24.1.2.2 Mongolian blue spots

These are large blue-grey patches, most common over the lumbosacral area and buttocks. They are very common in infants of oriental, Asian or black ethnic groups, but rare in white children. They gradually fade and are rarely visible by the age of 10.

 PRACTICE POINT

They may be mistaken for bruises and so raise child protection concerns – so document them when they are first noticed.

24.2 Rashes

24.2.1 Napkin rash

This is common in infants. An erythematous rash affects the convexities of the buttocks, inner thighs and genitalia. The skin creases, which do not come into contact with the nappy, are spared. At its simplest, it may merely be an irritant rash caused by wet nappies. Fresh urine does not injure the skin, but prolonged contact with stale urine which has broken down to form ammonia products does (ammoniacal dermatitis). In severe cases, papules and vesicles form which ulcerate, leaving a moist surface which easily becomes secondarily infected with either pyogenic organisms or *Candida*.

Infection with *Candida* usually involves the skin creases. It causes an erythematous rash with oval macules, a pimply margin and scattered satellite papules (Figure 24.4).

Nappy rashes do not mean poor care. Some babies have a more sensitive skin than others, and are prone to develop the rash. Explain this to parents to dispel needless guilt. Grossly ulcerated and chronic napkin rashes raise concerns about bad care, including infrequent changing.

 TREATMENT Treatment of napkin rash

- Frequent and prompt changing of wet nappies
- Wash and dry perineum carefully
- Barrier cream or benzalkonium cream to the napkin area.

If severe
- Leave nappies off for a few days to expose to a warm dry environment
- Use steroid cream to suppress inflammation
- Treat secondary infection with local bactericidal or fungicidal cream.

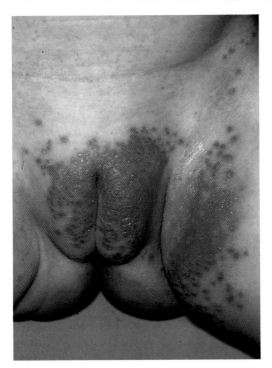

Figure 24.4 Candidal napkin rash.

whole skin surface. Skin cracks behind the pinnae are almost pathognomonic of infantile eczema. The rash is erythematous, scaly or weeping, and intensely itchy. Scratching frequently leads to secondary infection. The condition fluctuates: it resolves completely in half the children by the age of 2, but in others persists in a mild form or periodically recurs.

After infancy, flexural eczema is seen. Prolonged inflammation and scratching lead to thick lichenified skin and local lymph gland enlargement. The condition tends to improve, and becomes more manageable as the child becomes older (Figure 24.5).

 TREATMENT **Eczema treatments**

- Emollient creams/ointments
- Bath oil, aqueous emollient
- Topical steroids
- Bactericidal creams
- Antihistamines for itching
- Night gloves/mittens to limit scratching
- Wet wraps (damp tubigrip underlayer covered by a dry top layer)
- Occlusive dressings.

Add in this order according to severity

24.2.2 Cradle cap (seborrhoea)

Cradle cap is as common in infants as dandruff is in older children. It is a thick, light brown crust over the top of the scalp which may look quite difficult to remove, but which should not be picked off by carers. Baby oil, olive oil or infant medicated shampoo usually helps. Regular washing of the scalp helps to prevent recurrence.

24.2.3 Seborrhoeic dermatitis

This is a more generalized inflammatory skin reaction particularly affecting the groins, axillae and neck. Skin may be very red and macerated with greasy scaling, but it is not irritant and usually resolves within a few weeks. Secondary infection with bacteria or *Candida* may occur.

24.2.4 Eczema

Eczema is common and important. It is seen in atopic children whose families give a history of asthma, eczema, urticaria or hay fever, and the child is also at risk of asthma and hay fever. Atopic eczema affects 3% of pre-school children.

In infants, eczema may be restricted to two or three small lesions or may involve virtually the

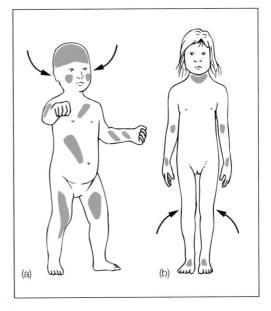

Figure 24.5 Distribution of eczema: (a) in infancy: cheeks, scalp, behind the ears and may be generalized: (b) in later childhood: skin flexures are affected, particularly antecubital and popliteal fossae.

PRACTICE POINT

Apply emollient liberally and often (so that the child shines)!

Consider environmental factors, including food intolerance. For children with severe eczema, an exclusion diet is worth trying. The child with eczema should avoid contact (particularly kissing) with someone who has herpes simplex (cold sore) because of the risk of developing widespread eczema herpeticum (a severe infection needing urgent treatment) (see Figure 24.6).

24.2.5 Psoriasis

Onset of this unsightly skin condition can occur in school children. It is genetically determined, and at all ages stress seems to be a provocative factor. The typical lesions are well circumscribed, red and raised with silvery scales on top. Most types affect extensor surfaces of the limbs and the scalp; they do not itch. Children are referred to the dermatologist. Coal tar

preparations, emollients, topical steroids, vitamin D (and analogues) and phototherapy are used. There may be associated arthritis, which often preceeds the rash. Guttate psoriasis, found mainly on the trunk, appears 2–3 weeks after a streptococcal infection such as tonsillitis.

24.2.6 Impetigo (Figure 24.7)

This skin infection is usually due to *Staphylococcus aureus*, though it is often complicated by *Streptococcus*. It commonly involves the face, around the mouth and nose, and the hands. It begins as a flaccid blister which rapidly ulcerates. The exudate produced dries in a golden brown crust over the red itching skin beneath. Spread may be rapid and scratching may spread it to other parts of the body or to other members of the family.

Impetigo is very contagious, so the child should be excluded from school until it is healed.

The lesions respond rapidly to bathing with cetrimide and water to remove the crusts, followed by antibiotic ointment and, if necessary, a course of oral antibiotic (flucloxacillin). The family must be warned about the risk of becoming infected themselves, and the affected child should use a separate towel and face cloth.

24.2.7 Urticaria (hives, nettle rash)

Urticaria is common in children, especially under the age of 5. It is characterized by red blotches and whitish weals that itch, and disappear and reappear over a period of hours or days. Sometimes sensitivity to a particular drug or food appears to be responsible.

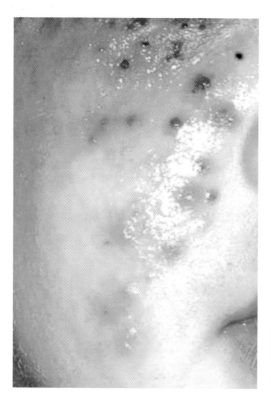

Figure 24.6 Eczema herpeticum.

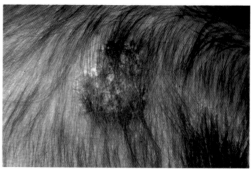

Figure 24.7 Impetigo on the scalp.

Oral antihistamines are effective. Anaphylaxis with angio-oedema of the face and mouth with airway compromise and shock is life threatening and needs urgent treatment with oxygen and adrenaline injection.

Papular urticaria consists of hard papules most often on the limbs. They appear in crops and itch so that secondary infection is common. In many children, they are associated with insect bites, fleas (including from pets), lice and bed bugs. Papular urticaria tends to recur for a few weeks each summer.

24.2.8 Erythema nodosum

These shiny red lumps are 1–3 cm in diameter and may be extremely tender (Figure 24.8). They are usually distributed symmetrically over the front of the shins, but do occur elsewhere. Initially purple and painful, they gradually subside and look like old bruises. They may occur at intervals in crops. Although they are thought to represent a hypersensitivity phenomenon, the stimulus is often not identified.

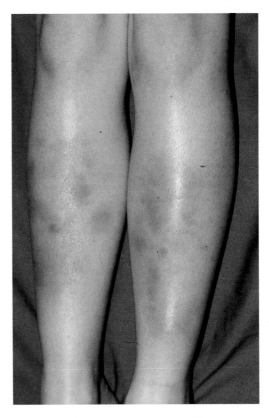

Figure 24.8 Erythema nodosum on the skin.

> **Erythema nodosum – causes**
>
> **Streptococcal infection**
> **Tuberculosis**
> **Drug reaction**
> **Diseases**
> • Inflammatory bowel disease
> • Lupus erythematosus
> • Sarcoidosis
> **Idiopathic**.

24.2.9 Molluscum contagiosum

This rash is common in school-age children. The pearly-white dome shaped lesions have a central dimple (umbilication). They are 3–5 mm in size and do not cause symptoms. They are due to infection with a pox virus, and are infectious. If left they will resolve spontaneously after many months or years, but occasionally they are treated by application of liquid nitrogen.

24.2.10 Erythema multiforme

This produces a dramatic red skin rash with varying skin lesions and characteristic target-shaped lesions (Figure 24.9). Often there is severe stomatitis and sometimes severe multi-system illness.

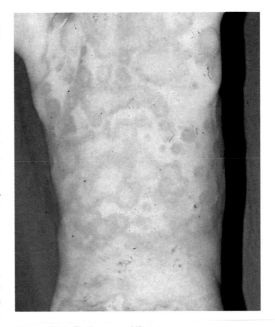

Figure 24.9 Erythema multiforme.

24.3 Warts

Warts are most common in childhood, probably because of spread of the responsible virus by contact. The average life of a wart is 9 months, so treatment is usually reserved for long-lasting warts. The variety of available treatments and magic cures is a fair indication of the therapeutic problem and the variable natural history. Topical keratolytics and cryotherapy can be used.

Warts are usually painless; however, a plantar wart (verruca) may be painful because the overlying hard skin presses into the foot on walking. Children with plantar warts should be allowed to use swimming baths, but should be advised to cover the wart with a waterproof plaster to lessen the chance of transmission.

24.4 Infestations

24.4.1 Pediculosis

The most common louse infestation in childhood is with the head louse (*Pediculosis capitis*). Head lice are most common at the age of 6–9 years and occur in all social classes. These parasites live close to the scalp and feed on blood which they obtain with their sucking mouth parts. This causes irritation, and the combination of the bites and frequent scratching may lead to impetigo and enlarged occipital and cervical lymph glands. The bites may resemble purpura confined to the neck and shoulders. Sometimes the lice can be seen, but more often just the tiny whitish eggs (nits) are seen attached singly to the hair. They can be identified with certainty beneath a microscope: they are ovoid with one blunt end and one pointed end by which they are stuck to the hair shaft. Regular use of a fine-toothed 'nit comb' on wet hair will remove eggs and is a simple, effective treatment. If necessary, anti-lice shampoo or scalp lotion is used by the whole family. Other members of the household should be examined for similar infestations.

24.4.2 Scabies

The mite *Sarcoptes scabiei* lays its eggs in burrows beneath the skin. The larva migrates and burrows into the skin, gradually developing into the adult mite, which re-emerges, becomes impregnated

and burrows to lay more eggs. After 2–6 weeks the child becomes sensitized and develops a very itchy papulo-vesicular rash. In older children, this is most marked in the interdigital spaces, wrist flexures and anterior axillary folds. In infants, any itchy rash may be scabetic.

The burrows can be seen as small, linear elevations of skin adjacent to a small vesicle, but they are often obscured by excoriation and secondary infection. Definitive diagnosis may be made by microscopic identification of a mite from one of the burrows. The infestation is transferred by bodily contact, so that other members of the family are usually affected, and all those living together should be treated at the same time. One or two applications of malathion or permethrin are required, and disinfestation of clothing and bedding is advised.

> **PRACTICE POINT**
>
> Think of scabies for any unexplained itching rash, and especially if another family member is affected.

24.5 Other skin problems covered elsewhere

24.5.1 Purpura and petechiae

These are non-blanching rashes (petechiae small dots, purpura larger blotches), and in a febrile or unwell child can indicate serious bacterial infection, especially meningococcal disease (Section 14.4.3.3, p. 133). Purpura on the legs and buttocks in a reasonably well child should make you think of Henoch Schonlein purpura (Section 23.3.5).

24.5.2 Exanthemata

This is the collective term for the common infectious diseases of childhood, which have characteristic rashes (Section 14.4.3). Kawasaki disease has a similar presentation (Section 14.4.3.4, p. 135). Children with viral infections present with non-specific rashes, such as fine pimples.

24.5.3 Neurodermatoses

These disorders affecting skin and nervous system include neurofibromatosis (Section 17.4) and tuberous sclerosis (Section 17.4).

24.5.4 Neonatal skin lesions

There are a number of lesions which are primarily seen in the neonatal period, such as erythema toxicum and milia (Section 7.4.1, p. 66).

 Summary

Birth marks are usually benign, need to be explained to the family, and occasionally have important health implications. Of all the chronic rashes, eczema most commonly requires medical attention and you should know the principles of management. Early recognition of meningococcal purpura can be life-saving.

 FOR YOUR LOG

- Management of eczema.
- Management of napkin rash.
- Child presenting with purpuric rash.

 OSCE TIP

- Stork mark, strawberry naevus, port wine stain, blue spots.
- Eczema, psoriasis, warts.
- Photographs of common skin conditions.

See EMQ 24.1 and EMQ 24.2 at the end of the book.

25

Haematology

Chapter map

Anaemia is quite common in childhood, and you should know the main differentials and be able to sensibly assess a patient. Coagulation disorders are less common, and sometimes present as purpura: know the important differential diagnoses.

25.1   The normal blood picture (Table 25.1)

Newborn infants at term have a haemoglobin of 17 g/dL (range 14–20) and a high mean cell volume (MCV). This falls until 3 months because of limited erythropoiesis and red cell survival.

The fetus and newborn have fetal haemoglobin - HbF. HbF is gradually replaced by HbA (adult) (Figure 25.1). Children have a high white cell count and lymphocyte count, particularly in the first year. Infection often provokes a marked neutrophil leukocytosis with immature white cells pouring out of the marrow. In infants, bacterial infection may produce a lymphocytic response. The platelet count is slightly reduced in the first months.

Table 25.1 Normal blood picture

Age	Haemoglobin (g/dL)	Type
Birth	17	HbF > HbA
1 year	12	HbA
12 years	14	HbA

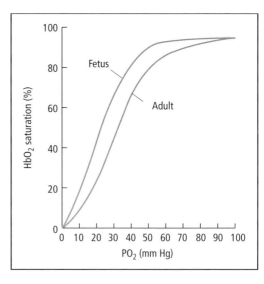

Figure 25.1 Fetal and adult oxyhaemoglobin dissociation curves. The fetus achieves a higher oxygen saturation at lower Pao₂. A small drop in Pao₂ will result in release of a large amount of oxygen to the tissues.

Paediatrics Lecture Notes, Ninth edition. Simon J. Newell and Jonathan C. Darling. © 2014 John Wiley & Sons, Ltd. Published 2014 by John Wiley & Sons, Ltd.

25.2 Anaemia

Anaemia is common in childhood, but does not usually lead to symptoms. Pallor is common and often not related to anaemia. Anaemia may cause tiredness and even breathlessness, but most tired children are not anaemic.

> Anaemia may be caused by:
> * Impaired production of red cells
> * Excessive breakdown of red cells
> * Blood loss.

PRACTICE POINT
Clinical approach to anaemia

History
* Dietary iron (consider dietetic assessment)
* Blood loss (e.g. periods)
* Malabsorption/diarrhoea
* Chronic illness
* Family history and ethnicity (inherited red cell disorders)

Examination
* Growth/failure to thrive
* Signs associated with anaemia (angular cheilosis, koilonychia)
* Jaundice (haemolysis)
* Lymphadenopathy, hepatosplenomegaly, bruising (leukaemia)
* Abdominal distension (malabsorption, coeliac)
* Signs of chronic illness e.g. clubbing

Investigations
* FBC with red cell indices and film (cells small, pale in iron deficiency, large in B12/folate deficiency)
* Reticulocytes (low in iron deficiency, rise within a few days of iron treatment; raised in haemolysis)
* Markers of iron deficiency (e.g. % hypochromic cells increased, low ferritin)
* Depending on clinical findings and results, consider haemoglobin electrophoresis, tests for haemolysis, other haematinics (folate, B12) and coeliac screen

Treatment
* Depends on cause; for iron deficiency anaemia treat with iron medication, attend to diet.

25.2.1 Impaired production of red cells

25.2.1.1 Deficiency anaemias

Iron-deficiency anaemia is by far the most common, with a hypochromic microcytic blood picture. MCV is low. It is usually dietary, but may occur because losses of iron or blood exceed intake. Iron-deficiency anaemia is more common in the following:

* Preterm babies and twins (Section 8.2.8).
* Infants fed mainly cow's milk who are late changing to iron-containing weaning foods – sometimes because the infant is late learning to chew solids, or simply prefers milk.
* Homes where poverty, ignorance or dietary restrictions prevent the child from receiving red meat, green vegetables, eggs and bread (which are the main sources of iron). Older infants and toddlers are most at risk.
* Chronic malabsorption such as coeliac disease (Section 21.2.5).
* Adolescent girls with rapid growth and menstrual losses.

PRACTICE POINT

Iron deficiency is common in socially deprived groups. It is associated with slowing of early child development in toddlers. Some foods (e.g. bread, cereals) and formula milks are iron fortified.

> **Red cell changes in anaemia**
>
> Hypochromia = pale cells. Mean cell haemoglobin (MCH) is low.
>
> Microcytosis = small cells. Mean cell volume (MCV) is low.

Pica, when children eat almost anything including soil or dirt, is associated with iron deficiency. Pica is the Latin name for magpie, a bird notorious for stealing and consuming almost anything. Other deficiency anaemias are uncommon. Folic acid deficiency is rare even in coeliac disease. Pernicious anaemia is extremely rare in children.

25.2.1.2 Bone marrow disturbance

Infiltration. Leukaemia (Section 26.1) is the most important. Secondary deposits from malignant tumours are less common. Aplastic anaemia may be drug related, post-viral (e.g. Epstein–Barr) or more commonly idiopathic.

25.2.1.3 Systemic disease

Chronic infection (e.g. cystic fibrosis), inflammatory disease (e.g. Crohn diease) and renal insufficiency depress haemopoiesis.

25.2.2 Excessive breakdown

Haemolytic anaemias are not common except in the newborn infant (Section 8.4.2.1). In paediatrics, haemolysis may have a cause specific to children or present mainly in childhood. Chronic or recurrent anaemia occurs with slight jaundice during periods of haemolysis. There is usually a reticulocytosis. If severe and sudden, it is called a 'haemolytic crisis': acute anaemia with jaundice, dark urine and dark stools seen. Splenomegaly is a feature of chronic cases.

25.2.2.1 Cellular abnormalities

These comprise abnormalities of red cell shape, red cell enzymes or haemoglobin structure.

PRACTICE POINT

Children who have sickle cell disease, or those who have had a splenectomy, are at high risk of pneumococcal infection. Make sure that they receive the pneumococcal immunization.

Red cell shape. The most important is *hereditary spherocytosis*. Red cells are small, spherical and show increased osmotic fragility. It is autosomal dominant, but one-third are new mutations. Splenectomy will help in severely affected children as one of the spleen's functions is the removal of faulty red cells from the circulation.

Enzyme defect. The most common is *glucose-6-phosphate dehydrogenase* (G6PD) *deficiency*. It is rare in Britain except in families of Mediterranean, African or Chinese origin. It is X-linked recessive.

Haemoglobinopathies. Haemoglobin synthesis is under genetic control. Some mutations prevent production of entire globin chains (e.g. β chains) so that the affected person lacks normal haemoglobin (e.g. β thalassaemia). Other mutations lead to substitution of one amino acid in the globin chain, producing an abnormal haemoglobin (e.g. HbS in sickle cell disease). Haemoglobin electrophoresis identifies abnormal haemoglobins and quantifies HbA and HbF.

Lead poisoning. Interferes with haemoglobin synthesis. May occur in children due to pica, especially if old paint ingested. Causes microcytic anaemia.

25.2.2.2 Thalassaemia

HbA is deficient and there is persistent preponderance of HbF.

Thalassaemia occurs in a broad belt extending from the Mediterranean countries through India to the Far East (Figure 25.2). The Mediterranean form is usually β thalassaemia. It is inherited as an autosomal recessive trait. Those with the heterozygous state have thalassaemia trait and are asymptomatic or have a mild microcytic anaemia (*thalassaemia minor*). Their red cells contain up to 20% HbF. Those with the homozygous state (*thalassaemia major*) have profound anaemia.

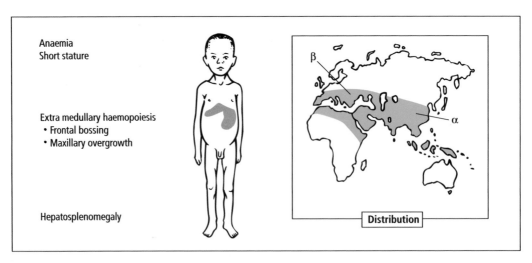

Figure 25.2 Thalassaemia major.

α Thalassaemia, which causes hydrops and perinatal death, occurs mainly in the Far East.

Diagnosis may follow family history, neonatal screening or severe anaemia at 6–12 months of age. Prenatal diagnosis and carrier detection are well established. Treatment involves regular blood transfusion every few weeks to prevent anaemia. Desferrioxamine by subcutaneous infusion helps prevent iron overload, and supplements of folic acid and vitamin C support red cell production. Hypersplenism may develop.

25.2.2.3 Sickle cell disease

This disorder occurs in Afro-Carribean families. HbS is present in place of HbA. At low oxygen tensions the cell becomes crescent- or sickle-shaped and is likely to haemolyse. Heterozygotes have about 30% HbS, may show sickling, but are usually well. Homozygotes develop recurrent episodes of haemolysis (crises) from infancy. Thromboses in mesenteric, intracranial or bone vessels produce severe pain (painful crisis), simulating acute abdominal emergencies, meningitis or arthritis.

Sickle cell disease

Anaemia
Acute crises
- Painful, vaso-occlusive
- Haemolytic
- Sequestration
- Aplastic (post-parvovirus)

Infection (e.g. pneumococcus)
Dactylitis (hand–foot syndrome).

 TREATMENT

Painful crises need:
- Analgesia
- Oxygen
- Hydration
- Warmth.

Death in late childhood or early adult life from infections, cardiac failure or thrombotic episodes is not uncommon. Outlook is better if general health and nutrition are good. DNA probes are available for prenatal diagnosis and carrier detection.

25.2.2.4 Extracellular abnormalities

Antibodies causing destruction of the red cell are usually associated with a positive Coombs' test. The only common example in childhood is haemolytic disease of the newborn (Section 8.4.2.1, p. 77). Rarer causes include severe poisoning or infection, malignancy and systemic lupus erythematosus.

25.2.3 Blood loss

Hidden blood loss is not common in childhood: peptic ulcers, piles and gastrointestinal malignancy are rare. Gastrointestinal bleeding from a Meckel's diverticulum or reflux oesophagitis is more likely to present with overt bleeding than unexplained anaemia.

25.3 Coagulation disorders

25.3.1 Haemophilia (Table 25.2)

Haemophilia A is over five times more common than B. Both are only seen in boys. Severity is related to the degree of deficiency of the relevant factor. In haemophilia A, symptoms occur with less than 10% of normal clotting activity. Severe disease occurs with <1%. Prolonged partial thromboplastin time leads to specific assay of the relevant coagulation factor. (Prothrombin time is normal.)

25.3.1.1 Presentation

- Excessive bruising as the boy learns to crawl and walk during the second year
- Prolonged bleeding following circumcision, blood sampling or tooth eruption.

25.3.1.2 Treatment

Bleeding episodes are treated and prevented by intravenous injection of factor concentrate; most families manage their own injections. Traumatic contact sports are forbidden, but an active, enjoyable life is encouraged. Haemarthroses (bleeding into a joint), especially of the ankle and knees, can lead to permanent joint damage. Haemorrhage after dental extraction and other surgical procedures can be avoided by factor replacement.

Table 25.2 Haemophilia

Haemophilia	Deficient factor	Inheritance
A	VIII	X-linked recessive
B (Christmas disease)	IX	X-linked recessive

Before 1985, some factor VIII was contaminated with HIV. Many haemophiliacs died of AIDS. Factor VIII is now treated to prevent transmission.

Haemophilia usually becomes less severe as an adult. Regional haemophilia centres provide expert care and provide a service for prenatal diagnosis and the identification of female carriers.

Von Willebrand syndrome affects both boys and girls, with autosomal dominant inheritance. Though there is a combination of factor VIII deficiency and platelet dysfunction, the degree of the bleeding disorder is usually mild.

25.3.2 Thrombocytopenia

The most common thrombocytopenic purpura of childhood is *idiopathic thrombocytopenic purpura* (ITP) (Table 25.3). The onset is acute, often occurring 1–3 weeks after an upper respiratory tract infection. A widespread petechial rash appears, developing into small purpuric spots (Figure 25.3). There may be bleeding from the nose or into the mucous membranes. Serious internal or intracranial bleeds are rare.

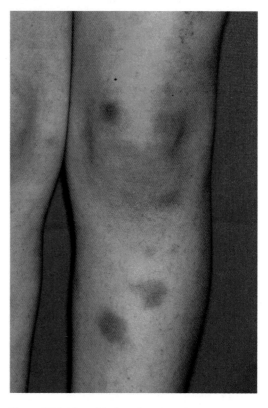

Figure 25.3 Idiopathic thrombocytopenic purpura.

ITP

Hb normal
WBC normal
Platelets low (<30 × 10⁹/L)
Marrow shows ↑ immature megakaryocytes.

Generally the outcome is good. Seventy-five per cent of children make a complete recovery within a month. Transfusions of platelets and blood are rarely needed. In severe cases with persistent bleeding, corticosteroids are given, usually after a bone marrow examination. Splenectomy is reserved for the small minority who have persistent or recurrent thrombocytopenia.

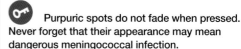 Purpuric spots do not fade when pressed. Never forget that their appearance may mean dangerous meningococcal infection.

Thrombocytopenia may be a feature of several systemic diseases, as well as leukaemia and other infiltrative diseases of the bone marrow and marrow aplasia.

Table 25.3 Main causes of purpura in children

Platelet count low (thrombocytopenia)	Platelet count normal
Idiopathic thrombocytopenic purpura	Septicaemia (particularly meningococcal)
Leukaemia (Chapter 26)	Henoch–Schönlein syndrome (Chapter 23)
Disseminated intravascular coagulation	Common viral infections
Toxic effect of drugs	

 PRACTICE POINT If you suspect a coagulation disorder

- Family history
- History of dental extraction, trauma, surgery
- Evidence of bleeding in different sites
- Initial investigations
  - Platelet count
  - Prothrombin time
  - Partial thromboplastin time
- Ask a haematologist.

25.3.3 Disseminated intravascular coagulation (DIC, consumption coagulopathy)

This syndrome is an important cause of bleeding and purpura. Examination of the blood shows haemolytic anaemia, fragmented red cells, thrombocytopenia and abnormal coagulation screen. In the neonate, it occurs as a result of severe hypoxia or massive infection. In older children, it may be associated with septicaemia and other severe illnesses.

Haemolysis is rare outside the neonatal period. Haemophilia is X-linked recessive, and is treated with factor replacement. ITP is a cause of purpura/bruising in childhood, and usually resolves within a month.

 FOR YOUR LOG

- Clerk a child presenting with anaemia
- Interpret full blood count results, reticulocytes and red cell indices in several patients
- Be able to recognize iron deficiency anaemia on blood film.

✓ Summary

Iron deficiency (usually dietary) is the commonest cause of anaemia in childhood, and causes a hypochromic, microcytic blood film picture. Haemoglobin disorders occur in certain ethnic groups and are diagnosed by electrophoresis of the haemoglobin. Look for any signs of leukaemia: do a blood film if doubt.

 OSCE TIP

- Assessment of bruising, anaemia (see OSCE station 25.1)
- Splenomegaly: spherocytosis, thalassaemia.

See EMQ 25.1 and EMQ 25.2 at the end of the book.

OSCE station 25.1: Assessment of bruising

Clinical approach:

Check
- Colour
- Anaemia
- Jaundice

Bruising
- Site
  ◦ Where are the bruises?
  ◦ Are they over bony prominences?
- Character
  ◦ Small petechiae
  ◦ Large bruised areas
  ◦ Does pattern suggest mode of injury?
- Age
  ◦ Bruises change appearance as they age
  ◦ Are these bruises of different ages?

Associated disease
- Coagulation disorders
  ◦ Previous bleeding into joints
  ◦ Medicalert bracelet
- Other haematological disorders
  ◦ Red cell problem — anaemia
  ◦ White cell problem — ill health, infection, treatment of malignancy
- If time allows or you are asked, examine for hepatosplenomegaly and lymphadenopathy

Sam is 5 years old. He has some marks on his skin. Please examine them

- Looks well and cheerful

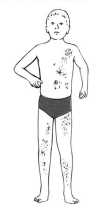

- Normal growth
- Widespread rash
- Non-blanching
- Varying size
  ◦ Petechiae and bruises
- No enlarged liver or spleen
- Normal cervical nodes

Sam has idiopathic thrombocytopenic purpura (ITP).

Never forget:

- Say hello and introduce yourself
- General health — is the child ill?
- Colour — ?pale/?jaundice
- Quickly assess growth, nutrition and development
- Mention the obvious (e.g. drip, hair loss from chemotherapy)

Look around for:

- Other injuries
- Features of neglect or abuse
- Treatment of associated disease
  ◦ Intravenous line
  ◦ Indwelling cannula

Special points

- Non-accidental injury (NAI) is suggested by the pattern, site and varied ages of bruises
- NAI is unusual in undergraduate examinations, but you might be asked why this child's bruises do not suggest NAI
- Accidental bruises are very common in childhood (usually on legs and forehead)
- Accidental bruising is rare before the infant walks

26

Neoplasia

Malignant disease is the second most common cause of death in childhood after accidents. Leukaemia has the highest incidence (Figure 26.1). With 1200 newly diagnosed UK cases a year, a child has a 1 in 600 chance of developing a malignancy before reaching adulthood. There has been steady improvement in outcome over the past decades due to ongoing treatment development, and the fact that most patients are entered into multicentre clinical trials. For the 0-14 year age-group, 5-year survival is 80% in Europe and the USA. Cure rates vary by tumour type, from around 60% for acute myeloid leukaemia, neuroblastoma and CNS tumours, to above 90% for Hodgkin's lymphoma.

26.1   Acute leukaemia, 257

26.2   Lymphomas, 258

26.3   Central nervous system tumours, 258

26.4   Neuroblastoma, 259

26.5   Wilms tumour (nephroblastoma), 259

26.6   Bone tumours, 259

26.7   Treatment of childhood malignancy, 260

Summary, 260

Reference, 260

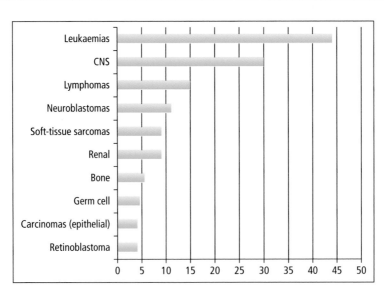

Figure 26.1 Incidence of childhood malignancy in Europe. New cases per million population. Source: adapted from data in Kaatsch (2010).

Paediatrics Lecture Notes, Ninth edition. Simon J. Newell and Jonathan C. Darling. © 2014 John Wiley & Sons, Ltd. Published 2014 by John Wiley & Sons, Ltd.

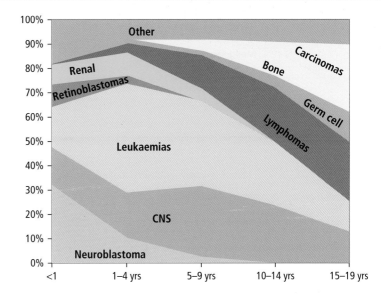

Figure 26.2 Relative incidence of malignancies through childhood.

Most common malignancies

- Leukaemia
- Lymphoma
- CNS tumours.

The relative frequency of different types of malignancy varies through childhood (Figure 26.2). In contrast to adult disease, childhood epithelial malignancies (e.g. carcinoma of the lung and gastrointestinal tract) are very rare. In children, the prognosis for malignancy is better than in adults (Table 26.1). Some genetic conditions increase the lifetime risk of cancer (e.g. Down syndrome, neurofibromatosis).

Early diagnosis improves outcomes. However, many of the initial presenting signs and symptoms are relatively common in the general population, so care is needed, and a high index of suspicion (Table 26.2). Early review, further investigation, or urgent referral should be considered.

26.1   Acute leukaemia

Leukaemia is characterized by the malignant proliferation of abnormal white cells (blasts) within the bone marrow. Acute lymphoblastic leukaemia accounts for 85% of cases. It is more common in boys and has a peak incidence between 2 and 5 years of age.

Leukaemia presentation

- Thrombocytopenia → bruising
- Anaemia → pallor
- Leucopenia → infection.

Also

- Bone pain
- Fever
- Lymphadenopathy
- Hepatosplenomegaly.

Table 26.1   5-year survival rates (%) for childhood malignancy

Malignancy	5 year survival rate (%)
Hodgkin's lymphoma	95
Wilm's tumour	84
Astrocytoma	83
Acute lymphoblastic leukaemia	84
Osteosarcoma	68
Neuroblastoma	73
All childhood malignancy	80

The diagnosis is confirmed by bone marrow examination. Blasts may also be seen within the peripheral blood. Children with a total white blood cell count less than 50×10^9/L at diagnosis have a good prognosis, whilst those with a count greater than 100×10^9/L have a worse outlook. Initial treatment consists of induction chemotherapy with the aim of achieving remission (defined as less than 5% blasts

Table 26.2 Common symptoms – when to worry

	Malignancy unlikely*	Malignancy more likely
Lymphadenopathy	Smooth, mobile, <2 cm Cervical or small inguinal Well child	Hard, craggy, tethered Bruising, pallor, fever Hepatosplenomegaly
Headaches	Typical migraine or stress headache Longstanding in older child No neurological signs or symptoms No other concerning symptoms (see section on central nervous system tumours below)	Present on waking Worse on coughing/sneezing Recent onset, worsening or persistent Any neurological signs/symptoms Any other concerning symptoms
Aches and pains	Vague, difficult to localize Well child No local signs	Localized pain Local signs (e.g. swelling and tenderness) Unusual pain (e.g. back pain in a toddler)

*Note that there may be other differential diagnoses for these symptoms.

on bone marrow examination). Within 1 month of commencing chemotherapy, 95% of children will achieve remission. Meningeal leukaemia is a common complication, so induction must be followed by intrathecal methotrexate, sometimes with cranial irradiation. Remission is maintained with intermittent cycles of chemotherapy for 2 years. With modern aggressive therapy, 85% of children will remain disease free 5 years after diagnosis. Relapse is rare after that time.

Children with acute myeloid leukaemia have a less favourable outcome. Remission can be achieved in 80% using intensive chemotherapy regimens, but relapse is common. For those in remission, bone marrow transplantation may offer the best chance of cure.

26.2 Lymphomas

Lymphomas present as painless and very enlarged lymph nodes, sometimes with fevers and drenching night sweats. They are classified into two groups based on their histological characteristics: Hodgkin's and non-Hodgkin diease. Hodgkin diease has a peak incidence in young adults. Treatment is with radiotherapy and/or chemotherapy depending on the extent of the disease. The 5-year survival rate is good (95%). Non-Hodgkin's lymphoma has a peak incidence between the ages of 7 and 10 years. It is almost always a generalized disease requiring treatment with intensive multiple drug chemotherapy; 70% of children will achieve prolonged remission.

26.3 Central nervous system tumours

These are most commonly gliomas: either astrocytomas or medulloblastomas. They are mainly infratentorial and present with cerebellar signs (ataxia, incoordination, nystagmus). Other presentations are due to raised intracranial pressure (vomiting, headache), or local effects (seizures, lethargy, behaviour change). Papilloedema is an important sign. Computer-assisted tomography (CAT) or magnetic resonance imaging (MRI) will identify the site and extent of the tumour (Figure 26.3). Treatment includes surgical excision, radiotherapy and chemotherapy. Astrocytomas have the best survival rates.

Brain tumour presentation by age

- Any age
  - Abnormal eye movements
  - Fits or seizures
  - Behaviour change (lethargy under 5)
  - Abnormal balance / walking / co-ordination
  - Persistent / recurrent vomiting
- Young children
  - Abnormal head position such as wry neck, head tilt or stiff neck
- Older children
  - Persistent / recurrent headache
  - Blurred or double vision
  - Delayed or arrested puberty.

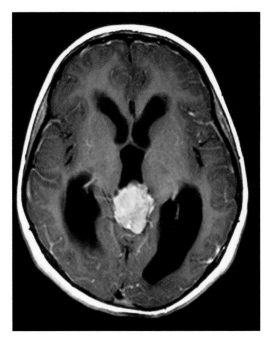

Figure 26.3 Pineal tumour (the white mass) presenting with headaches.

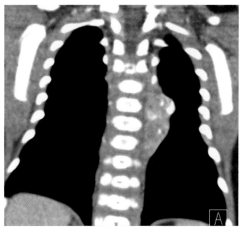

Figure 26.4 Neuroblastoma arising from the sympathetic chain in the chest shown on MRI scan.

> **RESOURCE**
>
> Headsmart is a UK project to increase awareness of symptoms of brain tumours in children and young people. See **www.headsmart.org.uk** for more information.

26.4 Neuroblastoma

This is a malignant tumour arising from the sympathetic nervous tissue. It commonly develops within the adrenal gland, but can arise from the cervical, thoracic or lumbar sympathetic chains (Figure 26.4). The most common presentation is with an abdominal mass. Early metastasis to bone, liver and skin often occurs. Urinary levels of catecholamine degradation products (e.g. VMA, HMMA) are usually raised.

Treatment comprises chemotherapy combined with radiotherapy and surgery. The outlook is poor except for those presenting with localized disease and for children aged less than 1 year.

26.5 Wilms tumour (nephroblastoma)

Nephroblastomas are embryonic renal tumours. Abdominal ultrasound is performed in the young child with an abdominal mass. Surgical excision and chemotherapy often achieve complete cure.

> **Wilms' tumour**
>
> - Unilateral abdominal mass
> - Solid and cystic
> - Microscopic haematuria.

26.6 Bone tumours

Ewing's sarcoma and osteosarcoma usually occur in the long bones and present with pain, swelling or a pathological fracture. Treatment is aimed at surgical excision of the tumour. The bone and joint can be replaced with an endoprosthesis, avoiding amputation. Chemotherapy is given before and after surgery. Radiotherapy may also be required. Around 65% children affected achieve long-term survival.

26.7 Treatment of childhood malignancy

Improvements in the treatment and survival of childhood malignancy have been dramatic over the last 30 years. As survival increases, the adverse effects of treatment become more apparent. Chemotherapy and radiotherapy may lead to bone marrow suppression, resulting in an increased risk of infection.

 Immunosuppession in malignancy

Febrile neutropenia – admit for urgent broad spectrum iv antibiotics

Avoid live vaccines

Varicella exposure – iv immunoglobulin, acyclovir if develop chickenpox.

A small proportion of survivors later develop a second primary tumour. Social and psychological problems for the child, their siblings and the family are inevitable. The diversity and complications of treatment mandate treatment in a specialized centre where there is a multidisciplinary team. Long-term follow up is important. For the child whose disease cannot be cured, every effort should be made for palliative care to be given at home or within a children's hospice.

Long-term complications

- Pituitary dysfunction
- Precocious puberty
- Growth failure
- Learning difficulties
- Cardiotoxicity
- Infertility.

 Summary

Childhood cancers are very different from adult malignancies both in type and prognosis. Although relatively rare, and with increasingly good outcomes, they are still the second commonest cause of death in childhood. Early diagnosis improves outcomes, but this can be challenging and requires awareness of the possibility and careful evaluation.

FOR YOUR LOG

- Visit a paediatric oncology ward or clinic.
- Follow up a child where malignancy is one of the differentials.

Reference

Kaatsch, P. (2010), Epidemiology of childhood cancer, *Cancer Treatment Reviews* **36**: 277–85.

27

Endocrine and metabolic disorders

Chapter map

Insulin-dependent diabetes mellitus is the most important endocrine condition in children. Other hormonal conditions, and inborn errors of metabolism, are relatively uncommon, and most are extremely rare. In general, they are characterized by their effects upon a child's growth and development. It is important, therefore, to include endocrine and metabolic disorders in the differential diagnosis of a wide variety of clinical presentations. Early recognition and appropriate management may confer long-lasting benefit.

27.1 Diabetes mellitus

27.1.1 Type 1 diabetes (insulin dependent)

Diabetes in children is nearly always Type 1. It has increased in frequency, now affecting around 1 : 500 children. Most present after the age of 2 years. Often there is no family history, although other members of the family may have diabetes or other autoimmune disease. Children who are genetically predisposed develop diabetes following an unknown trigger. Possible triggers include viral infection.

27.1.2 Presentation

 Presentation of diabetes

- Polydipsia/thirst
- Polyuria/enuresis
- Weight loss
- Dehydration/vomiting
- Ketoacidosis
- Altered consciousness/coma.

At presentation, children are often ill and have a markedly elevated blood glucose level

Paediatrics Lecture Notes, Ninth edition. Simon J. Newell and Jonathan C. Darling. © 2014 John Wiley & Sons, Ltd. Published 2014 by John Wiley & Sons, Ltd.

(>14 mmol/L), together with glycosuria and ketonuria. The glucose tolerance test is never needed to diagnose type 1 diabetes, but can be used to assess glucose control in other conditions. The HbA1C (percentage of glycosylated haemoglobin) is useful for diagnosis and monitoring, since it reflects recent blood sugar levels.

RESOURCE

The '4 Ts' is a national UK campaign to increase awareness of early symptoms of diabetes: Toilet, Thirsty, Tired, Thinner) – see **www.diabetes.org.uk/The4Ts**.

27.1.3 Management

TREATMENT Principles of acute management of ketoacidosis

- Rehydration
- Control of blood sugar with insulin
- Care of electrolyte status, especially potassium.

Longer term management involves principally the introduction of dietary regulation and insulin therapy, and an intensive programme of support and education for the child and their family.

TREATMENT Management of diabetes mellitus

Aims
- Regulated carbohydrate intake matching growth needs and activity
- Insulin regime designed around child and family's needs and abilities
- Continuous monitoring of control - usually home blood glucose.

Advice to family
- Understanding of blood sugar control
- Good control reduces likelihood of complications
- Diabetes management can usually be adjusted around lifestyle
- How to adjust diet/insulin with activity/illness
- Recognition, importance and treatment of hypoglycaemia ('hypos').

PRACTICE POINT

If you suspect diabetes mellitus, or glycosuria is found, check blood sugar with a stick test: if the blood sugar is elevated, refer to hospital immediately.

There are a wide variety of different insulin preparations. The traditional regime of twice-daily, mixed short- and medium-acting insulin is being increasingly replaced by multi-dose regimes delivered by pen device (Figure 28.2), or continuous variable insulin delivered subcutaneously by body-worn pump. These bring greater flexibility, adaptation to lifestyle and better glucose control. However they require a high level of understanding on the part of parents or older children and teenagers. Insulin is injected subcutaneously, rotating round sites including the arms, thighs and abdomen.

PRACTICE POINT

Whenever the child becomes acutely unwell, the administration of glucose or sugary food or drink is always the right thing to do. If it is a hypo, this action will save lives. If it is hyperglycaemia or another problem, the glucose or sugar given will make little difference.

Each child will get different early symptoms of hypoglycaemia. It is essential that they understand the importance of recognizing a 'hypo'. The child may wear a medical alert bracelet. The child, family, teachers and others caring for the child need to know what to do. If a child is unable to eat or drink, a glucose gel (*Hypostop*), sugar or jam can be smeared onto the buccal mucosa and is rapidly absorbed. The child's parents should know how to administer subcutaneous or intramuscular glucagon in emergencies.

Diabetic control can be difficult in children. Loss of control during infection, and difficulty in maintaining tight control during periods of rapid growth are characteristic.

27.1.4 Family support

All children with diabetes, and their families, require intensive support. Children should be encouraged, as soon as they are old enough, to take responsibility for their diabetes. Membership of Diabetes UK is a great asset. Self-help groups and the outreach children's nursing service can all help the child and the family to take diabetes in their stride, so that it is not a major interference with the normal way of life. Long-term complications, such as retinopathy and renal disease, are rare during childhood, but good glycaemic control is important to reduce their incidence in later life.

Chronic illness does not fit well into the teenage years. This is well known in diabetes, when depression and psychological disturbance become more common. The discipline of diabetes is particularly irksome at this age. Teenagers should be encouraged to become more independent of their parents, managing their own diabetes. Unfortunately they may frequently break dietary rules, cheat on tests or omit insulin.

27.1.5 Type 2 diabetes (insulin-resistant diabetes)

Previously very rare, this form of diabetes is increasingly recognized. The epidemic of childhood obesity largely explains the increase in type 2 diabetes. Family history is often positive. Unusual specific genetic forms are found. In the obese child with type 2 diabetes, weight loss and exercise are key. Oral drug treatments are used, and insulin depending upon control. Good control is important to reduce the risk of long-term complications.

27.2 Hypoglycaemia

> **PRACTICE POINT**
>
> Check for hypoglycaemia in all children with acute illness, collapse or fits. If low, save plasma in the freezer for further testing later.

Hypoglycaemia is most common in the newborn period. Symptoms are difficult to recognize in babies, and routine monitoring is indicated for those at high risk (Section 8.4.3). If hypoglycaemia is allowed to persist, permanent neurological damage may occur. This may lead to cerebral palsy, learning problems and epilepsy. In the collapsed child, intravenous dextrose is given. Investigation is complex.

> **Causes of hypoglycaemia**
>
> **Hormonal**
> - Excess insulin
> - Lack of cortisol (e.g. congenital adrenal hyperplasia).
>
> **Metabolic**
> - Ketotic hypoglycaemia
> - Liver disease
> - Glycogen storage disorders
> - Galactosaemia
> - Other inborn errors of metabolism.

27.3 Thyroid disease

Normal thyroid function is necessary for healthy physical and mental growth.

27.3.1 Congenital hypothyroidism

This is usually due to the absence of the thyroid gland. Occasionally a small or ectopic thyroid is present, or metabolic problems in the gland prevent production of thyroid hormone. Neonatal screening at the end of the first week of life measures thyroid-stimulating hormone (TSH), which is raised. Very rarely hypothyroidism is due to panhypopituitarism and TSH levels are normal or low.

This successful screening programme allows early instigation of lifelong hormone replacement therapy with oral thyroxine. The untreated child with very short stature, coarse features, scanty hair, an umbilical hernia and severe learning problems is now a feature of history.

27.3.2 Juvenile hypothyroidism

Later thyroid failure is more common in children with diabetes and in those with Down or Turner syndromes. The cardinal feature is a fall-off in physical growth (Section 13.1.2). Symptoms are very similar to those seen in the adult, with school failure and learning problems. Juvenile hypothyroidism is normally due to auto-immune disease, and auto-antibodies are present. Rarely it is of pituitary origin.

> Children with Down syndrome may be screened annually for hypothyroidism and coeliac disease as both are more common and difficult to recognize.

27.3.3 Hyperthyroidism and goitre

A transient form of this occurs in newborn infants who receive IgG transplacentally from a mother who has a history of *Graves' disease* (autoimmune hyperthyroidism often associated with exophthalmos).

Goitre may occur in adolescent girls who are euthyroid. Classical Graves' disease is unusual in children.

27.4 The adrenal glands

Disorders of the adrenal gland are uncommon in children. The least rare is congenital adrenal hyperplasia. *Addison diease* (hypoadrenalism), presenting later in life with growth failure and hyperpigmentation, is very rare. Cushing syndrome, the result of excess corticosteroid activity, is almost always the result of therapeutic use of steroids. Rarely, adrenal cortical tumours secrete androgens or oestrogens, with consequent early appearance of secondary sexual characteristics (adrenarche).

27.4.1 Congenital adrenal hyperplasia

This results from a metabolic block in the synthesis of hydrocortisone. The 21-hydroxylase enzyme is absent in children who are homozygous for an autosomal recessive gene mutation. There are two consequences:

- Absence of sufficient circulating corticosteroids and mineralocorticoids
- ↑ pituitary ACTH → adrenal cortical hypertrophy → ↑ androgens.

Clinical features depend on the child's sex. Girls are virilized with abnormal genitalia, enlarged clitoris and labia fusion, which may prevent accurate determination of sex at birth. Boys have normal genitalia. The majority of children with this condition lack mineralocorticoids, and present in the first weeks because of salt loss. Typically they have a history of vomiting and are markedly dehydrated. Some are severely ill and the condition is lethal if not recognized and treated.

Diagnosis is made by finding elevated levels of cortisone precursors (17-hydroxyprogesterone) and, in salt losers, a low serum sodium and an elevated potassium. Treatment is lifelong hormone replacement therapy. The dose must be increased at times of illness and stress. Girls may require genital plastic surgery.

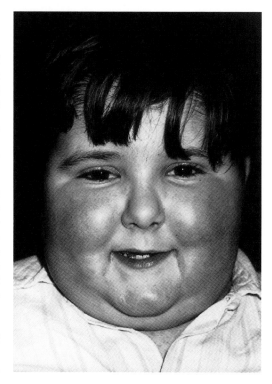

Figure 27.1 Steroid therapy has led to obesity, a round face and hirsuteness.

 PRACTICE POINT

If a newborn infant is not clearly male or female, do not assign the sex until clarified through further investigation. This is awkward, but better than discovering that a boy is in fact a girl.

27.4.2 Cushing syndrome

Features of Cushing syndrome

- Round, fat face
- Obesity
- Poor growth
- Hypertension
- Osteoporosis.

The effects of excess glucocorticoid are almost always due to steroid treatment (Figure 27.1). Long-term steroid therapy should only be used when it is essential. *Cushing diease* (primary excess steroid secretion by the child's own adrenals) and other causes of endogenous excess glucocorticoids are rare. The combination of obesity and reduced height/growth should raise suspicion.

 PRACTICE POINT

Short obese children are more likely to have an endocrine problem than those who are tall or of average height.

27.5 Growth hormone deficiency

Deficiency of growth hormone (GH) is an uncommon, but important, cause of growth failure. It may be isolated, or associated with deficiency of other pituitary hormones. It is sometimes secondary to an intracranial lesion.

Lack of response to stimulation of GH secretion is diagnostic. In the GH stimulation test, clonidine or glucagon is given and blood samples are taken over a few hours. Often, thyroid and pituitary function tests are done at the same time.

Genetically engineered human GH is given by injection, under expert supervision and close monitoring. GH is sometimes used to treat short children without deficiency (e.g. Turner syndrome, achondroplasia).

27.6 Diabetes insipidus

In this rare condition, antidiuretic hormone (ADH) is not produced or does not work. There is marked thirst, and the passage of large volumes of dilute urine of low osmolality. There is constant danger of serious water depletion, especially in hot weather.

Central diabetes insipidus

Hypothalamus not producing ADH.

Nephrogenic diabetes insipidus

Renal tubule not responding to ADH.

ADH deficiency can result from brain tumours, cysts, vascular accidents and meningitis. ADH replacement therapy is given. Nephrogenic diabetes insipidus is caused by an X-linked gene and therefore only occurs in males.

27.7 Inborn errors of metabolism

There are many hundreds of these disorders due to a metabolic block. Most are extremely rare, and most show autosomal recessive inheritance (Figure 27.2).

 PRACTICE POINT

Metabolic disorders are more common when parents are consanguinous (e.g. first cousins), so ask about this in the history when these are suspected.

 Symptoms suggesting an inborn error of metabolism

- Unexplained illness
- Fits, coma
- Hypoglycaemia, metabolic acidosis
- Acute liver disease; jaundice
- Failure to thrive
- Developmental delay.

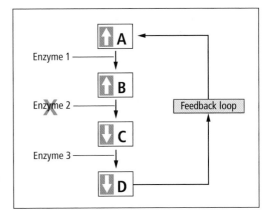

Figure 27.2 Schematic inborn error of metabolism. Enzyme 2 is non-functional. Low levels of D provide positive feedback driving the metabolic pathway. Clinical symptoms may result from low levels of C or D, OR the high levels of A or B. Diagnosis is usually made by measuring the high levels of A or B, or by determination of enzyme activity.

Diagnosis is made by collecting urine, preferably at the time of symptoms, for a 'metabolic screen'. Successful management usually depends upon dietary restriction or replacement of the missing metabolites. Many of the severe inborn errors of metabolism are untreatable and some are lethal.

27.7.1 Phenylketonuria (PKU)

This disorder affects 1 : 10 000–20 000 children born with a deficiency of the enzyme which converts phenylalanine to tyrosine. High levels of phenylalanine in the blood result in delayed development, poor growth and seizures (Table 27.1).

Children affected by PKU are detected in the neonatal screening programme (Section 7.4.1, p. 68). Early implementation of a strict low phenylalanine diet results in good outcome. Lifelong dietary restriction is recommended. In pregnant women with PKU, high phenylalanine levels cross the placenta, and may lead to fetal brain damage. In pregnancy, tight dietary control is mandatory.

27.7.2 Medium Chain Acyl-CoA Dehydrogenase deficiency (MCADD)

MCADD is an autosomal recessive inborn error which occurs in 1 in 10 000. The enzyme deficiency prevents

Table 27.1 Criteria for a good screening test: two examples

	Condition		
Screening test criteria	Hypothyroidism		Phenylketonuria
Identifiable disease	Absent thyroid		Enzyme deficiency
Natural history known	Learning difficulties Growth failure		Learning difficulties Seizures
Safe, acceptable test		Blood spot at 7 days of age	
Sensitive test		Positive when disease present	
Specific test		Negative when disease not present	
Recognized treatment	Thyroxine		Low phenylalanine diet
Benefit from diagnosis		Normal growth and development	

fatty acid oxidation, so that starvation results in potentially lethal hypoglycaemia, acidosis and collapse. Typically an apparently healthy child has a minor viral infection, does not feed and then collapses. The condition was recently added to the national UK newborn screening programme (Section 7.4.1, p. 68). Treatment is avoidance of starvation, and IV dextrose when nutrition cannot be taken orally.

27.7.3 Galactosaemia

A deficiency of the enzyme galactose-1-phosphate uridyl transferase leads to accumulation of galactose. Affected babies become ill almost as soon as they begin to drink milk. Typical presenting features in the first weeks of life include vomiting, weight loss, jaundice and severe infection. The infants have a low blood sugar and may have cataracts. If the diagnosis is considered, the enzyme level is easily measured on the red cells. Exclusion of lactose (galactose + glucose) from the diet is curative. A lactose-free milk is given.

 Summary

It is essential that you can recognize the cardinal symptoms of early diabetes (thirst, weight loss and polyuria) – you may prevent life-threatening diabetic

ketoacidosis (DKA). Know the key points of management of DKA, and of long-term diabetes. Other metabolic problems are rarer, but key messages are: check glucose in fits, faints or funny dos; check thyroid in a tired, cold child who has stopped growing; and do electrolytes, sugar and a metabolic screen in collapsed or acidotic infants.

 FOR YOUR LOG

- Sit in on a diabetes clinic.
- Take a history of a child presenting with DKA and review how the child was managed.
- Be familiar with insulin syringe, pen and pump.
- Be able to perform near-patient glucose testing (e.g. Bm stix).
- Observe newborn screening test.

 OSCE TIP

- Thyroid status and examination (see OSCE station 27.1).
- Video and lab results of child with diabetic ketoacidosis.

See EMQ 27.1 at the end of the book.

OSCE station 27.1: Examination of the neck

Clinical approach:

Check
- Colour
- Anaemia

Inspection
- Site
- Skin, scars
- Swelling
- Position of head

Palpation
- Position of trachea
- Swellings, masses
  - ◇ Anterior triangles
  - ◇ Posterior triangles
  - ◇ Suboccipital

If lymph nodes, consider:
- Size of nodes
- Are they mobile?
- Tenderness, signs of inflammation
- Local infection (skin, scalp, etc.)
- ENT examination (tonsils, otitis externa)
- Generalized lymphadenopathy
- Hepatosplenomegaly

If thyroid swelling, consider:
- Size and shape (?symmetry)
- Smooth/nodular
- Ask child to sip and swallow a drink
- Thyroid function
  - ◇ Growth and developmentf
  - ◇ Acial appearance
  - ◇ Clinical signs of hypo-orhyperthyroidism

Natalie is 13 years old. Please examine her neck

- Pleasant, chatty girl
- Early pubertal development

- Thyroid swelling
  - ◇ Smooth
  - ◇ Non tender
  - ◇ Symmetrical
  - ◇ Moves with swallowing
  - ◇ No bruit

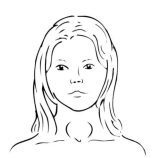

- No other abnormal findings
  - ◇ No exophthalmos
  - ◇ No tremor of outstretched hands

Natalie has a goitre. She is clinically euthyroid

Never forget:
- Say hello and introduce yourself
- General health — is the child ill?
- Quickly assess growth, nutrition, and development
- Mention the obvious (e.g. drip, tracheostomy)

Look around for:
- Medication
- Growth measurements

Special points
- Examine her neck gently, it can be uncomfortable
- Most children have palpable cervical nodes
- Lymph nodes are rarely malignant or tuberculous
- Goitres
  - ◇ Commonly auto-immune thyroiditis
  - ◇ Usually euthyroid, or hypothyroid
  - ◇ The cardinal feature of hypo-thyroidism is loss of height velocity
  - ◇ Classic signs of hypo- or hyper-thyroidism are unusual and appear late in thyroid disease

Part 4

After paediatrics

This chapter takes you beyond your paediatric placement. You will need to prepare for exams, and we give you tips and pointers for paediatric examinations in Chapter 28.

It won't be long before you are prescribing, including for children. It is worth keeping this in mind throughout your time in paediatrics. Prescribing for children has unique risks, and we highlight these in Chapter 29.

Chapter 30 gives some careers advice – we hope of interest to many readers!

Finally the section after Chapter 30 provides self-test questions (with answers and explanations) which we hope will be a useful way to review what you have learnt.

28

Preparing for clinical examinations in paediatrics and child health

Chapter map

Although we hope that you are learning about paediatrics and child health because it is an interesting and enjoyable subject, we know that you want to pass clinical examinations in the subject. The purpose of this chapter is to give you specific help with how to prepare for such examinations. There are currently many modes of assessment in under-graduate paediatric examinations, but they divide into written and clinical examinations.

28.1   Clinical examinations

Traditionally, these consisted of a long case and several short cases, but such formats have been criticized for lacking objectivity and reproducibility, and for inadequate sampling of students' skills. They are very close to what you will do in real practice, and encourage a thoughtful, integrative and patient-centred approach to clinical skills. In an OSCE (see below) you are asked to demonstrate a variety of clinical skills, but it is harder for examiners to make sure that you can put a whole series of skills together and make sense of the outcome. Some medical schools use an exam format that is part way between long and short cases, where you might be partly observed taking a history or examining a patient (or both) in a shortened time frame and then be asked questions about diagnosis and management.

28.1.1   Objective Structured Clinical Examinations (OSCEs)

These have become the most widely used method of assessing clinical skills, because they allow all students to be assessed performing the same tasks in the same or similar clinical situations, with objective marking criteria and wide sampling of skills. In an OSCE, candidates rotate around stations, with a pre-set time of between 5 and 20 min allowed for each (Figure 28.1). Stations will range over a variety of clinical skills.

Paediatrics Lecture Notes, Ninth edition. Simon J. Newell and Jonathan C. Darling. © 2014 John Wiley & Sons, Ltd. Published 2014 by John Wiley & Sons, Ltd.

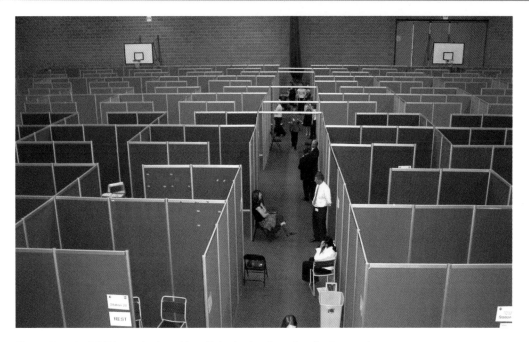

Figure 28.1 An OSCE examination with multiple circuits all running simultaneously.

The principle is simple. The examiners first determine what is required of the candidate. A standardized question is given to the candidate (e.g. please examine this 4-year-old boy's cardiovascular system), and the candidate is observed by the examiner, who ticks off or grades essential elements as they are performed. Further marks are given for general approach, rapport with the child and their parent (or proxy parent), and interpretation of the findings.

A badly written OSCE station will allow you to accumulate marks by a haphazard approach, where you do everything you can possibly think of in a thoughtless and random order. Such stations are now rare. To gain high marks in a good OSCE station, you need to demonstrate a logical approach, good communication and examination skills, and then show that you are able to synthesize and make sense of the clinical information.

> **OSCE TIP Examples of clinical skills tested in OSCE stations**
>
> **Communication (sometimes with a proxy parent)**
> - History-taking
> - History presentation and discussion
> - Counselling and explaining
>
> **Physical examination (with a patient, manikin, or video)**
> - Systems examination, e.g. CVS, respiratory, abdomen, joints, neurology (part), gait, squint, ENT (manikin), newborn hips (manikin)
> - Developmental assessment
> - Assessment of peak flow or use of asthma devices
>
> **Practical and emergency skills**
> - Practical tasks without a patient (dipstick testing of urine)
> - Resuscitation (manikin).

28.1.1.1 Communication stations

Here, an actor or member of staff will play the role of a parent. There are two main types of communication station.

History-taking

You may be observed taking a history about a particular presenting symptom. Histories will usually focus on common paediatric presenting symptoms. even if you think you know the diagnosis, it is important to consider differential diagnoses, and to ask relevant questions to help rule those in or out. At the end you may be asked to summarize. Get in the habit of writing and presenting a concise summary for every history you take. This will help you acquire this important clinical skill.

History presentation and discussion

You may have a linked, or stand-alone station, where you present and then discuss a history you have taken or are given. You may need to present this verbally (in person or over the telephone), in note form, or in a letter. The examiner may then ask you questions about the history, or about management.

 OSCE TIP OSCE history-taking tips

- Read the task carefully, and check it part way through to make sure you are doing what has been asked of you.
- Don't forget to introduce yourself and use the child's name.
- As with any good history, you need a balance of open questions that allow the parent or child to say what is the matter and how it is affecting them, combined with focused closed or follow-up questions, so that you have the necessary details.
- Spend most time on the history of the presenting complaint, and make sure you know exactly what has been happening, the impact on child and family, any treatments given (including names and doses), and their effect. This aspect is where students lose most marks.
- Use a problem-orientated, logical approach, where you generate your differential diagnosis early based on the presenting complaint, and then repeatedly test and refine this as you gather more information. Avoid blindly asking random questions!
- If you are going to present, summarize or be questioned on the history, try to allow yourself some time to think through the information, and decide on a problem list, differential diagnosis and management plan.

Counselling and explaining

Your task may be to explain a diagnosis, illness or a treatment to a parent or young person, offering the essential facts in a way that is easy to understand, while demonstrating appropriate empathy and good interpersonal skills. The parent may be primed to ask you certain questions. See the example OSCE station at the end of Chapter 2.

 RESOURCE

The following sites provide useful patient information:

- www.patient.co.uk
- www.cks.nhs.uk

 OSCE TIP OSCE counselling and explaining tips

- You cannot explain well if you don't have a good understanding yourself. Learn topics that are flagged as important/essential in your syllabus, or that are common and important.
- Read parent information leaflets (and websites), which are usually focused on such topics.
- Listen to consultations in clinics and on wards.
- Be clear about the task: Is any history taking included? – if not, keep to a minimum (although some checking questions can be an appropriate way in).
- Consider drawing a diagram if this helps to explain things more clearly.
- Avoid medical jargon.
- Use the child's name.
- Consider starting with 'ICE' – Ideas, Concerns and Expectations; and finishing with: a summary, asking if any further questions or concerns, and planning follow up (if appropriate).
- Parents will often want the following questions addressed: What is it? What does it mean for my child? What do I do in an acute attack? What do I do to prevent/treat?
- It is quite easy to prepare and practice realistic stations 1 or 2 colleagues. Video yourselves and review – it is easier to spot ways to improve.

28.1.1.2   Clinical examination stations

You may be asked to examine a system in an infant, child or young person. With some thought about your own examination system (particularly venue and number of students), you should be able to work out the sort of things that are unlikely to be examined in this format in real children. For example, children with acute problems are unlikely to be seen in examinations away from clinical areas, or involving large numbers of students. There is increasing use of video or DVD for such cases. Manikins may also be used for testing resuscitation skills, ear examination, hip examination, or auscultation skills. Stations may feature combinations of real patients or well children, manikins, video and audio. For example, you could be asked to peform a cardiovascular examination in a healthy child without a murmur, and then be asked to comment on an audio recording of a ventricular septal defect murmur. Make sure you can do practical tasks such as doing a peak flow measurement, making up a feed, putting on a urine bag or testing urine with a dipstick.

OSCE TIP **OSCE Approach**

There are three ways to approach the examination or development OSCE stations:

- **Section, then report**
  Here you will divide up the task into sections and report back to the examiner after each. This allows you to talk to the child. You can remember HIGHCOST (Section 3.1.2) and use this as a structure (e.g. you could begin with Hello–Introduce yourself–General inspection, and then tell the examiner about this before going on to Health and hands–Centiles–Obvious). In this way you can bank the points as you go through. Finish by mentioning anything that still needs to be done, and summarizing your findings briefly.
- **Finish and present**
  Here you will complete the task and the examination and present it to the examiner at the end. This can look very accomplished. It is difficult to do and you will only get the marks that you deserve if you remember to tell the examiner everything that you did or that needs to be done. If time prevents you from presenting, you may get very few marks.
- **Running commentary**
  Here you give a continuous account of what you are doing, why and what you find. It interferes with building any rapport with the child. It is also very tedious. It can confuse candidates who need to think as they go through.

Few exams tell you which approach to choose. It is up to you. Most students use the 'Section, then Report' approach, and we recommend this because it allows you to focus on the child and family without risking loss of many marks if you do not complete in time to present all your findings.

Review the OSCE stations and tips at the end of each chapter. These give you examples of typical OSCE stations in undergraduate examinations. Most chapters have a detailed example of a common OSCE station with helpful pointers.

 OSCE TIP **OSCE physical examination tips**

- Introduce yourself.
- Wash your hands or use alcohol wipes – if you do this outside the station, tell the examiner.
- Examiners may be told to say nothing to you – do not be put off.
- Don't forget to comment on growth: 'I would like to assess growth by measuring height and weight, plotting on a centile chart, and comparing to previous measurement plots if available.'
- Do **not** do anything to a child that could be painful, uncomfortable or embarrassing.
- If you do not do something (for any reason), state that it needs to be done (e.g. 'I would like to plot Billy on a growth chart'; 'I would normally check the blood pressure'; 'Would you like me to check the femoral pulses, only I do not want to embarrass Susan').
- If you do not do something, and you do not mention it, you will not get the marks for it!
- If you are having a bad OSCE station, stop, think, and then return to task. It is usually possible to recheck the instructions. You may explain to the examiner (e.g. I would have liked to start with gait, so I am going to do it now). Put the station behind you and remember each station is marked independently.
- When reporting your findings, include important negatives (e.g. no acute respiratory distress).

28.1.1.3 Data interpretation stations

Some undergraduate OSCEs also include stations where no examiner is present, with tasks such as interpretation of growth or laboratory data, and recognition and understanding of clinical photographs and radiology. These are essentially written paper-type questions, and are dealt with in the written paper section below.

 OSCE TIP **General OSCE preparation tips**

1. Spend plenty of time on the wards, in out-patients and in A&E, clerking in-patients and presenting them.
2. Practise and hone the skills that are likely to be tested in the OSCE format. OSCE examples are given throughout this book, and you can use these as a starting point for your practice. You can also use these to help you generate likely questions for other areas.
3. Make sure that you are able to take a problem-orientated paediatric history for common and important paediatric conditions.
4. Ensure you are proficient in the usual systems examinations, and that you can modify these according to age.
5. Practise child development assessment, and examination for squints.
6. For OSCE stations focused on a system examination, don't forget the 'HIGHCOST' approach (Chapter 3).
7. If you have access to a clinical skills lab, use it.
8. Ask teachers and peers to observe you taking histories and performing physical examinations and to give you constructive feedback. The only way you will convince an experienced examiner that you have performed a clinical skill many times before is to have performed it many times before!

28.1.2 Long case

This consists of a detailed history and examination of one patient (you might often have an hour unobserved to do this), followed by presentation of the 'case' to the examiners, who will then ask you questions about differential diagnosis, investigation and management. A shortened version may involve an observed history (15–20 minutes) followed by an abbreviated physical examination (for example, you may be asked to select the most appropriate system to examine).

> **? OSCE TIP Long case tips**
>
> - There is no substitute for clerking many patients and presenting them to teachers and colleagues.
> - The history-taking tips above all apply. Don't forget to ask about impact on the child and family.
> - 'Is there anything I have missed' is a reasonable question towards the end!
> - If the parent or child tells you the diagnosis early on, beware that you do not miss out questions that rule out other differentials.
> - Allow yourself at least 5 min at the end of the time you have been allotted with the patient and parent to gather your thoughts, construct a summary, list problems and a differential diagnosis, and consider an approach to investigation and management. This has the added advantage that if you have forgotten something important, you still have the chance to ask it.

28.1.3 Short cases

These are not commonly used in undergraduate examinations. You are taken by one or two examiners to see a series of children, and asked to examine them. Often there would be physical signs to elicit or abnormalities apparent on general inspection. At undergraduate level, the skills being tested in this format can be more appropriately assessed using an OSCE (see above).

28.2 Written examinations

> **Written question types**
>
> - Extended matching questions (for applied clinical knowledge)
> - Multiple choice questions (for factual knowledge)
> - Short answer questions
> - Clinical image questions
> - Essays.

28.2.1 How to do well in written exams

1. Get to grips with the knowledge base by knowing the contents of this book (or one like it).
2. Make sure that you have covered the ground in your core curriculum.
3. Spend time on the wards, in clinics and A&E, and learn from clinical experience.
4. Read questions carefully (they are not meant to trick you), and follow basic technique rules when answering questions.
5. Practise example questions provided by your course, and from other sources. Commit yourself to answers on paper, and take a break before reviewing the correct answers and any available discussion. Read up any areas that you feel unsure about.

28.2.2 Extended matching questions

There are few published EMQ practice questions, and in general students find them harder than multiple choice questions (MCQs). We have included samples towards the end of this book, which we hope will help in your preparation. In general, EMQs are about testing *applied* knowledge in real clinical situations. Time spent on the wards, in clinics and in the A&E department will help you do well in this exam format. Make it your habit to read about the clinical problems that you

> **? OSCE TIP Short case tips**
>
> - The physical examination tips above apply. As always, be kind, thoughtful, and child-friendly in your approach.
> - Although you are asked to examine a particular system, the initial stage of general inspection and looking for clues is particularly important, since this may give some context to any physical signs you find.
>
> - Comment on the obvious – this may be directly relevant to the underlying diagnosis.
> - Be clinically 'sensible' in trying to make sense of your findings: beware of starting with rarities, but work through broad categories of differentials, thinking what would be likely in real clinical practice.
> - Consider what would help you forward in making a diagnosis or management: particular questions (history); another system examination; investigations; symptom diary. This may well be the route further discussion will take.

see, in terms of both differential diagnosis of presenting symptoms (e.g. causes of wheeze) and specific illnesses. Whenever you have the opportunity, present your findings to supervising doctors, your tutors and your peers, and discuss differential diagnoses and management.

Example EMQ

(Theme): Causes of cough
(Option list):

A Asthma
B Bronchiolitis
C Croup
D Cystic fibrosis
E Habit
F Normal
G Pneumonia
H Upper respiratory tract infection
I Whooping cough (pertussis).

(Lead-in): For the following children presenting with cough, select the most likely diagnosis from the list above:
(Stems):

1. A 2-year-old boy is seen in clinic with chronic cough which he has had since a few months of age. It has been worse since his admission 2 months ago with his third episode of pneumonia. On examination, he appears thin, and his weight is on the 0.4th centile, compared with the 25th centile 1 year ago. He is afebrile and there is no respiratory distress. He has crepitations in the right lower zone.

2. A 4-year-old girl is brought for review because she coughs frequently, especially at night, and this is bad enough to wake her. During these episodes she often seems short of breath and her breathing is noisy. She has mild eczema. On examination, she appears well, her growth is good, and her chest is clear.

3. A 6-month-old boy with a noisy cough for 3 days is increasingly short of breath. He is hardly taking any of his feeds. He had a bad cough 6 weeks ago when he had a runny nose. On examination, he is well grown, but displays intercostal recession and a respiratory rate of 50 per minute. He has wheezes audible on auscultation throughout the chest. There are also a few inspiratory crepitations.
   Correct answers are given at the end of the chapter. See the respiratory chapter for help with this question (Chapter 19).

The *options* are based around a particular *theme*, which can be diagnoses, investigations and treatments. Options are usually presented in alphabetical order, and there may be 16 or more listed. There will then be a *lead-in* statement which will usually ask you to select the most likely diagnosis or option for each patient or clinical scenario. A number of *stems* will follow, describing patients who present with the problem given in the theme. Question banks will often contain stems that correspond to each option in the option list, although when the question is featured in an exam, only a small number of the stems may be presented. The description given in the stem should be such that if you have gained reasonable clinical experience of that problem, you will be able to state the correct answer *without looking at the option list*.

EMQ tips

1. Read the theme, lead-in and first stem, but not the option list initially.
2. Imagine yourself in the clinical situation given, for example seeing a child on the ward, in outpatients or in A&E, and try and decide what the most likely answer would be in that setting.
3. Now look at the option list and see if your answer features there.
4. Check the other options to see if any others would be a reasonable alternative answer and if so decide which of these is the most likely.
5. If you cannot come up with the answer without looking at the option list, then work through them and see if you can work out the correct option by a process of exclusion.
6. You may notice that several of the options could not apply.

28.2.3 Multiple choice questions

This has been a common question format for years, and there are many sources of example questions. MCQs test your factual knowledge over a broad area in a short space of time. A number of tips can allow you to benefit from flaws in question writing. However, increasingly, such flaws are recognized by question reviewers and will be edited out before the question gets to you. Then you have to depend on your factual knowledge, which is how it should be. Don't forget to read questions carefully and avoid jumping to conclusions.

MCQ tips

• Responses that state the something 'never' occurs or 'always' occurs are unlikely to be correct.
• Responses that don't follow grammatically from the stem are more likely to be incorrect.
• Options that are significantly longer than the rest are more likely to be correct.
• Options that repeat words from the stem are more likely to be correct.

28.2.4 Clinical image questions

These may be questions based on pictures projected as slides or printed in a question book. The questions may be in short answer format or you may be asked to select the best option from many, particularly for computer-marked exams. Where there are follow-on questions, there may well be clues to the answers of previous questions. Therefore, it is worth reading the whole question set before committing yourself on paper. This sort of question type has often been a feature of paediatric OSCE examinations where you may be presented with a piece of equipment, a picture of a patient or an X-ray and asked to answer questions about it. Most such questions can be converted into a written paper, computer-marked format.

> **Clinical image tips**
> - Being regularly around clinical areas will help you in your preparation for such papers.
> - Make sure you are familiar with all common pieces of equipment and other items used in the care of children that you might see on the wards or in out-patients (see Figure 5.2).
> - Look through paediatric atlases, focusing particularly on common and important problems that manifest in a way that can be photographed.

28.2.5 Short answer questions and data interpretation

In this question format, you may be presented with some data (e.g. a set of results, or a pedigree), or a clinical image with some background clinical information. You are then asked a series of questions to which there are succinct answers, for example 'What

> **Short answer tips**
> 1. If three options are asked for, give exactly three, and never more.
> 2. Keep your answers precise and clear.
> 3. Imagine yourself dealing with the real clinical problem in out-patients or A&E.
> 4. Make a list of the various categories that can cause disease (sometimes called a 'surgical sieve' – see box below). Go through each category and decide whether it could contain an explanation to the problem.
> 5. Look carefully at *all* the clinical information you have (including later questions).
> 6. Look for a single diagnosis that will explain all the features.

> **PRACTICE POINT A 'sieve' for aetiology**
>
> **Vitamin CDEFG**
> | | |
> |---|---|
> | **V** | Vascular |
> | **I** | Inflammatory/infective |
> | **T** | Traumatic |
> | **A** | Autoimmune |
> | **M** | Metabolic/metastatic |
> | **I** | Iatrogenic/idiopathic |
> | **N** | Neoplastic |
> | **C** | Congenital |
> | **D** | Dysplastic |
> | **E** | Endocrine |
> | **F** | Functional/psychosomatic |
> | **G** | Genetic. |

is the most likely diagnosis?', or 'Suggest the three most appropriate next investigations'. Again, take time to read the whole question. If you think you know the answers, be as precise as you can (e.g. '*left upper lobe* pneumonia', not just 'pneumonia').

28.2.6 Essays

These are an unusual feature of undergraduate examination in paediatrics, because marking is less objective and more time consuming. Some courses use 'modified-essay' questions, for example where you are asked to write short notes on a topic in 15 min. These are good for testing your approach to complex but important clinical situations, for example 'Describe key aspects of the management of the a child with diabetic ketoacidosis'. They can also be used to test areas that do not lend themselves to testing in computer-marked formats, for example 'Describe the potential ill-effects of admitting a 3-year-old child to hospital for a 3-day course of intravenous antibiotics for a urine infection, and how these may be minimized'. Those marking your responses are likely to have a pre-prepared scheme with key points for which they will award marks. It is well worth jotting down as many key points as you can before you start formally answering the question. Vague answers that keep repeating the same points will not do well.

 # Summary

Paediatrics is a clinical subject, and to do well in examinations you need to do plenty of clinical practice. You need a basic grounding of factual knowledge, which you will find in a textbook such as this one, but you need to take every opportunity to put that knowledge into practice in real clinical situations. Once you have become proficient in all the basic paediatric clinical skills through frequent practice, you are likely to improve your examination outcomes further through attention to technique, and practice that is specifically targeted at the exam format used in your undergraduate course.

Answer to EMQ example earlier in this chapter: 1D, 2A, 3B

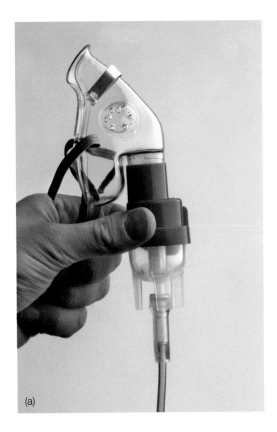

(a)

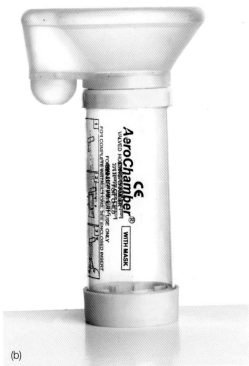

(b)

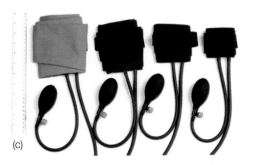

(c)

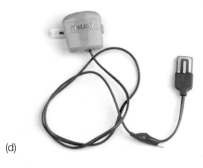

(d)

Figure 28.2 Identify the objects a–i in Figure 28.2 (answers at the end of this chapter in OSCE station 28.1).

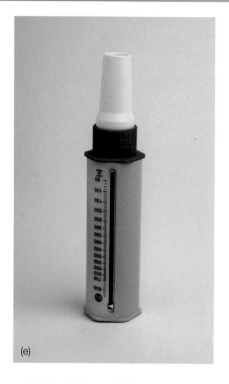

(e)

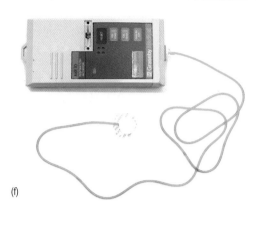

(f)

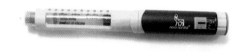

(g)

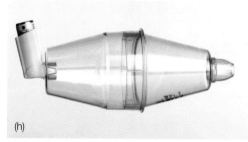

(h)

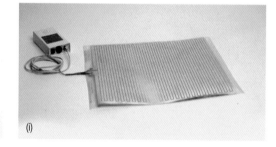

(i)

Figure 28.2 *Continued*

OSCE station 28.1: Equipment

You may be shown equipment commonly used in paediatric practice. Some examples are given in Figure 28.2. You should be able to recognize them and know how they are used. Answers are given below!

a Nebulizer
b Aerochamber (Chapter 19)
c Blood pressure cuffs of different sizes (Chapter 3)
d Body-worn enuresis alarm (Chapter 11)
e Peak flow meter (Chapter 19)
f Apnoea alarm (Chapter 15)
g Insulin pen (Chapter 27)
h Spacer device with aerosol (Chapter 19)
i Pad and buzzer enuresis alarm (Chapter 11)

29

Safe prescribing

Chapter map

The next time you work on paediatric wards after your medical student placement may be as a foundation doctor or specialty trainee with responsibility to prescribe. This brief chapter is to remind you that prescribing for children has special challenges and risks. Take an interest in prescribing while you are doing paediatrics – it will help you when you come to do it for real.

Prescription errors are important and avoidable. Error rates vary from 1 to 10%, they are greater in children's wards and intensive care units, and up to a third involve drug dose. A similar proportion have the potential to harm.

 No-one should prescribe for babies or children without training.

In children, the most difficult decision is deciding which drug to give when. This is beyond the scope of this book and is a skill learned in training in practice.

Prescriptions should be clearly written and include your name and contact details. The child's details must include age, date of birth and current weight (kg). Complete the drug allergies and adverse reactions box. You should know if the child is on any other medication. In the newborn or breastfeeding infant, you should be aware of the drugs mother is on, or has received recently.

Generic drug names should usually be used. Make numbers clear and legible, avoiding decimal points if possible (e.g. write 500 micrograms instead of 0.5 mg). 'g', 'mg', and 'mL' are used but other units should be written out in full. Be clear which formulation to use, and how it is to be given (oral, IV, IM, SC, etc). Often the duration or number of doses should be recorded and this is important for antimicrobials.

Liquids, suspensions and syrup preparations vary in strength. The medication should usually be prescribed in mg, and the recommended strength noted.

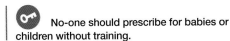 **TREATMENT Prescribing for children is different:**

- Drug choice will vary with:
  - disease
  - maturity
  - pharmacology
- Dose calculated on one of:
  - age
  - weight
  - surface area
- Administration must suit child, e.g.:
  - oral versus IV
  - inhaler versus nebuilizer
  - tablet versus syrup.

> β_2 agonists like salbutamol often do not work below 18 months of age and may even make wheeze worse.

> The fit young person of 14 years needs a different dose from the preterm infant of 500g birthweight.

> Teaching a child to take tablets saves money, teeth and time, and helps them take their dose at school.

Paediatrics Lecture Notes, Ninth edition. Simon J. Newell and Jonathan C. Darling. © 2014 John Wiley & Sons, Ltd. Published 2014 by John Wiley & Sons, Ltd.

PRACTICE POINT

A 5-year-old boy, who weighs 20 kg is admitted. He takes sodium valproate 300 mg bd.

He should be prescibed his dose of 300 mg, specifying the strength of his medication (200 mg/5 mL).

It is good practice to also note the volume of his dose (7.5 mL).

Prescribing is a team event. If you are the presciber, welcome comments from parents and colleagues ranging from the convenience of the timing to 'that seems a big dose'. The check by the pharmacist has saved many potential errors.

The BNF for Children is indispensable. Find out if your unit has its own local prescibing policy. Make yourself familiar with the local prescription chart. Above all, if in doubt ask.

The Royal College of Paediatrics and Child Health offers a free guide to prescribing tool with tips and a scenario.

RESOURCE

- Paediatric Prescribing Tool: **www.rcpch .ac.uk/training-examinations-professional-development/examinations/assessment-tools/safe-prescribing-tool/p**
- See **www.bnf.org** for the British National Formulary (BNF) BNF for Children (BNFC).

OSCE station 29.1: Safe prescribing—otitis media and fever.

Amanda has had a febrile convulsion (see Chapter 17). She is unwell with severe otitis media (see Chapter 18). She is to have Amoxicillin and regular paracetamol.

Please write the prescription. Amanda has no allergies.

Amanda Hall	**Hospital number AA1234**	
DoB 10.10.08	**Age 4.5 years**	**Current weight 19.0 kg**

BNFC

Amoxicillin for otitis media	**By mouth**	**Formulation**
Child 1 month–18 years	40 mg/kg daily in 3 divided doses (max. 1.5 g daily in 3 divided doses)	Oral suspension 250 mg/5 mL
Paracetamol for fever	**By mouth**	
Child 4-6 years	240 mg every 4-6 hours (maximum 4 doses in 24 hours)	Oral suspension 120 mg/5 mL

Approach

- Make sure you know what medication you are giving and which child it is for.
- Take care to write legibly, and begin with the child's names and hospital number.
- Use the NHS number if you have it.
- All children should have current weight and age/date of birth.
- Use the BNF for Children provided to work out the dose and frequency
- Calculate the dose using the child's weight or age [calculator provided].
- Avoid decimals if you can (500 mg is better than 0.5 g)
- Units are written in full except 'g', 'mg' and 'mL'.
- Ensure route of administration is clear – oral, IV, IM., etc

Never forget:
- The right drug, the right patient, the right dose, and the right route
- Everyone should be able to read what you have written.
- Check with parents and young people, they know about their medications.
- Check with colleagues. Listen to advice. If in doubt, ask.

Look around for:
- BNF for Children
- Local drug policies and formularies
- Locally approved sites on web on intranet
- Your local prescription sheet or system

Special points

- Some drugs are calculated using surface area (use table in BNFC)
- Some doses differ by different routes of administration.
- Intrathecal medications are very dangerous, do not use without supervision.

(next page)

(continued)

The prescription should look like this. Try the calculations and see.
The 6 hourly paracetamol is adjusted to give the late dose at the same time as the amoxicillin.

Allergies and Adverse Drug Reactions – List the medicines or substances & the nature of the reaction (write NKDA if none)				First name	Surname			
It is mandatory to complete this section				Amanda	Hall			
Medicine / Substance		Reaction		Hospital No:			DOB:	
NKDA					AA1234		10.10.08	
				NHS No:				
Sign	Print NAME		Date	Date	Consultant		Ward	Hosp
Sue Harvey	SUE HARVEY		01.04.13	01.04.13	JONES		40	LGI
Allergy status unconfirmed Authority to administer medicines ceases after 24 hours.	Sign (Print NAME)		Time & Date	Date	Consultant		Ward	Hosp
Self Administration Level	Level	Date	Sign (and Print NAME)	Age(if<18)	Weight	Height	Surface Area	
				4.5 y	19.0 kg			

Drug (1)	Dose		1/04				
Amoxicillin	250mg	(6)	X				
Additional Instructions 250mg/5mL Review 5 days	Route oral	8					
		12					
Print Name & Contact SUE HARVEY bleep 6543	Date 01.04.13	(14)					
		18					
Sign Sue Harvey	Pharm	Supply (22)					

Drug (2)	Dose		X				
Paracetamol	240mg	(6)					
Additional Instructions 120mg/5mL for fever	Route oral	8					
		12					
Print Name & Contact SUE HARVEY bleep 6543	Date 01.04.13	(14)					
		(18)					
Sign Sue Harvey	Pharm	Supply (22)					

Careers in paediatrics

Chapter map

If you enjoy working with children and families, we hope you will consider a career in paediatrics and child health. There are many career options, from preventative, community and public health work, to work in acute tertiary specialty. Every area has its challenges and rewards, and the satisfaction of making a difference for children and their families.

30.1   Why consider paediatrics?

30.1.1   Early training jobs

Even if you're not sure you want to be a paediatrician, it's worth considering a foundation programme job, because this will stand you in good stead for the many career pathways that involve work with children. These include many surgical specialties (such as ENT, orthopaedics, plastics), primary care, emergency medicine and anaesthetics. You will be well supported and supervised in paediatric job, and will gain confidence and practical skills useful in other areas of medicine. It will allow you to test out whether the specialty is for you, and the experience gained will help you in interviews for paediatric training.

30.1.2   Career

A paediatric career is all about making a difference for children and their families. It is both rewarding and challenging whether dealing acutely with a child admitted with meningococcal sepsis, or working long-term in the community with the child with learning difficulties and epilepsy. Most paediatricians have a community and preventative perspective to their role, even if they are primarily hospital-based. Paediatric skills are particularly useful in developing countries, where the largest burden of childhood morbidity and mortality remains.

30.2   Is paediatrics for me?

Personal qualities which suit paediatrics
- Patience, sensitivity, emotional resilience
- Communication skills
- Team working
- Informality
- Sense of humour
- Flexible, opportunistic
- Committed to child health

Hopefully the experience of being part of paediatric services in hospital and the community will have given you insight into what the specialty involves, and whether you have the right personal qualities. It is

---

Paediatrics Lecture Notes, Ninth edition. Simon J. Newell and Jonathan C. Darling. © 2014 John Wiley & Sons, Ltd. Published 2014 by John Wiley & Sons, Ltd.

obviously important to enjoy working with children, and most jobs require a combination of flexibility and attention to detail.

30.3 Career options

Paediatrics is one of the few careers when you can still be a generalist. Most paediatricians have a special interest, and there is a huge range of subspecialties, which are usually based in tertiary centres.

Careers in paediatrics

- General paediatrician (district general or teaching hospital)
- Community paediatrician
- Neonatologist
- Subspecialty paediatrician
  - Cardiology
  - Child mental health
  - Clinical pharmacology and therapeutics
  - Diabetes and endocrinology
  - Emergency medicine
  - Gastroenterology, hepatology and nutrition
  - Haematology
  - Immunology, infectious disease (IID) and allergy
  - Inherited metabolic medicine
  - Intensive care
  - Nephrology
  - Neurodisability
  - Neurology
  - Oncology
  - Palliative medicine
  - Respiratory medicine
  - Rheumatology

30.4 Training and exams

In the UK, paediatric training is 'run-through', in that once you enter the program you will proceed through to completion of training, providing you pass the necessary exams. It currently lasts 8 years, and most enter straight after foundation. The Membership of the Royal College of Paediatrics and Child Health (MRCPCH) exam is usually completed within the first three years, and then trainees enter registrar

level training which will contain a mix of core areas (general community and neonates) and subspecialties, depending on final career destination. Towards the end of training, a detailed formal assessment provides feedback to trainees on their readiness for a consultant post.

30.5 Developing your interest

At medical school, look out for other options to develop and maintain your interest. These may include special projects, an elective or intercalated degree. Your medical school may have paediatric club or society and if not you may consider setting one up. Do take the chance to talk to paediatric consultants and trainees about the specialty. The Royal College of Paediatrics and Child Health provides careers advice on its website, runs its own career fair, supports careers events at medical schools, and offers free student membership. In addition, a number of prizes are available.

 RESOURCE

Go to **www.rcpch.ac.uk** and search for 'Careers', 'Medical students' or 'Prizes'. A summary of the Paediatric Training Pathway can be found at www.rcpch.ac.uk/system/files/protected/page/Paediatric%20Training%20Pathway.pdf

 Summary

Paediatrics is a great specialty, but don't just take our word for it – we hope you have found this out for yourself!

 FOR YOUR LOG

- Talk to consultants and trainees about careers in paediatrics
- Look at the RCPCH website careers section, and become a student member.

Extended matching questions

For each question, select the single most likely option, unless otherwise stated. Options may be used once, more than once or not at all.

Emergency paediatrics (Chapter 4)

EMQ 4.1 Management of emergencies

A. Abdominal X-ray
B. Antibiotics
C. Chest X-ray
D. Intravenous saline bolus
E. Intubation and mechanical ventilation
F. Lumbar puncture
G. Oral rehydration therapy
H. Oxygen by face mask
I. Paracetamol, oral
J. Stool culture

In each case, select the most important next step in immediate management:

1. Sian is an 8-month-old child admitted with bronchiolitis. She has had upper respiratory tract symptoms for 3 days and has become worse. She is moved to the ward, given facial oxygen, but keeps having episodes of apnoea and going blue. O/E she is quiet and at times agitated. Respiratory rate 10 bpm. Her circulation is good. Blood glucose 7.3 mmol/L.

2. Danny is 16 months old. He is brought to A&E by his distraught mother, who feared he was dying. He has had a 3 min seizure at home while he was watching TV with his sister. On arrival he appears flushed but is lively and alert. He has a temperature of 39.5 °C and an inflamed throat.

3. Anchelle is 7 months old. She has a 2-day history of diarrhoea and today she is vomiting all that she is given. Her mother is concerned that Anchelle is hardly responding to her. Anchelle's respiratory rate is 45 bpm, she is mottled, pulse 180 bpm and capillary refill time 5 s. She has cool hands and feet. Blood glucose 6.2 mmol/L.

EMQ 4.2 Basic life support

A. 15 chest compressions, 2 rescue breaths
B. 5 rescue breaths
C. Call for help
D. Check circulation
E. Ensure that you can approach child safely
F. Look, listen and feel for breathing
G. Open airway
H. Stimulate and see if responsive

A man rushes into the supermarket, saying that a 3-year-old child has collapsed outside. There is no reason to suspect trauma. In each sequence, choose the next action:

4. Outside you find the child on the pavement. Traffic has stopped and it is safe. Two people tell you that the ambulance is on its way. You are unable to elicit any response from the child. You turn her onto her back, and apply head tilt, chin lift.

5. Outside is a pedestrian precinct. The child is surrounded by a number of desperately worried shoppers. You approach the child who is not moving, and does not respond to stimulation.

6. Outside a little boy is lying in the car park. He is unresponsive. A man is sending cars away and it is safe. You can hear the ambulance on its way. The airway is open with head lift and chin tilt, you look, listen and feel and there is no breathing.

EMQ 4.3 Maintaining the airway

A. Back blows and abdominal thrusts
B. Chin lift, jaw thrust
C. Head tilt, chin lift
D. Mouth-to-mouth ventilation
E. Oral airway
F. Tracheal intubation and ventilation

In each of the following cases, select the most appropriate airway procedure. Assume all the equipment needed for each procedure is to hand:

7. A newborn infant needs resuscitation. He is given bag and mask ventilation, but his pulse remains <100 bpm, he is pale and not breathing.

8. A 2-year-old is admitted in status epilepticus. Fits are terminated with intravenous lorazepam. As the fits stop, the child makes some croaking sounds, his chest continues to move, but he is becoming blue.

9. On her 3rd birthday a child suddenly becomes distressed at her party, while playing a game with sweets. She runs to her mother looking terrified, and is clearly not breathing.

10. A 10-year-old boy is knocked off his bike at traffic lights. You see him go through the air and land on the road. When you get there he is not breathing.

Fetal medicine (Chapter 6)

EMQ 6.1 Fetal diagnoses

A. Down syndrome
B. Hydrops fetalis
C. Intrauterine growth restriction (IUGR)
D. Macrosomia (growth greater than 95th centile)
E. Tracheo-oesophageal fistula
F. Urethral valves

For each of the following, choose which fetal condition is most likely:

11. A woman has pregnancy-induced hypertension with proteinuria and oedema (pre-eclampsia). There is placental insufficiency, and ultrasound shows oligohydramnios (reduced amniotic liquor).

12. Fetal ultrasound shows reduced liquor and dilated urinary tract with a full bladder. The baby needs to be delivered in a centre which can provide surgery.

13. A woman is found to have polyhydramnios (excess liquor). Fetal growth is normal. At birth the infant is in good condition, but is bubbly and mucousy and needs oral suction twice.

14. A woman of 37 years is pregnant. Fetal ultrasound at 17 weeks shows thickening of the back of the neck (nuchal fold). The fetus appears otherwise normal.

15. A 28-year-old woman has gestational diabetes. Her diabetic control is less good in the third trimester and her fundal height (size of uterus) is large for dates.

16. In her third pregnancy a woman is found to have anti-Rhesus D antibodies in her blood. Fetal ultrasound shows ascites. Arrangements are made for fetal blood transfusion because the fetus has become anaemic.

Birth and the newborn infant (Chapter 7)

EMQ 7.1 Examination of the newborn

A. Cephalhaematoma
B. Erythema toxicum
C. Stork mark
D. Strawberry naevus
E. Subaponeurotic haemorrhage
F. Traumatic cyanosis

For each of the following, choose the most likely diagnosis:

17. At 2 days of age, a baby has a widespread red rash, which has appeared rapidly. Each spot has a yellow centre. Some of the spots present this morning are no longer visible.

18. A baby's mother is concerned about a red mark between her daughter's eyebrows. It is more visible when the baby cries and goes onto the upper eyelids.

19. A newborn baby has a swelling over the left side of his head. He appears generally well.

20. A 6-week-old infant had no birthmarks at birth. Mother has now noticed a bright red, pea-sized lump over the upper arm. It is getting bigger.

21. After ventouse vacuum delivery, this infant is found to be unwell at 8 h. She is pale, and quiet, with a raised respiratory rate. Her head feels boggy all over.

EMQ 7.2 Management of neonatal problems

A. Admit the baby to the neonatal unit
B. Reassure and arrange community or outpatient follow up
C. Reassure but arrange to review the infant next day
D. Reassure the mother, no action is needed
E. Refer to the surgeon

For each of the following choose the most appropriate management:

22. A 12-h-old baby is noted to have a full fontanelle when he cries. Otherwise he is well and the fontanelle feels normal when he is quiet.

23. A newborn baby boy has an abnormal foreskin, which is gathered round the dorsal surface of the glans.

24. A 4-h-old girl has a respiratory rate of 75/min and has a quiet expiratory grunt. Examination otherwise is entirely normal.

25. A 1-day-old girl has numerous small white spots over her nose.

26. At the routine examination, you notice that a baby's head circumference is 1 cm over the 99.8th centile.

Disorders of the newborn (Chapter 8)

EMQ 8.1 Definitions used in neonatal medicine

A. Appropriate weight for gestational age
B. Large for gestational age
C. Low birth weight
D. Postmature
E. Preterm
F. Small for gestational age
G. Term
H. Very low birth weight

Classify each of the following using one or more of the definitions above. You will need to use the growth chart (Chapter 8, Figure 8.1). **More than one of the terms above may apply to each infant.**

27. An infant born at 34 weeks gestation with a weight of 1.6 kg.

28. An infant born at 41 weeks gestation with a weight of 3.7 kg.

29. An infant born at 29 weeks gestation with a weight of 1.2 kg.

EMQ 8.2 Respiratory problems in the newborn

A. Congenital diaphragmatic hernia
B. Congenital heart malformation
C. Group B streptococcal pneumonia
D. Meconium aspiration syndrome
E. Pneumothorax
F. Respiratory distress syndrome
G. Transient tachypnoea of the newborn

For each of the following, choose the most likely diagnosis:

30. Peter is 1.9 kg at 31 weeks gestation. He is tachypnoeic at 2 h of age, needing 40% oxygen to maintain good oxygen saturation.

31. Catherine was born at term, 28 h after rupture of membranes. She appeared well, but now at 6 h the midwife notes a raised respiratory rate, and Catherine is not interested in feeding.

32. Lawrence was delivered by elective caesarean section at 39 weeks. He was tachypnoeic 20 min after delivery, but on review 25 min later he has less respiratory distress.

33. Simon is born at term. He has respiratory distress with cyanosis from birth. Air entry is difficult to hear on the left side and his abdomen is very flat. He becomes pink with oxygen.

EMQ 8.3 Neonatal problems

A. Preterm infant, appropriate for gestational age
B. Small for gestational age infant born at term
C. Term infant after intrapartum asphyxia
D. Term infant of a mother with diabetes
E. Term infant who is small for gestational age

Which infant or infants are most likely to have the following problems (more than one option may be appropriate)?

34. At 7 h, this infant is increasingly jittery. She is pale, sweaty and floppy, and will not feed.

35. At 6 h, this infant begins to have fits and appears floppy and unresponsive.

36. This infant's mother was unwell in the first trimester. At term after birth, he is noted to have cataracts and microcephaly.

37. This infant has a birthweight of 1.3 kg, and after 7 days of intensive care for respiratory distress syndrome, the baby deteriorates. A loud systolic murmur is heard and her pulses are bounding.

EMQ 8.4 Management of neonatal jaundice

A. Double phototherapy and prepare for exchange transfusion
B. Investigate for biliary atresia
C. Phototherapy and repeat bilirubin
D. Reassure parents and observe

For each infant, choose the most appropriate management:

38. James is 3 days old and has visible jaundice; he appears well. His bilirubin level is above the line for phototherapy on the chart.

39. Billy is 12 days old, appears healthy and is breast feeding well. He is still jaundiced. His stools are normal.

40. At 4 h, Sally is jaundiced. Her mother had raised anti-D antibody levels. Sally's haemoglobin is 8 g/dL and her bilirubin is high.

41. Marie is 18 days old, and she is still jaundiced. She appears well, taking regular formula feeds. Her stools are pale off-white.

Child development and how to assess it (Chapter 9)

EMQ 9.1 Types of developmental delay

A. Normal
B. Gross motor delay
C. Fine motor delay
D. Language delay
E. Gross motor and fine motor delay
F. Gross motor and language delay
G. Fine motor and language delay
H. Global delay

For each child, select the most appropriate description.

42. A 20-month-old boy is cruising round furniture but not yet taking any steps. He can pull to stand, and has been sitting on his own since about age 12 months. He has about 20 clear words, and some two-word sentences. He understands simple commands and his parents have no concerns about his hearing. He can scribble with a crayon, but cannot copy a line. He can build a tower of four cubes.

43. A 4-year-old walked at age 19 months, and falls often when he tries to run. He cannot kick a ball, ride a trike or jump. He can copy a line, but not a circle or a cross. He cannot copy a three-brick 'gate' or six-brick 'steps', but can copy a four-brick 'train'. He knows about 300 words, and speaks in sentences of 5–10 words.

44. A 9-month-old girl sat unaided at 8 months, and is now pulling to stand and cruising round furniture. She is not taking any steps on her own, but crawls on all fours. She reaches out for objects, which she grasps with a mature palmar grasp and transfers from hand to hand. She uses a pincer grip to pick up a sultana. She babbles constantly but has no clear words.

45. A 6-month-old boy has head lag when pulled to sit, and when held sitting has curved spine and little head control. When placed prone, he lifts his head (but not his chest) briefly, and does not attempt to roll over or crawl. He does not reach out for objects, although he fixes and follows them with his eyes. He cries when hungry, and makes occasional 'ooh' sounds. He smiles, but not in response to his parents' smiles.

EMQ 9.2 Causes of developmental delay 1

A. Cerebral palsy
B. Chronic illness
C. Deafness

D. Down syndrome
E. Fragile X
F. Hypothyroidism
G. Neglect
H. Phenylketonuria (PKU)
I. Prematurity
J. Tuberous sclerosis

For each of these children, select the most likely cause of their developmental delay:

46. A 2-year-old girl who is the first of triplets attends a hospital clinic for review of previous laser treatment. She wears glasses, and from above her head appears long and narrow from front to back.

47. A 3-year-old boy particularly enjoys the music and singing at his nursery, and is an affectionate child. On examination, he has a sternotomy scar that is well healed, the back of his head is rather flat, and he is small for his age. He is hypotonic, and has an unusual face.

48. A 12-month-old girl's parents are taking legal action because a routine blood spot sample was mislaid by the laboratory, and so her condition was not diagnosed until late. She takes a normal diet, and is on a single medication, which she takes daily. She has global delay.

49. A baby girl is admitted acutely at 8 months of age with irritability and fever, and is treated for 7 days with intravenous cefotaxime. Several family members receive rifampicin. She makes a good recovery. Two months later she has a test that was arranged at the time of discharge. Her parents are disappointed but not surprised that it is abnormal.

Learning problems (Chapter 10)

EMQ 10.1 Conditions associated with developmental delay

A. Cerebral palsy
B. Congenital viral infection
C. Down syndrome
D. Emotional neglect
E. Fragile X syndrome
F. Hypothyroidism
G. Idiopathic global developmental delay
H. Tuberous sclerosis

For each of the children, choose the most likely condition:

50. Mark is 9 years old. His teacher notes his difficulty learning to express himself and with reading. He has a number of learning problems. His face is unusual with a prominent jaw and big forehead. His motor function is good.

51. Gary is 8 years old. Age 4 months he had infantile spasms. He now has complex partial seizures. He has moderately severe learning problems. On examination he has a number of pale elliptic patches of skin on his trunk and limbs. He has abnormal finger nails.

52. Sophie is just 6 h old. She has been well since delivery, but she is very floppy and her mother thinks her face looks unusual. She has short fingers and single palmar creases.

53. Susie is 2 years old. She sat unaided at 13 months and walked at 22 months. She walks on tiptoe with her knees and hips flexed. Tone and reflexes in her lower limbs are increased. Otherwise her development and neurology are normal.

Nutrition (Chapter 12)

EMQ 12.1 Management of nutritional problems

A. Admit to hospital and observe weight gain
B. Give an iron supplement, check diet and follow up
C. High-energy, high-fat diet with variety of other foods
D. Reassure and explain that there is nothing to worry about
E. Reduce energy intake by cutting down on fatty and high-energy foods while eating a wide variety of foods

For each of the following choose the most appropriate management:

54. A baby born at term weighed 2.8 kg (2nd centile) but appeared well. At 9 months he remains on the 2nd centile for weight and 2nd–10th centile for length. His parents are convinced that he is well. His development is normal.

55. Jason is 2 years old. He presented with chest infections, diarrhoea and offensive stools. A sweat test is abnormal, and he is homozygous for DF508. His chest is now better but his weight is on the 2nd centile, height 10th–25th centile.

56. At 17 months of age, Anjali is pale but growing normally along the 50th–75th centile. Haemoglobin is 10.2 g/dL (reference >11 g/dL) with a hypochromic microcytic picture.

EMQ 12.2 Nutritional advice

A. Add thickeners to the milk
B. Advise against breast feeding
C. Advise that breast feeding is the best option
D. Prescribe a cow's milk-free formula
E. Stop milk and give glucose electrolyte solution (e.g. Dioralyte)

For each of the following, choose the most appropriate advice:

57. Mrs Phillips has her second child. The first was bottle fed and has cow's milk allergy with some eczema.

58. Ms Johnson is soon to deliver. She is receiving treatment for HIV.

59. Mrs Passoudi is breast feeding her 2-month-old son, adding one feed of artificial formula each day. He has diarrhoea but is well.

60. Ms Williams has a 5-month-old with a 2-day history of diarrhoea with occasional vomiting. The baby is not clinically dehydrated and does not appear ill.

EMQ 12.3 Causes of failure to thrive 1

A. Chronic disease
B. Inadequate intake
C. Malabsorption
D. Nutritional or emotional deprivation
E. Vomiting

For each of the following children, choose the most likely explanation:

61. Sian is 8 months old. She has mild cerebral palsy. Feeding takes a long time, and she is not keen on solids.

62. McKenzie is 10 months old. There is concern about her growth. She gains weight well for the first time while she is staying with her aunt. Her mother is in hospital after preterm delivery of her sibling.

63. Mustafa is 9 months old. His weight has fallen from the 50th to the 2nd centile. He eats very well, and is fully weaned. He has offensive diarrhoea.

Abnormal growth and sex development (Chapter 13)

EMQ 13.1 Causes of failure to thrive 2

A. Coeliac disease
B. Cystic fibrosis
C. Emotional and nutritional neglect
D. Gastro-oesophageal reflux
E. Heart failure
F. Inadequate intake of calories and protein
G. Normal small child
H. Pyloric stenosis

In each of the following cases, choose the most likely cause of growth failure:

64. Alice was born at term weighing 2.3 kg. This was her mother's fourth pregnancy, and was uneventful. She is now 18 weeks of age and her mother says she is well. Her weight is increasing just below and parallel to the 2nd centile.

65. Hannah age 25 months has fallen across the weight centiles from the 50th to the 2nd in the last 9 months. Her grandmother tells you that Hannah had begun to talk, but now she is less confident, and still only has a few words. She has no other symptoms. On examination, she is thin, and unhappy, but there are no other abnormal findings.

66. Sam is 13 weeks of age. Born on the 90th centile he is now on the 25th. His parents tell you he is generally well, he smiles and is attentive. He is bottle feeding, appears hungry, but then only takes about 2 fl oz (50 mL), before he stops feeding. After a feed, he breathes quickly and is sweaty. He is not vomiting, and has no diarrhoea.

EMQ 13.2   Causes of short stature

A. Achondroplasia
B. Chronic renal failure
C. Constitutional
D. Hypothryoidism
E. Normal delayed puberty
F. Normal early puberty
G. Turner syndrome

For each child, select the most likely cause:

67. Neil is 13 years of age. He has always played in the school football team. Now his family are worried that he is not as tall as his peers. He is well and examination is normal. He has no evidence of pubertal development.

68. Manuella is 12 years of age. She thinks she is not growing and her height now is the same as it was when she started secondary school 15 months earlier. She is otherwise well, although she tends to be tired. Her periods, which began at 10.5 years, have become irregular. She has normal pubertal development.

69. Robbie is 15 years of age. His growth chart from school shows that he was on the 97th centile at 11 years, but that since he has fallen to the 50th. He first developed some pubic hair at the age of 10. He is concerned that he is not as tall as he would like to be.

On examination he has stage 4 pubic hair and penile development. He occasionally has to shave.

70. Eniola is 14 years of age. Her height is just below the 0.4th centile, and weight is appropriate for height. She is generally well. She has had no periods. On examination she has some stage 2 breast development, and a fold of skin on each side of her neck down onto her shoulders.

Immunization and infections (Chapter 14)

EMQ 14.1   Valid and invalid contraindications to immunization

A. No contraindication
B. Acute illness
C. Depressed immunity
D. Eczema
E. Egg allergy
F. Family history of egg allergy
G. Hypersensitivity to antibiotics
H. Major reaction to previous vaccine
I. Mild reaction to previous vaccine
J. Minor infection without fever
K. Previous seizures
L. Risk to other family member
M. Too old for this immunization

For the following scenarios, select the option that best describes whether there is any valid contraindication to immunization and its nature:

71. A 4-month-old baby is brought for his third set of primary immunizations. After the last set, he had a temperature of 37.8 °C and was irritable for a few hours. One of the injection sites had some redness the size of a 10 pence piece. Today he has a cough and runny nose, but is quite well and not febrile.

72. A 4-year-old boy has arrived from overseas, and has never been immunized. He is brought for the first primary set of immunizations. He has had two febrile convulsions in the past. His development is normal for age. He had a 3-day course of oral prednisolone for asthma 2 weeks ago and is on low-dose inhaled steroids. He gets a rash when given penicillin.

73. A 3-month-old baby is due to have a second set of primary immunizations at the GP surgery. After the first set she had a fever of 39.5 °C for about 12 h, with a prolonged high-pitched cry, and the whole of the right thigh was swollen and red. She has been fine since. Her sister is strongly allergic to egg. Today she has a cough and runny nose, but is quite well and not febrile.

74. A 2-year-old is brought for his first MMR immunization. His mother is worried because he is allergic to egg and has eczema. He gets coughs and colds frequently, at least once a month, and she feels there is something wrong with his immunity. He had a low-grade fever after his last immunizations.

Accidents and non-accidents (Chapter 15)

EMQ 15.1 Likelihood of injury being non-accidental

A. Almost certainly NAI
B. Very likely to be NAI
C. 50/50 NAI or accidental
D. Likely to be accidental, but consider NAI
E. Almost certainly accidental

Select the best description for the likelihood of NAI, based on the information available:

75. A 3-month-old is admitted with six bruises on the ribs, all between 0.5 and 1.0 cm in size. There is no history of any injury. A skeletal survey shows three rib fractures of different ages (two of which correspond with the bruises). There are three retinal haemorrhages on examination of the fundi. The CT head scan shows a subdural haemorrhage on the right.

76. A 2-year-old is brought to A&E having ingested two mouthfuls of white spirit, which her father had put in a lemonade bottle while painting a bedroom. The parents are upset and anxious, but the child is well. Growth is normal, examination is normal.

77. A 6-month-old baby boy is brought to A&E with a 5 cm swelling over the right parietal region. There is a 5 cm skull fracture. His bouncy chair toppled off the table onto a laminate floor 45 min earlier. He is well grown, and there are no other findings on examination. He is now well.

Neurology (Chapter 17)

EMQ 17.1 Headache

A. Acute otitis media
B. Dental abscess
C. Eye strain
D. Hypertension
E. Meningitis

F. Migraine
G. Sinusitis
H. Space-occupying lesion
I. Stress headache

For the following children, select the most likely cause of their headache:

78. Matthew, age 12, presents to out-patients with a 6-month history of right-sided, frontal, throbbing headaches which last 12–24 h, and are associated with nausea and photophobia. They are made worse by movement and noise, and are sometimes helped by paracetamol and lying in a darkened room. BP is 105/65. Examination is normal.

79. Kylie, age 7, has been absent from school for more than half the time this term with headaches and abdominal pains. The headaches are 'all over' the head, 'like a constant ache', and she has had them for a year. The abdominal pains are central. She has been bullied at school over the last few months. BP is 80/50. Examination is normal.

80. Henry, age 9, has a 5-week history of increasingly severe headaches, which are right-sided and present on waking most mornings. He complains of double vision, and had vomited five times in the last week. BP is 95/63. Examination is normal except that the margin of his right optic disc is indistinct.

EMQ 17.2 Fits and 'funny dos'

A. Complex partial seizures (temporal lobe epilepsy)
B. Faint (syncope)
C. Febrile convulsions
D. Infantile spasm
E. Normal myoclonus (physiological myoclonus)
F. Simple absences (petit mal)
G. Symptomatic epilepsy secondary to meningitis
H. Tonic clonic (grand mal)

81. The mother of a 4-month-old tells you that her baby keeps jerking in her arms. The infant tenses up suddenly bringing his head forward. This happens several times in a few minutes. He then cries and goes back to sleep.

82. A 4-year-old girl's father has noted odd movements sometimes when he is reading to her at bedtime. At times, as she falls asleep, she has sudden violent movements of her legs and sometimes her arms. Her colour does not change. The episode lasts a few seconds and then his daughter sleeps normally.

83. A 2-month-old child has become gradually less well, is not feeding and has been irritable. He has a high temperature and presents after a short fit involving all four limbs; 45 min later he is pale, and lethargic. His fontanelle is bulging.

84. An 8-year-old boy collapses at the school concert while he is standing quietly with his friends in the choir. He was pale and said he felt sick and dizzy. He slowly recovered when placed in the recovery position by his teacher. One hour later in A&E, he looks well.

85. A 6-year-old girl attends the clinic with a history of about 12 episodes over the last 5 months that have concerned her parents. On each occasion she appears agitated, then vacant. After up to 3 min, she twitches in her left arm and does not seem to know she is doing it. Afterwards she cries a little and has a mild headache; 30–60 min later she appears well.

EMQ 17.3 Difficulty walking

A. Acute post-infectious polyneuropathy (Guillain–Barré)
B. Congenital dislocation of the hip
C. Duchenne muscular dystrophy
D. Global developmental delay
E. Normal late walking
F. Perthe diease
G. Spastic cerebral palsy

For each of the following choose the most likely diagnosis from the list:

86. A two-and-a-half-year-old boy is having difficulty walking. He was cruising at 13 months and beginning to walk at 16 months. Now his parents think he is less strong, and is no longer able to get up the stairs. You notice he is able to walk if helped onto his feet, but waddles with a lumbar lordosis.

87. A 7-year-old boy was previously healthy. He now attends with a severe left-sided limp and pain when he tries to bear weight on his left leg. His leg looks normal but neurological examination is difficult.

88. A 22-month-old girl is not walking. In her development of posture and movement she sat up unsupported at 7 months and crawled at 11 months. She will weight bear on her legs, but when left prefers to get about by shuffling on her bottom. Her muscle tone and reflexes seem normal. Her father first walked at 18–20 months.

89. A 22-month-old girl is not walking. In her development of posture and movement she sat up unsupported at 13 months and will now crawl, but tends to drag her legs behind her. She gets about by rolling over. At rest, her legs are extended and crossed over. If helped, she will bear weight on her tip toes but will not stand

90. A 12-year-old boy develops pain in his legs, 2 weeks after an episode of 'flu'. The pain is followed by weakness and now he cannot walk well. He is able to sit up. He has also noticed tingling and abnormal sensation in his feet. He appears generally well, but his legs are weak, muscle tone is reduced and you cannot elicit leg tendon reflexes.

EMQ 17.4 Lumbar puncture results

All the following children had neck stiffness and a lumbar puncture (LP). For each one, blood glucose was 5.6 mmol/L. Results of culture are awaited. For each of the scenarios, choose the most likely LP result from the table below.

91. An Asian boy of 11 years presents with 8 weeks of being tired and losing weight. Headache has been present for 2 weeks, and now he has had two fits and remains drowsy. His grandmother is receiving treatment for tuberculosis.

92. An 18-month-old has a fit associated with fever. He is a little sleepy afterwards and febrile, but examination is normal. It is difficult to hold him during the LP and he jumps as the needle is inserted.

93. A 5-year-old girl is rushed in. She had become very ill during the day, and her mother noticed a non-blanching red/purple rash. She is quiet, pale and very unwell. The rash has spread since she left home.

94. A 4-year-old girl has a 2-day history of sore throat and fever. She has tonsillitis on examination. She is otherwise alert and responsive.

EMQ 17.5 Causes of developmental delay 2

A. Congenital sensorineural deafness
B. Down syndrome
C. Emotional and physical neglect
D. Spastic diplegia with mild learning problems
E. Spastic quadriplegia with severe learning difficulties

For each clinical scenario, choose the most likely diagnosis:

95. A 20-month-old boy is not able to walk well. He can use 2–3 words and appears miserable when you talk to him. Growth: weight 0.4–2nd centile; height 10th–25th centile; head circumference 25th centile. After a week on the ward he is much more cheerful, talking more and beginning to walk.

96. A 2-year-old suffered severe birth asphyxia. He now shows little progress in development since birth although he smiles occasionally and has some head control. His limbs are stiff with brisk reflexes in arms and legs.

97. A 15-month-old child has little language development. He walks well, and is able to use a pencil to scribble. His parents have difficulty in getting him to respond and he has never developed babbling or speech.

98. A 4-year-old child was born at 26 weeks gestation. He had intensive care for 5 weeks. He is soon to go to school. He tends to be unsteady and trips easily. There is increased tone in his legs. He has good fine motor function in his hands.

Ear, nose and throat (Chapter 18)

EMQ 18.1   **ENT problems**

A. Congenital stridor
B. Croup
C. Epiglottitis
D. Foreign body
E. Infectious mononucleosis
F. Obstructive sleep apnoea
G. Quinsy
H. Streptococcal tonsillitis

For each of the following children, choose the most likely diagnosis:

99. Georgia, a 3-year-old, at a wedding party suddenly appears distressed, is making no noise and becoming cyanosed.

100. Mark is 14 years old, and has been unwell for 2 weeks. He is very tired and has marked lymphadenopathy. His tonsils are entirely coated in a thick white discharge.

101. Rosie is 3 years old and presents at 2 a.m. with noisy breathing in inspiration, distress and not feeding. She is relaxed and quiet on her father's knee, but the noise returns when you try and examine her.

102. Nick is 7 years old. He had a sore throat that got better a week ago. Now it has come back and he is ill and febrile. His left tonsil is pushed towards his uvula, and his left neck is tender.

Respiratory medicine (Chapter 19)

EMQ 19.1   **Causes of cough**

A. Asthma
B. Bronchiolitis
C. Croup
D. Cystic fibrosis
E. Habit
F. Normal
G. Pneumonia
H. Upper respiratory tract infection
I. Whooping cough (pertussis)

For each of the following children, select the most likely cause of the cough:

103. A 2-year-old boy has had a chronic cough since a few months of age. It has been worse since his admission 2 months ago with his third episode of pneumonia. On examination, he appears thin, and his weight is on the 0.4th centile, compared with the 25th centile 1 year ago. He is afebrile and there is no respiratory distress. He has crepitations in the right lower zone.

104. A 4-year-old girl is brought for review because she coughs frequently, especially at night, and this is bad enough to wake her. During these episodes she often seems short of breath and her breathing is noisy. She has mild eczema. On examination, she appears well, her growth is good and her chest is clear.

	Cells × 10⁶/L	Cell differential	Protein g/L	Glucose mmol/L	Microscopy
Normal	<5		0.2–0.4	3–6	
A	<5	all lymphocytes	0.2	4.7	Nil
B	80	80% lymphocytes	0.6	5.1	Gram stain negative
C	650	90% lymphocytes	2.5	1.9	Gram stain negative
D	1200	90% neutrophils	2.7	2.1	Gram neg diplococci
E	Heavily blood-stained specimen. Microscopy and biochemistry not possible. Second specimen less heavily blood stained than first.				

105. A 6-month-old boy presents in winter with a noisy and unpleasant cough for 3 days, and increasing shortness of breath. He is hardly taking feeds. He is well grown, but has intercostal recession, respiratory rate of 50/min, and wheezes and inspiratory crepitations throughout the lung fields.

EMQ 19.2 Abnormal or noisy breathing

A. Apnoea
B. Asthma
C. Bronchiolitis
D. Croup
E. Epiglottitis
F. Foreign body
G. Upper respiratory tract infection

Select the most likely diagnosis for each of the following:

106. A 2-year-old presents with a 1-day history of noisy breathing and barking cough. On examination, he has a quiet inspiratory monophonic noise from the upper airway audible at rest. He looks quite well. There is some intercostal and subcostal recession, and his respiratory rate is 40/min. His chest is clear.

107. A 2-year-old with noisy breathing for 1 day looks frightened, and is drooling, toxic and unwell. He is leaning forward, has intercostal and subcostal recession, respiratory rate 40/min and an inspiratory stridor.

108. A 16-month-old girl has a 4 h history of noisy breathing and cough, which started while playing with her brother's Lego set. She looks anxious, with inspiratory stridor and intercostal recession. She is afebrile. Respiratory rate is 50/min, and her chest is clear.

EMQ 19.3 Management of acute respiratory problems in hospital

A. Intubate and ventilate
B. IV antibiotics
C. Bronchodilators and oral steroids
D. Nebulized saline
E. Oral antibiotics
F. Oxygen
G. Pleural tap

Select the most appropriate management for the following children:

109. An 8-year-old girl has had cough for 7 days, productive of green sputum, and fever. She is currently quite well with no respiratory distress and an oxygen saturation of 94%. She has bronchial breathing and crepitations in the right middle zone.

110. A 5-month-old boy, who has been previously well, has a 3-day history of runny nose, increasingly severe cough and shortness of breath. He is still managing to feed quite well. On examination, his respiratory rate is 65/min, and he has widespread wheezes and inspiratory crepitations in his chest. His oxygen saturation is 89%.

111. A 4-year-old boy has had cough, shortness of breath and wheeze for 12 h. He had several previous similar episodes, although has never been admitted. His respiratory rate is 50/min. He is unable to talk in sentences. Oxygen saturation is 95%.

Cardiology (Chapter 20)

EMQ 20.1 Cardiac problems

A. Aortic stenosis
B. Atrial septal defect
C. Coarctation
D. Patent ductus arteriosus
E. Pulmonary stenosis
F. Tetralogy of Fallot
G. Transposition of the great arteries
H. Ventricular septal defect

What is the most likely diagnosis for the following children:

112. You see a 6-year-old child in clinic. She sees the paediatric cardiologist for a cardiac murmur which is likely to resolve, and no treatment is needed. On auscultation, there is a grade 3 harsh systolic murmur loudest at the left sternal edge. The rest of the examination is normal.

113. A 4-day-old baby suddenly becomes blue, breathless and extremely ill. Septic screen is negative. There is no cardiac murmur, but the cardiac shadow on his X-ray is abnormal like 'an egg on the side'. He is taken to the cardiac catheter lab for an emergency procedure.

114. On routine paediatric examination prior to a minor surgical procedure, a 9-year-old girl is found to be hypertensive (BP right arm 180/120). She has a systolic murmur, loudest between the shoulder blades, and there is radio-femoral delay.

115. A 4-month-old baby is failing to thrive, sweaty with feeds, and has a smooth liver edge 3 cm below the costal margin. He has a harsh systolic murmur all over the precordium, but loudest at the left sternal edge.

116. A 3-year-old boy who has moved to this country has never seen a doctor. He has recurrent episodes of sudden breathlessness and cyanosis, and squats down when it happens. He has a systolic murmur at the upper left sternal edge.

EMQ 20.2 Management of cardiac symptoms and signs

A. Bag valve mask ventilation with oxygen
B. Blood cultures (several sets) and IV antibiotics
C. Diuretics
D. Immunoglobulin (IV) and aspirin
E. Oxygen by face mask
F. Reassure that it is normal or physiological and no action is needed
G. Review again in a week or so
H. Vagal stimulation and oxygen

Select the most appropriate next step in management of the following children:

117. Adam, a 3-year-old boy, has a 2-day, history of viral upper respiratory infection. Adam is febrile (38.0 °C), and there is a grade 2/6 soft systolic murmur loudest at the upper left sternal edge. The murmur has not been noted when Adam had chesty symptoms on two previous occasions in the past year. The rest of the cardiovascular examination is normal but there is rhinitis and an inflamed throat.

118. A 4-year-old girl has a continuous grade 1/6 blowing murmur below the right clavicle, which disappears when she turns her head to look at her toddler brother.

119. A 4-year-old has been febrile and irritable for 6 days, and now has a fine macular rash on the trunk, non-purulent conjunctivitis, large cervical lymph nodes, very red, cracked lips and peeling of the finger tips. There is a grade 1/6 soft murmur in the pulmonary area.

120. A term baby is born by emergency caesarean section because of placental abruption. At delivery, he is very pale, with little respiratory effort and a heart rate of 40 bpm.

121. A 6-month-old baby has been off his feeds for 24 h and is mottled and unwell looking, but conscious. His heart rate is 300 bpm, and ECG shows narrow QRS complexes.

EMQ 20.3 Cardiac murmurs

Select the description of a murmur that would best fit the following scenarios:

Site	where loudest	Character	Systolic or diastolic
A	2nd left intercostal space	Soft	Systolic
B	2nd right intercostal space	Harsh	Systolic
C	Apex	Soft	Diastolic
D	Back	Soft	Systolic
E	Lower left sternal edge	Harsh	Continuous
F	Under one of the clavicles	Blowing	Continuous
G	Under left clavicle	Machinery	Both

122. A 4-year-old well boy attends his GP with an upper respiratory infection, and the GP notices a grade 1 cardiac murmur as an incidental finding. The boy has been previously well and there are no other findings of note. He arranges to listen again a week later, and the murmur has gone.

123. A 7-year-old child has been found to have hypertension when his blood pressure was checked in the left arm. Blood pressure in the legs is normal, and the femoral pulses are delayed compared with the brachial. A grade 2 murmur is heard.

124. A 3-year-old child is reviewed in cardiology clinic. His murmur was first heard at his postnatal check, and he has remained well since then. The murmur has got louder since the last visit 6 months ago, and the cardiologist informs the parents that the problem will resolve.

125. A 3-year-old boy has a murmur which disappears when he lies down, or when his neck is pressed. He is otherwise well.

126. A 10-year-old boy has presented with three episodes of dizziness and then syncope on exercise. He has a grade 3 cardiac murmur which radiates to his neck and is awaiting surgery.

Gastroenterology (Chapter 21)

EMQ 21.1   Abdominal pain

A. Appendicitis
B. Constipation
C. Duodenal ulcer
D. Gastroenteritis
E. Henoch–Schönlein purpura
F. Inflammatory bowel disease
G. Intussusception
H. Mesenteric adenitis
I. Pneumonia
J. Stress-related
K. Urinary tract infection

For the following children with abdominal pain, select the most likely cause:

127. Ellie age 3 has had vague lower abdominal pain for the past 5 days and a low-grade fever. She has started wetting day and night having been dry for 6 months.

128. Alan age 14 months appears to have colicky abdominal pain, which started 12 h ago. He screams in pain for several minutes and looks very pale and sweaty, but then settles for a similar length of time. His stools are dark red in colour.

129. Terry age 10 has had recurrent abdominal pain for a year. His parents demand that it be solved quickly, because otherwise it may affect his chances in his school admission exam. The pain is central, and it tends to come daily for several days, and then not at all for a few weeks. Examination is normal (including growth). He has had some blood in his stool on one occasion 3 months ago after a hard stool, but usually his stools are soft, formed and passed daily.

EMQ 21.2   Vomiting

A. Cow's milk protein intolerance
B. Gastroenteritis
C. Gastro-oesophageal reflux
D. Pneumonia
E. Pyloric stenosis
F. Tonsillitis
G. Urinary tract infection
H. Volvulus due to malrotation

For each of the following children, choose the most likely cause of their vomiting:

130. Jo is 10 months old and her parents report that she vomits day in day out. It does not seem to bother Jo, who is generally well and growing nicely. Her bowels are opened normally.

131. Javed is 14 months old and has been a bit unwell for a few days. He is now febrile, miserable and unwell, and started vomiting earlier today. He looks pale and has cold hands and feet. Capillary refill is 6 s. (You may select more than one option for this question.)

132. Jayne is 9 months old. She started vomiting 6 h ago, and is now bringing up bile-stained vomitus every 20 min. She is distressed and her abdomen is full but not distended, and a little tender.

133. James is 5 months old and his mother has left him with the child minder for the first time. He fed well then started vomiting, and has developed a red rash which is blotchy and blanches on pressure.

EMQ 21.3   Management of gastrointestinal problems

A. Air contrast enema, and surgery if unsuccessful
B. Consider steroids or dietary therapy and try to avoid surgery
C. Delay surgery until blood electrolytes are corrected
D. Give a balanced glucose electrolyte solution
E. Reassure and expect resolution
F. Refer to surgeons now

For each of the following choose the most appropriate step(s):

134. Alex is a 1-year-old who was born preterm. He has been vomiting and had diarrhoea for a day and is mildly dehydrated. On examination, he has an easily reduced inguinal hernia. (You may select more than one option.)

135. Charlie is 7 months. She has a large round umbilical hernia.

136. Sean has been well until 5 months old. Yesterday he began to vomit and was fretful. He has passed some blood PR. He has a distended abdomen. (You may select more than one option.)

137. Stephanie is 12 years old and has had diarrhoea, with blood and mucus on and off for 6 months. She is tired and run down. Her weight has fallen from the 50th to the 10th centile. She has an anal fissure.

138. Patrick is 5 weeks old. His vomiting is getting worse. He now has projectile vomiting after each feed, and then is still hungry.

EMQ 21.4   Urgency of referral for surgical management

A. Arrange routine surgical clinic appointment in 8 weeks
B. Ask surgeons to see in the next week

C. No action other than reassurance
D. Reassure and advise surgery unlikely to be necessary
E. Reassure and arrange clinic review in 1 year
F. Refer urgently to the surgeon on call

For each of the following, choose the best management:

139. Jemal is 6 years old. He presents with a painful swollen left testis. It is very tender.

140. Hayden was born at 28 weeks' gestation. He is now 2 months post-term and has a large left-sided inguinal swelling. He is generally well and the swelling may be reduced into the inguinal canal, but then reappears.

141. Emily is 3 months old. She has a 4–5 cm swelling over her umbilicus. It is readily reduced into the abdomen.

142. Ben is 2 years old. He has moderately severe cerebral palsy. He has persistent and distressing regurgitation which has not responded to medical therapy aimed at the gastro-oesophageal reflux demonstrated on a barium study.

143. Casey is 4 days old. She is vomiting green, bile-stained fluid. Her abdomen is distended but not clearly tender. She is slightly dehydrated.

Urinary tract and Genitalia (Chapter 22)

EMQ 22.1 Treatment of continence problems in children

A. Address maintaining factors
B. Avoid reinforcement
C. Avoid triggers
D. Timer alarm set to ring 1–2 hourly, with star chart
E. Desmopressin
F. Enuresis alarm with star chart
G. Explain and reassure only
H. Imipramine
I. Laxatives with star chart

For each of the scenarios below, select the most appropriate measure to use first:

144. An 8-year-old has presented with primary nocturnal enuresis most nights for which there are no obvious triggers or maintaining factors, and no other associated symptoms. He is going on a cub camp in 2 weeks' time and he and his mother are desperate for something to help him be dry for that weekend.

145. A 6-year-old wets the bed nearly every night, and his parents have found that the easiest solution is to let him get into their bed after he wets, and then sort the wet bed out in the morning. There are no obvious triggers or maintaining factors, and no other associated symptoms.

146. A 5-year-old girl has been passing loose stools into her pants for 6 months. However, she struggles to pass stool on the toilet, and passes a large hard stool every week or so. She seems happy at home and at school. She has occasional daytime wetting, but is dry at night.

147. A 3-year-old is brought to clinic because of frequent night-time wetting, combined with occasional daytime wetting ever since he came out of nappies a year ago. He is happy and well, and there are no other symptoms.

EMQ 22.2 Urine result interpretation

A. Contaminant
B. Diabetes mellitus
C. Glomerulonephritis
D. Nephrotic syndrome
E. Normal
F. Possible urinary tract infection
G. Urinary tract infection

In each of the following situations, select the best interpretation:

148. Vicky is three and a half years old. She presents with vomiting and facial swelling. Urine output is low. She is hypertensive.

pH 7.0   blood ++   protein +++   nitrites neg

leucocytes +

microscopy: white cells 28×10^9/L red cell casts

culture sterile.

149. Frazer is 16 months old. He presents with vomiting and fever.

pH 5.5   blood +   protein +++   nitrites ++

leucocytes ++

microscopy: white cells 45×10^9/L no casts

culture *E. coli* $> 10^5$ organisms/mL.

150. Ian is 4 years old. He has chronic constipation and is on laxatives.

pH 6.0   blood neg   protein neg   nitrites +

leucocytes neg

microscopy: white cells $< 10 \times 10^9$/L no casts

culture no significant growth.

151. Shaun is 4 years old. He presents with facial swelling. Urine output is low. He is normotensive.

pH 5.5   blood neg   protein ++++   nitrites neg

leucocytes neg

microscopy: white cells $<10 \times 10^9$/L hyaline casts

culture mixed growth $<10^5$ organisms/mL.

152. Leanne is 24 months old. She presents with acute illness and abdominal pain.

pH 6.0   blood neg   protein ++   nitrites ++

leucocytes neg

microscopy: white cells 15×10^9/L no casts

culture mixed growth $>10^5$ organisms/mL.

EMQ 22.3   Causes of haematuria

A. Drugs
B. Glomerulonephritis
C. Haemophilia
D. Idiopathic thrombocytopenia
E. Trauma to urinary tract
F. Urinary stones
G. Urinary tract infection

Each child has haematuria on testing. For each child, choose the most likely cause of haematuria:

153. A 7-year-old girl presents with nose bleeds. She has bruises on her legs and arms for which there is no explanation. She is otherwise well.

154. An 8-year-old girl presents with a history of episodes of severe abdominal pain over 3 and a half weeks. She is now in severe pain. Her father, who no longer lives in the house, had a history of an operation on his kidney age 15 years.

155. A 6-week-old boy presents with episodes of apnoea and appears very unwell with a fever. On examination he is ill and has poor capillary refill.

Bones and joints (Chapter 23)

EMQ 23.1   Joint and bone pain

A. Acute lymphoblastic leukaemia
B. Henoch–Schönlein purpura
C. Irritable hip (transient synovitis)
D. Non-accidental injury
E. Osteomyelitis
F. Perthe diease
G. Trauma/fracture

For each of the following select the most likely cause:

156. Michael, 3 years, presents with pain and a left sided limp. He has had a recent viral upper respiratory tract infection. He is afebrile, but there is limited rotation and abduction of his leg.

157. Ellie, 6 years, has a purpuric rash over her buttocks and legs, and pain in both knees and ankles. She also has abdominal pain.

158. Peter, 7 years, has had pain in his right hip for 10 days and a worsening limp. He is otherwise well. X-ray shows a flattening of his femoral capital epiphysis.

159. Janine, 2 years, has had pain and limited movement of her right knee. Her parents give no history of trauma. She has fresh bruising around her ankle and old bruises across her right pinna.

Skin (Chapter 24)

EMQ 24.1   Skin lesions

A. Ash leaf macule
B. Café-au-lait spots
C. Mongolian blue spots
D. Port wine stain
E. Stork mark
F. Strawberry naevus

Select the most appropriate option from the list:

160. A 3-year-old child has a red, raised lesion on the right forearm, which is 2 cm in diameter and has an irregular surface. It was hardly noticeable at birth, but then gradually enlarged until about 1 year of age. Since then it has become smaller.

161. You are examining a 3-week-old baby and notice two red lesions with irregular edges, one just above the bridge of the nose and the other on the nape of the neck. They are not palpable, and have been present since birth.

162. A 6-year-old boy has seven brown macules on his trunk and limbs each measuring about 1 cm in diameter. Two were present at birth (but smaller), and the others have gradually appeared over the past 3 years. His father has similar lesions.

163. A 1-year-old girl has had seizures for the past 2 weeks and is found to have several flat pale oval skin lesions, which are more obvious under ultraviolet light.

164. A 10-year-old boy is admitted with an episode of hemiplegia, which resolves over a few days. He has a prominent dark red lesion on the left side of his face.

165. A 2-week-old Asian baby is referred because his health visitor is concerned about non-accidental injury to his back. When the hospital notes are obtained, it is found that the lesions in question had been recorded as being present when the postnatal check was performed at 1 day of age.

EMQ 24.2 Rashes

A. Chickenpox
B. Eczema
C. Henoch–Schönlein purpura
D. Herpes simplex
E. Impetigo
F. Kawasaki disease
G. Measles
H. Meningococcal sepsis
I. Molluscum contagiosum
J. Scabies
K. Urticaria

Select the most likely cause of the child's rash:

166. A 10-year-old boy has had painful ankles for 2 days and has a rash on his buttocks. He is otherwise well.

167. A 3-year-old girl with red eyes and sore lips has been febrile for a week. She has some peeling of her fingertips.

168. A 4-year-old boy has had a cough and cold for a few days, along with rather red eyes. He has now developed a maculopapular rash which started behind his ears and is spreading over his trunk.

169. A 7-year-old girl has developed an intensely itchy rash on her trunk. New spots keep appearing, evolving from macules to papules, which then develop a central vesicle containing fluid.

170. A 7-year-old boy has pearly-white dome-shaped lesions 3–5 mm in diameter all over his trunk. Each has a small central dimple. They are not troubling him, but his parents are concerned that they should be treated.

171. A febrile 2-year-old has developed dark red spots over his trunk in the past 2 h and is lethargic and irritable.

172. Twin 5-year-old boys are brought with several erythematous lesions on their faces and arms, which have a golden crust.

Haematology (Chapter 25)

EMQ 25.1 Anaemia

A. Acute lymphoblastic leukaemia
B. Blood loss
C. Chronic disease
D. Haemolysis

E. Iron deficiency
F. Physiological
G. Sickle cell disease
H. Beta thalassaemia trait

For each of the following children, select the most likely cause of their anaemia:

173. Billy is a 2-year-old white Caucasian boy, who 'lives on crisps, milk and pop'. His stools are often rather loose with some undigested vegetable matter. His height and weight are on the 50th centile. He is pale but there are no other findings on examination. On full blood count, his Hb is 8.0 g/dL, WBC 9×10^9/L, platelets 400×10^9/L, MCV 60 fL (normal range 75–87) and MCH is 23 pg (normal range 27–32).

174. Isobel had a full blood count done at birth (for suspected sepsis) with the following results: Hb 14.0 g/dL; WBC 11×10^9/L; platelets 357×10^9/L. A second full blood count was performed by her GP at 2 months, because her parents thought she looked pale. The results are as follows: Hb 9.4 g/dL; WBC 8.2 $\times 10^9$/L; platelets 294×10^9/L. She has otherwise been well, is breast fed, and growing nicely. Examination is normal.

175. Baraka age 4, originally from Tanzania, has painful swollen fingers for the fourth time this year. Three episodes occurred when he was unwell with an upper respiratory infection. He has just had diarrhoea and vomiting for 3 days. He looks pale, and his spleen is palpable 2 cm below the left costal margin. His full blood count is as follows: Hb 7.3 g/dL; WBC 9.1×10^9/L; platelets 312×10^9/L.

EMQ 25.2 Bruising

A. Accidental injury
B. Acute lymphoblastic leukaemia
C. Disseminated intravascular coagulation
D. Haemophilia
E. Henoch–Schönlein purpura
F. Idiopathic thrombocytopenic purpura
G. Non-accidental injury
H. von Willebrand diease

Select the most likely cause of these children's bruising:

176. James age 8 has developed large bruises over his legs, arms and trunk, which are noticed after he played a game of football for his school team. He had a cold last week, from which he has recovered. There is no family history of anything similar. Examination is otherwise normal. His full blood count is as follows: Hb 12.4 g/dL; WBC 8.1×10^9/L; platelets 20×10^9/L.

177. Tanya age 11 months has two bruises each measuring 4–5 cm on either side of her forehead, some scratches on her nose, and a few petechiae behind the right ear. Her parents say she has climbed out of her cot (the sides were up) and bumped her head on the carpeted floor. There is no family history of note. The bruises were not present when she went to bed, and there is no history of any other injury. Her full blood count is as follows: Hb 10.4 g/dL; WBC 7.1×10^9/L; platelets 167×10^9/L.

178. David age 1 has a swollen tender right knee joint with bruising around it. He has had several similar episodes since the age of 3 months, involving both knees and his right elbow. There is no history of any injury. He has no other bruising. His uncle has had a similar problem.

Endocrine and metabolic disorders (Chapter 27)

EMQ 27.1 Problems of glucose metabolism

A. Diabetes insipidus
B. Galactosaemia
C. Renal glycosuria
D. Type 1 insulin-dependent diabetes
E. Type 2 non-insulin-dependent diabetes

In each of the following children, choose the most likely diagnosis:

179. James is 8 years old. He is obese and is found to have glycosuria on some days but not on others. His blood glucose levels vary between normal and high.

180. Susan is 5 years old. Glycosuria is found on routine testing. Her blood glucose level is normal and on fasting urine there is no glycosuria.

181. Marie is 10 days old and presents unwell with vomiting, weight loss and jaundice. She is hypoglycaemic. Milk feeds are replaced with intravenous dextrose and electrolytes, and she improves.

182. John is 6 years old and presents with a 1-week history of being very thirsty. His mother thinks he has lost weight. His GP finds a random blood glucose of 18 mmol/L.

Answers to extended matching questions

References are given to the appropriate chapter.

EMQ 4.1 Management of emergencies (see Chapter 4)

1. E. Sian is in respiratory failure. Call for help, she will need ventilation.
2. I. Danny has had a febrile fit (Section 17.1.1). Bring down the temperature. His infection is probably viral.
3. D. Anchelle is dehydrated with hypovolaemia (Table 21.1). She has an altered level of consciousness.

EMQ 4.2 Basic life support (see Chapter 4)

4. F. Check breathing, by looking, listening and feeling with your head bent over the child's face, looking down their chest.
5. C. It sounds safe to approach, so ask at least two of the onlookers to call an ambulance on 999. Do they know where they are? In a few minutes, make sure they have done it.
6. B. Mouth-to-mouth. If after five breaths, he is still unresponsive, then check circulation: you may need to do cardiac massage and mouth-to-mouth.

(Note: if this is an easy question for you, good. If it is not, go back to the chapter and learn it now.)

EMQ 4.3 Maintaining the airway (see Chapter 4)

7. F. This newborn has failed with bag and mask. Ensure airway and ventilation and he will get better.
8. C. A simple manoeuvre will open the airway and hopefully he will maintain his respiratory effort.
9. A. Foreign body history and the child is conscious (Section 19.5.4).
10. B. Avoid movement of the cervical spine in trauma.

EMQ 6.1 Fetal diagnoses (see Chapter 6)

11. C. IUGR occurs because of placental insufficiency. The compromised fetus produces less urine (oligohydramnios) and will have poor growth, and abnormal Doppler's. (You should cover this in obstetrics.)
12. F. Fetal diagnosis can guide fetal management and preparation for delivery.
13. E. In oesophageal atresia, polyhydramnios occurs because the fetus cannot swallow the liquor. Always pass a nasogastric tube in any newborn with polyhydramnios. If this baby is fed milk, it will go straight into his lungs (Figure 21.6).
14. A. This finding is not diagnostic. The couple may decide to have a diagnostic amniocentesis for chromosomes. Risk of Down syndrome increases with maternal age, but most children with this condition have young mothers (Section 10.3.1).
15. D. Diabetes in pregnancy is important. Good control prevents problems (Section 8.4.3.1).
16. B. Hydrops fetalis (generalized fetal oedema with ascites) occurs for many reasons. Fetal anaemia is an important cause due here to Rhesus disease. Therapy is intrauterine blood transfusion in a specialized centre (Section 8.4.2.2).

EMQ 7.1 Examination of the newborn (see Chapter 7)

17. B. The red rash with yellow spots comes and goes.
18. C. The most common birthmark. It fades over weeks. There is often another on the nape of the neck (Figure 24.1).
19. A. This never crosses the midline (Figure 7.5).
20. D. Strawberries get bigger in the first weeks and then gradually get smaller (Figure 24.3).
21. E. This is a dangerous emergency. Blood loss can be major and needs urgent transfusion (Section 7.5.3 and Section 7.5.3.2).

EMQ 7.2 Management of neonatal problems (see Chapter 7)

22. D. This is normal. A full fontanelle at rest is abnormal and may indicate raised intracranial pressure in meningitis or hydrocephalus.

Paediatrics Lecture Notes, Ninth edition. Simon J. Newell and Jonathan C. Darling. © 2014 John Wiley & Sons, Ltd. Published 2014 by John Wiley & Sons, Ltd.

23. E. This is a mild form of hypospadias (Figure 22.3). He must not have a circumcision.

24. A. This baby is tachypnoeic (rate over 60/min). The major concern is life-threatening group B streptococcal infection (Section 8.4.4 and Section 8.4.4.2).

25. D. Milia (Figure 7.4).

26. B. Most babies with big heads are normal; often the family have big heads.

EMQ 8.1 Definitions used in neonatal medicine (*see Chapter 8*)

This is not rocket science, but it is very important, allowing anticipation of likely problems. Learn these and the definitions of the mortality rates. They are favourites for examination questions!

27. E, C, F.

28. G, A.

29. E, H, A.

EMQ 8.2 Respiratory problems in the newborn (*see Chapter 8*)

30. F. With prematurity, surfactant deficiency is most likely. He may need surfactant and ventilation.

31. C. Vitally important, never miss it. Antibiotics at this stage are life saving.

32. G. More common after caesarean section. He will need to be reviewed and should continue to improve as lung fluid clears.

33. A. His abdominal contents have herniated into his chest (Section 21.2.3 and Section 21.2.3.2). He could have a cardiac problem, but those with cyanotic congenital heart disease do usually go pink with oxygen.

EMQ 8.3 Neonatal problems (*see Chapter 8*)

34. B or D. This is likely to be hypoglycaemia. D will be macrosomic. Treatment of symptomatic hypoglycaemia is needed urgently.

35. C. Fits have many causes. Intrapartum asphyxia is an important cause.

36. B. This is congenital rubella syndrome, and should be prevented by immunization (Figure 8.10).

37. A. This preterm infant has developed symptoms due to a patent ductus arteriosus (Figure 8.4, Section 20.5.2 and Section 20.5.2.2).

EMQ 8.4 Management of neonatal jaundice (*see Chapter 8*)

38. C. This is common physiological jaundice (Chapter 8).

39. D. Probably breast milk jaundice. If the jaundice is still present at 14–21 days, investigate to exclude biliary atresia.

40. A. Rhesus haemolytic disease.

41. B. This may be biliary atresia. If a baby is still jaundiced at 14 days, do not forget to consider this and refer for investigation.

EMQ 9.1 Types of developmental delay (*See Chapter 9*)

42. B. Not walking by 20 months is significant gross motor delay. Consider causes such as muscular dystrophy (Section 17.11 and Section 17.11.2) and developmental dysplasia of the hip(s) (Chapter 23).

43. E. This boy is around age 2 for fine and gross motor skills, but his language is normal or even advanced.

44. A.

45. H. The global delay is significant.

EMQ 9.2 Causes of developmental delay 1 (*see Chapter 9*)

46. I. The laser treatment (to her eyes), the fact she is triplet and the head shape all suggest prematurity.

47. D. Although the classic features are not described, this description (including the scar from cardiac surgery) fits well with Down syndrome (Section 10.3 and Section 10.3.1).

48. F. The blood spot is the Guthrie card, which screens for several conditions in the neonatal period (Section 7.4). PKU would require a special diet (Section 27.7 and Section 27.7.1). This child is on thyroxine (Section 27.3 and Section 27.3.1).

49. C. Meningitis can cause deafness (Section 17.5 and Section 17.5.1).

EMQ 10.1 Conditions associated with developmental delay (*see Chapter 10*)

50. E. In learning difficulties with language problems and other behavioural problems, do not forget fragile X.

51. H. One of the neurodermatoses: infantile spasms are typical. He has ash leaf patches and abnormal nails (Figure 17.4).

52. C. Expert review and chromosome analysis will be needed to make the diagnosis. Explaining the diagnosis to the family is difficult and taxing.

53. A. Susie has a diplegia with spasticity in her legs (Section 17.8). Spastic diplegia is more common in infants born preterm.

EMQ 12.1 Management of nutritional problems (*see Chapter 12*)

54. D. You can be reassured by the normal growth velocity.
55. C. He has cystic fibrosis (Section 19.8).
56. B. This is classic iron deficiency (Section 8.2.8, Section 12.1.5 and Section 25.2.1.1). Is he drinking too much milk?
See Chapter 12

EMQ 12.2 Nutritional advice (*see Chapter 12*)

57. C. If formula was necessary, you might use a cow's milk-free feed.
58. B. Breast feeding may transmit HIV. It is still recommended in the developing world (Section 12.1.2, p. 111 and Section 14.4.3.2, p. 132).
59. C. The diarrhoea may not be linked to the diet.
60. C. In gastroenteritis, breast feeding should continue (Section 21.2.4 and Section 21.2.4.1). Add glucose–electrolyte solution if there is dehydration.

EMQ 12.3 Causes of failure to thrive 1 (*see Chapter 12*)

61. B. This is common in children with neuro-developmental problems.
62. D. You can see the cycle of deprivation turning.
63. C. Coeliac disease (Section 21.2.5 and Section 21.2.5.1).

EMQ 13.1 Causes of failure to thrive 2 (*see Chapter 13*)

64. G. Careful history and examination is important. Continue to monitor growth. It is most likely that Alice is a small normal child and was a small normal fetus.
65. C. An important cause of failure to thrive. It may or may not be associated with physical abuse. Does Hannah grow when she is given adequate calories?
66. E. Breathlessness after feeding is typical of heart failure. Sam has a VSD. Failure occurs as the shunt increases due to falling pulmonary pressure after birth (Figure 20.3).

EMQ 13.2 Causes of short stature (*see Chapter 13*)

67. E. Neil may well have a family history of late puberty. He is reassured and told that in the end his stature will be normal.
68. D. Hypothyroidism is a difficult diagnosis. It seldom presents with classical features (Section 27.3).

69. F. Robbie went into normal early puberty. After accelerated early growth, he has now stopped growing.
70. G. Some girls with Turner syndrome do not have classic features. Check chromosomes in girls with short stature or delayed pubertal development (Figure 13.4).

EMQ 14.1 Valid and invalid contraindications to immunization (*see Chapter 14*)

71. A. The last reaction is a typical mild reaction and is not a contraindication to further immunization, and neither is his current mild illness.
72. A. Children are never too old to start the immunization programme, and immunization should be encouraged. The previous seizures are not a contraindication, nor is his exposure to either the short course of oral steroids, or ongoing low-dose inhaled steroids. A longer course of oral steroids (over a week) would be a contraindication to giving a live vaccine, which should then be deferred for 3 months. However, none of the primary-course vaccines are live, and so history of steroid use is irrelevant here. Reaction to antibiotics is not relevant to any of the killed vaccines, and in any case would need to be extreme to count as a valid contraindication.
73. H. This child has had a major reaction to a previous vaccine. The sister's egg allergy and the current minor illness are not relevant.
74. A. Although he has been brought late for his first MMR (should be 13 months), that is no contraindication, and neither is his allergy to egg or his eczema. The coughs and colds are actually around average frequency, particularly if there is a school-age child in the house. He has had a mild previous reaction.

EMQ 15.1 Likelihood of injury being non-accidental (*see Chapter 15*)

75. A. This picture describes shaken baby syndrome.
76. E.
77. D. Young babies with skull fractures should be thoroughly assessed, and the possibility of NAI considered. Here, the injury fits with the history, the child has been brought promptly and, on the brief information given, it seems likely this is accidental. A CT head scan is needed (Chapter 15).

EMQ 17.1 Headache (*see Chapter 17*)

78. F. This is typical migraine (Section 17.9 and Section 17.9.2).
79. I. Significant school absence is worrying in any child. The vague symptoms and bullying point to stress headaches (Section 17.9).

80. H. This is a space-occupying lesion (Section 17.10) until proved otherwise, and he needs brain imaging within a few days. He has early papilloedema.

EMQ 17.2 Fits and 'funny dos' (see Chapter 17)

81. D. Infantile spasms are typically flexor, and occur in runs of a few spasms.

82. E. The occasional myoclonic jerk as someone falls asleep is normal.

83. G. The history of being generally unwell and the bulging fontanelle suggest meningitis. Remember the fontanelle is often normal in this condition.

84. B.

85. A. This focal seizure is complex because consciousness is affected.

EMQ 17.3 Difficulty walking (see Chapter 17)

86. C. Progressive weakness with waddling and a lordosis.

87. F. Also consider infections: irritable hip and osteomyelitis (Chapter 23).

88. E. Bottom shufflers are amusing to watch, but will go on to walk normally (Chapter 9). Note the family history.

89. G. Late motor development. Her legs show toe pointing and scissoring indicating spasticity (upper motor neurone: increased tone and brisk reflexes).

90. A. Progressive motor and sensory problems starting in the legs and moving up the body after an infection.

EMQ 17.4 Lumbar puncture results (see Chapter 17)

You should know how to interpret CSF results, it is important and often urgent Table 17.4.

91. C. TB is becoming more common. Note the long history (Chapter 14).

92. E. The CSF is clearer in the second specimen. You cannot interpret it.

93. D. Meningococcal meningitis–recognition and urgent treatment is lifesaving, if you can see the rash (Figure 14.5).

94. A. URTI can give neck stiffness and no meningitis.

EMQ 17.5 Causes of developmental delay 2 (see Chapter 17)

95. C. A very important cause. Improvement in changed circumstances (e.g. admission or foster care) is an important pointer.

96. E.

97. A. All babies are now screened for deafness to prevent this problem (Section 10.4.5).

98. D. Diplegia predominantly affects legs and is more common after preterm brain injury (Chapter 8).

EMQ 18.1 ENT problems (see Chapter 18)

99. D. You should know how to give first aid in this emergency (Chapter 4). This story could also be anaphylaxis.

100. E. Epstein–Barr viral infection can be protracted and severe in teenagers (Section 14.4.3.2, p. 131).

101. B. Intervention to protect the airway is rarely needed in croup. Don't provoke her.

102. G. Antibiotics, analgesia and urgent ENT review are needed. He may need surgical drainage.

EMQ 19.1 Causes of cough (see Chapter 19)

103. D. Children with chronic respiratory problems and poor growth should have a sweat test.

104. A. These symptoms are typical of asthma, and the eczema is a further pointer. Ask about wheeze and auscultate for it.

105. B.

EMQ 19.2 Abnormal or noisy breathing (see Chapter 19)

106. D. Chapter 18.

107. E. Chapter 18. Don't try to examine his throat!

108. F. Chapter 19. Sometimes the episode of inhalation is not obvious, so remember to ask.

EMQ 19.3 Management of acute respiratory problems in hospital (see Chapter 19)

109. E. She has a right sided chest infection, but is well enough to be treated with oral antibiotics.

110. F. He has bronchiolitis. Oxygen is usually given for saturations less than 93%.

111. C. He has an acute exacerbation of asthma.

EMQ 20.1 Cardiac problems (see Chapter 20)

112. H. The murmur is typical of a VSD. This is a small VSD: she is well, there are no other signs, it is expected to resolve.

113. G. When there is sudden deterioration in the first few days of age, especially with cyanosis, consider a cardiac cause (there doesn't have to be a murmur). It happens when the ductus arteriosus closes. This child has a TGA and is going for a balloon septostomy.

114. C. The murmur, hypertension and radio-femoral delay are all due to coarctation of the aorta. Look for signs of Turner syndrome.

115. H. This baby is in cardiac failure due to a large VSD.

116. F. Think of Fallot's in any child with cyanotic spells. In Europe, surgery is performed by 1 year.

EMQ 20.2 Management of cardiac symptoms and signs (*see Chapter 20*)

117. G. Almost certainly a pulmonary flow murmur because Adam is unwell with a fever. It should disappear (or be quieter) when he is well.

118. F. This is a venous hum due to blood cascading down the internal jugular vein. Pressure on that side of the neck, turning of the head or lying down will make the murmur disappear.

119. D. He has Kawasaki disease (Section 14.4.3.4). Coronary artery aneurysms occur but do not cause a murmur. Treat with immunoglobulins and aspirin urgently.

120. A. This baby is bradycardic because he is hypoxic. He needs neonatal resuscitation (Chapter 7). With ventilation and oxygenation, he will improve.

121. H. This is acute supraventricular tachycardia (SVT). The rate is too fast to count. If oxygen and vagal stimulation do not work, use adenosine and/or cardioversion (Section 20.8 and Section 20.8.1).

EMQ 20.3 Cardiac murmurs (*see Chapter 20*)

122. A. This is a typical pulmonary flow murmur, often heard when children are unwell or febrile.

123. D. This is a coarctation murmur, hence the higher BP in the arms and the delayed femorals.

124. E. A small VSD causes a murmur that often gets louder as the VSD slowly closes, and then disappears.

125. F. This is a venous hum. It disappears when he lies down.

126. B. The harsh murmur radiating to the neck is aortic stenosis, and is the cause of his syncope.

EMQ 21.1 Abdominal pain (*see Chapter 21*)

127. K. Urine infections may not be that obvious clinically in young children, but are important to diagnose and treat promptly to prevent renal damage (Chapter 22).

128. G. A sausage-shaped lump detected on palpation made this diagnosis even more likely, and it was confirmed on ultrasound. Unfortunately, it could not be reduced with air enema, and he had to have surgery with resection of part of the small bowel (Section 21.2.2.2, p. 212).

129. J. The description of the pain, and the implied pressure on Terry, make a stress-related pain most likely (Section 11.5.1.1).

EMQ 21.2 Vomiting (*see Chapter 21*)

130. C. A chronic history of effortless vomiting in a young child who is well is typical. Monitor growth and expect resolution.

131. B, D, F, G. All you can tell is that he is ill and probably has an infection. Often the site of infection is not clear in young children. If you cannot tell on examination, he needs an infection screen.

132. H. Bile-stained, persistent vomiting suggests obstruction. This could be any cause, check for hernia and remember intussusception.

133. A. He has had a cow's milk formula instead of breast milk. The urticarial rash is a helpful clue.

EMQ 21.3 Management of gastrointestinal problems (*see Chapter 21*)

134. D and F. Fluid replacement with ORS in gastro-enteritis. The hernia is not the cause of problems now, but needs referral.

135. E.

136. A and F. Intussusception is more likely to respond to air enema if performed early.

137. B. Crohn disease.

138. C. The metabolic alkalosis must be corrected before operating for pyloric stenosis.

EMQ 21.4 Urgency of referral for surgical management (*see Chapter 21*)

139. F. Jemal probably has testicular torsion, a surgical emergency.

140. B. Around 10% of preterm infants develop a hernia. Complications are common and surgery should not be delayed (Section 21.2.3.3).

141. D. This is an umbilical hernia. Almost all resolve. If still unsightly over 2 years, some are operated upon (Section 21.2.3.1).

142. A. Reflux is common in cerebral palsy. Fundoplication (wrapping the top of the stomach around the bottom of the oesophagus) can be used (Section 21.1.1.1).

143. F. All bile-stained vomiting is obstruction until proven otherwise. Casey had a malrotation and volvulus (Section 21.2.2).

EMQ 22.1 Treatment of continence problems in children (*see Chapter 22*)

144. E. Desmopressin is the treatment of choice for short-term control of enuresis. Alarms and charts will take longer to be effective (Section 22.6).

145. B. The parents are inadvertently giving positive reinforcement to the wetting behaviour.

146. I. She is constipated and, along with the laxatives to soften her stools, needs help in establishing a routine for defaecation using the star chart (Section 21.1.5).

147. G. He is normal (Section 22.6).

EMQ 22.2 Urine result interpretation (*see Chapter 22*)

148. C. Note hypertension, haematuria and red cell casts. She has a recent history of sore throat.

149. G. Frazer needs antibiotics for UTI.

150. E. A normal result.

151. D. Shaun has heavy proteinuria, oedema and will have a low blood albumin.

152. F. You cannot tell because the growth is mixed and there is no significant pyuria. Certainly Leanne needs a repeat urine.

EMQ 22.3 Causes of haematuria (*see Chapter 22*)

153. D. Bleeding in more than one place suggests a bleeding diathesis. In a girl, haemophilia is very rare.

154. F. Stones may be familial. Save any stone that is passed for analysis, and refer for investigation.

155. G. UTI can be life threatening in young children. Signs are seldom specific. Never forget the possibility in the child with sepsis.

EMQ 23.1 Joint and bone pain (*see Chapter 23*)

156. C. Typical history. Differentiation from osteomyelitis is difficult at times.

157. B. HSP is a multisystem disorder, note the rash.

158. F. Note insidious onset of hip pain or limp in a boy.

159. D or G. The absence of history and the presence of bruising of different ages raises the suspicion of abuse (Section 15.2 and Section 15.2.1).

EMQ 24.1 Skin lesions (*see Chapter 24*)

160. F. The gradual enlargement followed by resolution is key. The majority resolve by age 5, 95% by age 9.

161. E. Typical location of stork marks.

162. B. Café-au-lait spots are seen in neurofibromatosis type 1, which is an autosomal dominant condition (Figure 17.3). They increase in number and size with age.

163. A. Ultraviolet light (the Wood's light) is used to make the hypopigmented lesions of tuberous sclerosis more visible (Figure 17.4). The classic lesion is shaped like an ash leaf (round at one end and pointed at the other). The condition may cause fits and developmental delay.

164. D. This is the Sturge–Weber syndrome where the port wine stain is associated with an intracranial hemangioma (Figure 24.2).

165. C. This is why it is important to document the existence of Mongolian blue spots.

EMQ 24.2 Rashes (*see Chapter 24*)

166. C. The classic distribution of the rash is on the buttocks and extensor surfaces of the legs. Three other systems are involved: renal, gut and joints (Figure 23.5).

167. F. The peeling is a late feature of Kawasaki disease. The most important complication is coronary artery aneurysm (Figure 14.7).

168. G. Remember the three Cs of the measles prodrome: cough, conjunctivitis and coryza. The rash typically begins behind the ears (Table 14.3).

169. A. The evolution through the phases described and the intense itchiness are typical of chickenpox (Table 14.3).

170. I. Molluscum contagiosum is benign, common and needs no treatment.

171. H. This description should immediately make you think of meningococcal disease. The rash will be non-blanching. The child needs urgent antibiotic treatment and admission to hospital (Figure 14.5).

172. E. Impetigo is contagious and so it is not surprising that both boys have it. The golden crusting is the important clue (Figure 14.7).

EMQ 25.1 Anaemia (*see Chapter 25*)

173. E. Note the low MCV (microcytosis — small cell size) and low MCH (hypochromia — pale cells). The loose stools may be toddler diarrhoea.

174. F. This is the normal physiological fall in haemoglobin that occurs over the first 2 months or so in all babies (Chapter 8).

175. G. He has dactylitis. Repeated splenic infarctions may in future years render him asplenic.

EMQ 25.2 Bruising (*see Chapter 25*)

176. F.

177. G. The pattern of injury does not fit the history. A single bruise would be expected (Section 15.2 and Section 15.2.1).

178. D.

EMQ 27.1 Problems of glucose metabolism (*see Chapter 27*)

179. E. This used to be rare in children. It remains unusual and usually occurs in children with obesity.

180. C. Note the normal blood glucose and effect of fasting. Susan's renal threshold is low and she has glycosuria at normal blood glucose levels. No action is needed once diabetes has been excluded.

181. B. This is a rare inborn error of metabolism.

182. D. Classic presentation demanding immediate action to prevent John progressing to diabetic ketoacidosis.

Paediatric symptom sorter

> **'I am about to see a child with...'**
>
> This section lists common presentations and their causes, according to whether you would
> see them in the resuscitation room (emergencies), acute paediatric unit, or out-patient clinic.
> The lists are not comprehensive, and often will vary with age, or if there is a pre-existing
> diagnosis. However, they give you a quick starting point as to what conditions should
> feature in your differential diagnoses when you start your history and examination.
>
> Conditions commonly causing that presentation are given in **bold**, while rare causes are
> in *italics*. Conditions highlighted with a red flag (►) are easy to miss, and may have serious
> consequences if you do.
>
> There is some overlap between acute and clinic presentations, so check both lists. Page
> numbers direct you to where to find main relevant information in the book. Check the index
> for a complete listing.

Emergencies	Respiratory failure[43, 178]	**Asthma**[182]; **pneumonia**[180]; **bronchiolitis**[180]; croup[175]; *pneumothorax* ►[186]; *foreign body* ►[45, 181]; *neurological (e.g. head injury*[140]*, raised intracranial pressure*[163]*); poisoning*[142]
	Circulatory failure/shock[43]	**D&V**[207]; **sepsis**[133]; DKA[262]; cardiac failure[262]; anaphylaxis ►[128]; haemorrhage/trauma (including NAI[143]), burns[141], *poisoning*[142]
	Collapse/ convulsions[43, 158]	**Prolonged febrile convulsion**[157]; **epilepsy**[158]; **meningitis**[162]; encephalitis[163]; brain tumour[258]; raised intra-cranial pressure[163]; head injury[140]; *hypoglycaemia* ►[263]; *hypocalcaemia* ►[116]; *poisoning*[142]; *inborn error* ►[265]
	Child death[4]	SIDS[146]; any of the above

 Visit **www.lecturenoteseries.com/paediatrics** to download and view this
symptom sorter on your tablet or mobile device.

Acute presentations	Abdo pain[205]	**Constipation**[207]**; mesenteric adenitis**[205]**; gastroenteritis**[213]; pyelonephritis[226]; appendicitis[206]; intussusception ►[212]; recurrent benign[206]; migraine[206]; stress-related[103]; *Henoch Schonlein*[238]; *pneumonia* ►[180]; *DKA* ►[262]

	Bleeding	**Low platelets**[254]**; other bleeding diathesis**[253]; NAI ►[143]
		- in vomit (haematemesis)[205]
		   Mallory-Weiss[205]; cracked nipple[205]; oesophagitis[205]; *varices*[205]
		- in stool[208]
		   constipation[207]; invasive gastroenteritis[213]; *inflammatory bowel disease*[216]; *Meckel's*[208]
		- in urine (haematuria)[224]
		   UTI[226], glomerulonephritis[224], recurrent[224]; trauma; stone[226]; *tumour*[224]

	Breathless/ noisy breathing/ cough[178]	**Asthma**[182]**; URTI**[178]**; bronchiolitis**[180]**; pneumonia**[180]**; croup**[175]; foreign body ►[181]; *epiglottitis* ►[175]; *cardiac failure*[201]; *DKA* ►[262]
	Bruising/ non-blanching rash[248]	**Trauma**[144]**;** viral; meningococcal ►[133]; Henoch-Schonlein[238]; *low platelets* ►[254]; *other bleeding diathesis*[253]
	Fever[46]	**Viral infection**[131]**;** bacterial infection (ENT[172], chest[180], urine[226], blood[133], brain[162], joint[236], other abscess). If prolonged: Kawasaki ►[135]; occult abscess; *TB*[134]; *malignancy*[257]; *systemic arthritis*[237]
	Fit, faint, funny do, collapse[157]	**Syncope**[161]**; febrile convulsion**[157]**; epilepsy**[158]**; reflex anoxic seizure**[160]**; breath-holding**[161]; meningitis[162]; encephalitis[163]; tics[160]; night terrors[105]; behavioural[100]; *hypoglycaemia* ►[263]; *cardiac arrhythmia* ►[201]
	Headache[167]	**Migraine**[168]**; meningitis**[162]**; trauma**[140]**;** stress-related[103]; poor visual acuity[95]; dental[209]; *brain tumour* ►[258]; *brain abscess*[168]; *hypertension* ►[202]; *carbon monoxide poisoning*
	Joint pain/ swelling/limp/ off legs[237]	**Trauma; reactive arthritis**[237]**; irritable hip**[237]; arthritis[237]; septic arthritis ►[237]; slipped upper femoral epiphysis ►[240]; Perthe's[239]; fracture; NAI ►[143]; rickets[115]; Henoch Schonlein[238]; *malignancy* ►[259]; *haemophilia*[253]
	Lethargy	**Viral infection**[131]**; UTI**[226]; gastroenteritis[213]; meningitis ►[162]; septicaemia[133]; DKA[262]; *hypoglycaemia* ►[263]; *brain tumour* ►[258]; *hypothyroid*[263]
	Rash[244]	**Infection**[130] **(any viral or some bacterial (esp strep and staph);** impetigo[246]**; drug-related; urticaria/allergic**[246]**;** eczema[245]; *meningococcal infection* ►[133]; *Henoch Schonlein* ►[238]; *low platelets*[254]; *eczema herpeticum* ►[246]; *bruising/NAI*[143]; *erythema nodosum*[247]; *erythema multiforme*[247]; *scabies*[248]
	Swelling or oedema	**Nephrotic syndrome**[224]**;** congestive cardiac failure[201]; malnutrition[115]
	Vomiting[204]	**Overfeeding; GO-reflux; gastroenteritis**[213]**;** protein intolerance[216]; appendicitis[206]; bowel obstruction ►[210]; pyloric stenosis ►[212]; viral infection[131]; acute otitis[172]; UTI[226]; sepsis ►[133]; meningitis ►[162]; *poisioning*[142]; *space-occupying brain lesion* ►[168]

Clinic presentations

Symptom	Causes
Abdo pains– recurrent[205]	**Constipation[207]; stress-related[103]; recurrent abdo pain of childhood[206]; migraine[206]; UTIs[226]; GO-reflux** oesophagitis[205]; irritable bowel[206]; *inflammatory bowel disease[216]*
Abnormal skin[243]	**Birthmarks (inc strawberry naevus)[161]; eczema[245];** neonatal lesions[66]; other rashes[244]; infestations[248]; bruises[144]; *purpura*►[248]; *NAI*►[143]; *neurodermatoses[161]*
Development/ learning delayed or abnormal[89]	**Normal variation[81];** specific learning problem[91]; Down Syndrome[92]; cerebral palsy[165]; hip dysplasia►[235]; *neurodegenerative disorders[169]; Duchenne*►[169]; *autism spectrum[106]*
Fits, faints and funny dos[157]	see under acute
Growth excessive[118]	**Obesity[114];** precocious puberty[122]; syndromes (Klinefelter[121], Marfan[121]); cushingoid (steroids)[264]; *Cushings[264]*
Growth poor[118]	**Failure to thrive[123]; constitutional small stature[120]; delayed puberty[122];** chronic illness; coeliac disease►[215]; genetic sydromes (Turner[121], Down[92]); renal failure[226]; hypothyroid[263]; neglect[142]; malnutrition[115]
Headaches[167]	**Migraine[168]; stress-related[103];** dental; poor vision; sinusitis[173]; *hypertension*►[202]; *brain tumour*►[258]
Head shape/size abnormal[168]	**Plagiocephaly[168]; familial large head;** *craniosynostosis*►[168]; *microcephaly[94]; hydrocephalus[164]*
Infections – frequent[128]	**Normal frequency for age[129];** immunodeficiency[129]; cystic fibrosis[186]; HIV[132]; *malnutrition[115]*
Loose stools[207]	**Constipation with overflow[207]; toddler diarrhoea[207]; food allergy[216];** coeliac disease[215]; inflammatory bowel disease►[216]; malabsorption[214]
Musculoskeletal problems[234]	**Intoeing[235]; genu valgum/varum[235];** rickets[115]; arthritis[237]; scoliosis[235]; club feet[235]; cerebral palsy[165]; hip dysplasia[235]; spina bifida[165]
Respiratory symptoms – recurrent[177]	**Asthma[182]; normal URTIs[178];** post-viral cough[179]; G-O-reflux[205]; *cystic fibrosis[186]; inhaled foreign body*►[181]; *immunodeficiency[129]; congenital lung problem[76]*
Tired/pale/ lethargic	**Behavioural[100]; anaemia[251]; post-viral;** diabetes►[261]; chronic illness; *coeliac[215]; hypothyroid*►[263]; *Crohn's*►[216]; *renal failure*►[226]; *liver disease[217]; leukaemia*►[257]; *malignancy[256]; chronic fatigue[151]*
Vomiting[204]	**G-O-Reflux[205]; overfeeding[205]; cows milk protein intolerance[216]; food allergy[216];** behavioural[103]; *coeliac disease[215]; recurrent obstruction[210]; space-occupying brain lesion*►[168]
Wetting problems[229]	**Delayed dryness but normal[229]; urine infections[226]; constipation[207]; overactive bladder[230]; primary nocturnal enuresis[229];** *diabetes mellitus[261]; diabetes inspidus[265]*

Index

Main entries for a topic are listed in **bold**.